Mental Health and Substance Use Disorders

A Growing Crisis

snova
New York

Mental Illnesses and Treatments Series

Hoarding Disorder: Insights and Implications for Health and Safety
Paul M. Singleton (Editor)
ISBN: 979-8-89530-506-5
eBook ISBN: 979-8-89530-521-8

A Desperate Asylum: Crisis in a Canadian Psychiatric Hospital During Wartime
Anne Marie Creamer, PhD
ISBN: 979-8-88697-696-0
eBook ISBN: 979-8-88697-863-6

The Training and Practice of Psychotherapy in Post-Apartheid South Africa: Case Studies, Controversies and Contemplations
Zelda G. Knight (Editor)
ISBN: 979-8-88697-782-0

Brain-Based Treatment: A New Approach or a Well-Forgotten Old One? Neuropsychology and Psychotherapy
Vanya Matanova, PhD, DSc, Martin Kolev, PhD, Pia Tohme, PhD and Zlatomira Kostova, PhD
ISBN: 978-1-53616-951-5
eBook ISBN: 978-1-53616-952-2

More information about this series can be found at
https://novapublishers.com/product-category/series/mental-illnesses-and-treatments/

Darren D. Stewart
Editor

Mental Health and Substance Use Disorders

A Growing Crisis

snova
New York

NOTICE TO THE READER

The Publisher has taken reasonable care in the preparation of this book, but makes no expressed or implied warranty of any kind and assumes no responsibility for any errors or omissions. No liability is assumed for incidental or consequential damages in connection with or arising out of information contained in this book. The Publisher shall not be liable for any special, consequential, or exemplary damages resulting, in whole or in part, from the readers' use of, or reliance upon, this material. Any parts of this book based on government reports are so indicated and copyright is claimed for those parts to the extent applicable to compilations of such works.

Independent verification should be sought for any data, advice or recommendations contained in this book. In addition, no responsibility is assumed by the Publisher for any injury and/or damage to persons or property arising from any methods, products, instructions, ideas or otherwise contained in this publication.

The Publisher assumes no responsibility for any statements of fact or opinion expressed in the published contents.

This publication is designed to provide accurate and authoritative information with regard to the subject matter covered herein. It is sold with the clear understanding that the Publisher is not engaged in rendering legal or any other professional services. If legal or any other expert assistance is required, the services of a competent person should be sought. FROM A DECLARATION OF PARTICIPANTS JOINTLY ADOPTED BY A COMMITTEE OF THE AMERICAN BAR ASSOCIATION AND A COMMITTEE OF PUBLISHERS.

Additional color graphics may be available in the e-book version of this book.

Library of Congress Cataloging-in-Publication Data

ISBN: 979-8-89530-699-4 (Hardcover)
ISBN: 979-8-89530-825-7 (eBook)

Published by Nova Science Publishers, Inc. † New York

Contents

Preface

Mental health and substance use disorders touch lives across all demographics, transcending age, race, and socioeconomic status. These conditions are not only prevalent and recurrent but also severe, yet there is hope in their treatability. In the past year, over 106,000 lives were tragically lost due to drug overdoses. Alarmingly, the CDC has reported a more than threefold increase in overdose deaths involving fentanyl over the last five years. Emergency room visits for opioid-related overdoses surged by 41 percent among boys and 10 percent among girls aged 12 to 17. Despite these harrowing statistics, a staggering 94 percent of individuals aged 12 and older with substance use disorders remain untreated.

The situation is equally dire for those facing mental health challenges. With over one in five adults in the United States experiencing a mental health disorder, there remains a significant gap in care, as evidenced by the over 10 million individuals reporting an unmet need for mental health services.

This book delves into the pressing necessity for an improved system of care, one that adequately addresses the intertwined crises of mental health and substance use disorders. By examining current gaps and proposing comprehensive solutions, we hope to illuminate a path toward a more equitable and effective approach to mental health and substance use disorder care.

Chapter 1

A Crisis in Mental Health and Substance Use Disorder Care: Closing Gaps in Access by Bringing Care and Prevention to Communities*

Committee on Health, Education, Labor, and Pensions

Wednesday, May 17, 2023
U.S. Senate, Committee on Health, Education, Labor, and Pensions,
Washington, DC.

The Subcommittee met, pursuant to notice, at 10 a.m., in room 430, Dirksen Senate Office Building, Hon. Edward Markey, Chairman of the Subcommittee, presiding.

Present: Senators Markey [presiding], Baldwin, Hickenlooper, Marshall, Murkowski, and Tuberville.

Opening Statement of Senator Markey

Senator MARKEY. Thank you all for joining us today for the first Primary Health and Retirement Subcommittee hearing on mental health and behavioral health for the 118th Congress.

---

* This is an edited, reformatted and augmented version of Hearing Before the Subcommittee on Primary Health and Retirement Security of the Committee on Health, Education, Labor, and Pensions, United States Senate, One Hundred Eighteenth Congress, First Session, Publication No. S. HRG. 118–200, dated May 17, 2023.

In: Mental Health and Substance Use Disorders: A Growing Crisis
Editor: Darren D. Stewart
ISBN: 979-8-89530-699-4

Thank you to Senator Marshall for your shared commitment to addressing the mental health and substance use crisis in the United States. There are many people at home who will watch this hearing and recognize the realities they face every day.

They call for help and are met with long wait times or an hour-long commute to care. They have lost a friend, or a loved one, to mental illness or a substance use disorder. But support and services aren't accessible. They know when they need help, but they don't know where to go to get it.

Let me start by saying, you are not alone. The reason we are here today is to identify those challenges and chart a path toward a future where help is there when you need it. On health—Senate Health, Education, Labor, and Pensions Committee it is our responsibility to take up the fight for a better mental health and substance use disorder care system that meets people where they are with dignity.

But today we are losing that fight. Last year, over 106,000 people died from an overdose. The CDC reported just last week that overdose deaths involving fentanyl had more than tripled in the last 5 years. Emergency department visits for opioid related overdoses increased by 41 percent for boys, and 10 percent for girls age 12 to 17 in the fall of 2022, compared to the year before.

Yet, 94 percent of people age 12 and older with substance use disorders did not receive treatment. The prospects for people facing mental health challenges are equally distressing. More than one in five adults in the United States has a mental health disability, yet over 10 million people report an unmet need for mental health services.

One in five highschoolers have seriously considered attempting suicide. For LGBTQ youth, the number was closer to one in two. Yet over 2 million adolescents who needed care did not receive it.

The cause is complex. Pharmaceutical companies supercharged an opioid pandemic by overprescribing oxycodone, ultimately hooking people on heroin and fentanyl. Big tech serves toxic content that grabs young people's attention, and fuels depression, anxiety, and eating disorders.

Childhood trauma and toxic stress linked to violence, poverty, racism, and housing instability create invisible scars that weigh heavily on caregivers' children and seniors. And as a growing number experience mental health conditions, our health system has not been able to keep up. People are looking for an open door to care, and instead they are locked out.

But these invisible scars continue to grow, and thousands of people find themselves in the emergency departments hoping for placement in treatment programs, or they leave, and without anywhere to go, we lose them to suicide and overdose.

Yes, the challenges are complex, but the solution is simple, affordable, accessible, mental and substance use care for any and all that need it, when they need it, and where they need it. This is easier said than done, but there is hope to be found in the everyday heroes who have rolled up their sleeves, looked into people's eyes, and offered a helping hand.

A few of those people are with us today, addiction medicine physicians, child psychiatrists, and providers from community health centers and certified community behavioral health clinics. They are the better angels of our health care system, and right now we need an army of angels.

We can build a system that treats people with dignity and doesn't price patients out of the care. We can invest in community health providers. We can pass legislation to break down antiquated barriers to medication, treatment for opioid use disorder.

We can support local communities, public health response to rising overdoses and mental health needs. And we can make sure that big pharma doesn't charge big bucks for life saving prescriptions. We can create a system that puts patients over profits.

I am proud that so many of our fiercest advocates for these efforts are in this room today, and we thank you for all of your work. And with that, I turn to the Ranking Member, Senator Marshall, for his opening statement.

Opening Statement of Senator Marshall

Senator MARSHALL. Well, thank you, Mr. Chairman. I also want to appreciate your dedication to addressing the mental health crisis and for holding our first Subcommittee hearing. I know our colleagues on both sides of the aisle interested in reauthorizing several expiring programs.

We also want to look for new ways to tackle this crisis. Our witnesses today will show us how they are using existing Federal programs and their own ingenuity to reshape their communities. It has been 5 years since Congress passed the Support for Patients and Community Act, the largest, most comprehensive legislative package that directs Federal resources and statutory changes toward prevention, treatment, and recovery.

The Support Act encourages payers and providers to utilize alternative treatments for pain. It increased patient education and awareness across many markets. Modernizing prescribing to detect and prevent fraudulent prescriptions.

The expanded safe disposal of unused prescription drugs, including at home deactivation packets. And finally, it helped people get on the road to recovery through various inpatient and outpatient services.

Let's talk about prevention first, where we are seeing great progress. Notably, substance use disorder related deaths as a result of prescription opioids are decreasing because physicians and nurses are increasing patient awareness and utilizing other treatments for pain. However, Chairman Markey and I in this Committee, our aim is to prevent addiction by moving away from addictive medicines.

The Support Act required the FDA to help address biopharmaceutical challenges in developing non-addictive pain therapies, but the agency has not successfully carried this out. We will hold the FDA accountable so patients can one day have access to innovative, non-addictive prescription drugs.

On treatment, we will hear from our witnesses on the successes of expanded access to medication assisted treatment, telehealth, and novel coordinated care models, including certified community behavioral health clinics, or CCBHCs, which I am a very strong advocate for. We have all witnessed too many people experiencing mental health crises in the wrong setting and receiving the wrong type of care.

While still new, the data looks promising. People who receive care at a CCBHC spend 60 less—60 percent less time in jail, 70 percent less time in the hospital, and are much likely—much more likely to have access to a primary care provider.

CCBHCs also contributed to a 41 percent reduction in homelessness. Congratulations, and I will look forward to Mr. Denny's testimony to share some more of those stats again. For all the good the witnesses are providing,

Congress must work to ensure that they can deliver timely access to care by addressing mental health parity issues. They need our help to eliminate unnecessary delays and denials from prior authorization, the No. 1 administrative burden across all clinicians and other health care providers.

On recovery, the Support Act provided peer recovery support services and other programs that are helping people help themselves become independent, stable, and healthy. In addition to the Support Act, I hope this Committee will work with us on developing solutions to address some of the root causes of the mental health crises in America's youth. Do the lockdowns result in isolation?

Kids increase their reliance on social media, shifting their habits beyond a casual pastime. In fact, experts have found that overuse of social media rewires their brains to constantly seek out immediate gratification. This leads to obsessive, compulsive, and addictive behaviors. Studies have linked heavy social media use increased risk for depression, anxiety, loneliness, self-harm, and even suicide ideation.

This year, the CDC released a new survey finding that nearly 60 percent of young girls reported a mental health issue, with 30 percent seriously considering suicide, double the rate there was among boys and up to almost 60 percent from a decade ago. We know social media companies are aware of this based upon their own similar findings. There is no silver bullet in solving the mental crisis.

We must continue to bolster efforts on prevention, treatment, and recovery. In doing so, we should value what we measure and measure what we value. As we consider reauthorizing expiring programs and exploring new ideas, they should be patient centered, outcome driven, cost effective.

They must be backed by data. Mr. Chairman, thank you again for calling this hearing, and I yield back.

Senator MARKEY. Thank you, Senator, so much. And we will turn to our first witness, Dr. Maria Celli, a Psychologist and Deputy CEO of Brockton Neighborhood Health Center in Brockton, Massachusetts.

She has worked at the Brockton Neighborhood Health Center since 2016 and has worked in community health centers since 2010. Dr. Celli launched the Brockton Behavioral Health Task Force to promote collaboration between behavioral health providers across the city's behavioral health and substance use services ecosystem.

Welcome, doctor, whenever you are ready, please begin.

Statement of Maria Celli, Deputy CEO, Brockton Neighborhood Health Center, Brockton, MA

Dr. CELLI. Good morning, Chairman Markey, Ranking Member Marshall, and Members of the Committee. Thank you for the opportunity to testify on the critical topic of mental health and substance use disorders and access to community-based prevention and services.

As Senator Markey noted, my name is Maria Celli, and I am a Psychologist and the Deputy CEO at Brockton Neighborhood Health Center, a federally qualified health center located in Brockton, Massachusetts.

In my role, I have witnessed the negative impact that the pandemic has had on the mental health of our patients and the community. The demand for behavioral health services is enormous, outstripping our community wide supply of resources. This morning, I am coming on behalf of our providers and patients I have the privilege to serve to propose four opportunities for support to improve community level access to behavioral health and substance use disorder services.

Those four are, increasing support for integrated care team models, leveraging mobile medical units and continued use of telehealth services, including audio only services when appropriate, prioritizing pediatrics, and workforce development and wellness.

Like many other community health centers across the country, Brockton Neighborhood Health Center employs integrated, multi-disciplinary teams to serve patients holistically. That means we address everything from food insecurity and housing insecurity to disease management.

Our patients are universally screened for health-related social needs, depression, and risky substance use. We make screening for mental health and substance use disorder a standard part of primary care.

By doing so, we reduce stigma and create easy and seamless access to mental health and addiction services. Additionally, we have found that primary care behavioral health integrated teams can reduce costs to the medical system, and I will give one example.

Recently, we had a 21-year-old male who was new to our adult medical department. This individual had significant medical complications and was in and out of the hospital frequently, very frequently, like seven times in a couple of weeks.

Concerned about his mental status, the primary care provider at the NHC engaged one of the integrated behavioral health clinicians who was able to meet with this individual and begin to build trust.

Since the team of the integrated primary care—the integrated clinician and the primary care provider has started to work with this patient, he has significantly reduced his emergency room visits and has begun to make good progress with his medical care addition.

Additionally, in addition to primary care, behavioral health integrated models of care, I propose increasing access through mobile units and telehealth services. We have found at Brockton Neighborhood Health Center through our first mobile unit that this is an effective way to reach vulnerable populations, and I will highlight three in particular.

In 2020, Brockton Neighborhood Health Center leveraged grant funding to launch our first mobile unit, which provides services specifically to those experiencing homelessness and people who use drugs. We have observed that overdose deaths have increased significantly in our town, and nationally that is the same.

The services on this mobile unit have undoubtedly saved lives. However, we have also observed a rise in mental health needs in both pediatrics and seniors within our community. That is why Brockton Neighborhood Health Center is working hard to acquire mobile units that can be deployed to provide integrated care at schools, at senior housing sites, etcetera, to meet our patients in the community that has the need where they are.

I am so appreciative that last year this Committee recognized the value of mobile care units when it passed the Mobile Health Care Act by unanimous consent to make it easier for health centers to finance mobile health units.

Additional new access point funding will help health centers like ours take advantage of this opportunity to create easier access to patients who need it. In addition to launching the mobile clinical unit, leveraging strategic use of telehealth is essential to address this crisis, and I strongly support permanently extending the telehealth flexibilities implemented during the COVID–19 public health emergency.

Of course, none of our work in addressing this crisis is possible without robust and well staffing. The NHC has designed and launched a number of grants funded professional pipeline projects, including one designed for the training, recruitment, and retention of behavioral health clinicians.

We would love for this Committee to provide more flexible funding to support projects like ours. Another priority for our workforce is wellness programing to mitigate employment related stress. I appreciate that last year the HELP Committee passed the Lorna Breen Act, which authorized funding for provider burnout, and we genuinely appreciate any support that our staff can receive to remain well in these roles as they continue to work daily to save lives.

Health centers like Brockton Neighborhood Health Center need long term, sustainable, and predictable funding to continue to address this behavioral health and substance use disorder crisis.

Chairman Markey, Ranking Member Marshall, and Members of the Committee, thank you for allowing me to share some of the great work that my team at the NHC is doing to fight the mental health and substance use disorder crisis in this country.

With this Committee's support, we will continue to find new ways to provide affordable, accessible, and high-quality care to the communities we serve. I look forward to your questions.

[The prepared statement of Dr. Celli follows:]

Prepared Statement of Maria Celli

Chairman Markey, Ranking Member Marshall, and Members of the Committee, thank you for the opportunity to testify on the critical topic of mental health and substance use disorders. My name is Maria Celli, and I am a psychologist and the Deputy CEO at Brockton Neighborhood Health Center, a federally qualified health center located in Brockton, MA, a city 24 miles south of Boston. BNHC serves over 37,000 unique patients and conducted over 200,000 visits in 2022.

While I am currently the Deputy CEO of BNHC, I have previously served as a COO and Director of Behavioral Health and Social Services at BNHC and as a Director of Behavioral Health at a Boston-based FQHC. As a psychologist, my areas of clinical work have focused on behavioral health-primary care integration and working with individuals who have experienced trauma. I have trained in early childhood mental health and perinatal care, and I continue to be attentive to the needs of our youngest patients because they are our future, and I am aware that the ills I see in our adult patients were, in many ways, impacted by their experiences as young children. I am eager to promote the well-being of children to reduce their risk of developing pathologies later in life.

From my clinical care and administrative perspectives, I have observed the current state of behavioral health and substance use needs and care access from the patient level through to systems level. In Massachusetts, we are fortunate that the state's Executive Office of Health and Human Services has committed to improving access to behavioral health and substance use disorder services, through the development of a Behavioral Health Roadmap, which is a blueprint for creating accessible and equitable access to behavioral health and substance use disorder services across the state. Introduced in 2021 and implemented in 2023, this roadmap included the design and launch of 24 Community Behavioral Health Centers across the commonwealth. We, at BNHC, are thankful that one of the 24 CBHC's is located within the city of Brockton; and we leverage this and every other resource in Brockton's behavioral health ecosystem to try to address our patients' and community's needs. Despite these improvements in access, we are still witnessing a demand for services that exceed our supply of resources. We were concerned about our staff and community's mental health and wellness prior to COVID. However, the needs have risen throughout the pandemic and remain high.

I have professionally witnessed the negative impact that the pandemic had on the mental health and well-being of our patient population. More specifically, the trauma of COVID has triggered exacerbations of what were once subthreshold mental health conditions. The demand for behavioral health services is enormous—outstripping our community-wide supply of resources. Unfortunately, the acuity of patient needs is also worse, meaning that patients who might have once sufficed with outpatient therapy, are now reporting symptoms requiring more intensive or even inpatient care due to imminent risk concerns.

From my own professional experience, and as the representative on behalf of providers and patients whose voices are not here, I propose four opportunities for continued or additional support to improve community-level access to behavioral health and substance use disorder services:

1) *Increasing support for integrated care team models:* Integrated primary care team models co-locate and integrate licensed behavioral health clinicians, Community Health Workers, Peer Recovery Coaches, and sometimes other disciplines to work alongside primary care providers so that health-related social needs and behavioral health screenings and treatment are universally available to any patient as part of their general medical care. This model of care is foundational to how FQHCs' practice and its expansion is essential to improving access.
2) *Leveraging Mobile Medical Units and continued use of Telehealth Services:* I propose support for care for hard-to-reach patients through support for unique and flexible models of care, including mobile medical units that can strategically deliver integrated primary care services to vulnerable individuals who are not engaging in their primary health care such as those struggling with homelessness, seniors and individuals with transportation or mobility barriers. Similarly, it is essential to continue to strategically use telehealth services for otherwise hard-to- reach populations.
3) *Prioritizing Pediatrics:* We must ensure that all pediatric patients have universal access to behavioral health screenings, assessments,

and treatments throughout their development, especially in their first 5 years of life.

4) *Workforce Development:* Finally, we must continue to invest in developing the healthcare workforce to serve these behavioral health and substance use disorder needs, through support for existing professional pipeline projects.

Increasing Community Access through Primary Care-Behavioral Health Integration

BNHC operates four clinical sites (including one in a homeless shelter and one mobile unit). BNHC provides the full spectrum of primary care services including adult medical, behavioral health, OB/GYN, pediatrics, nutrition, oral health, optometry, cancer screenings, onsite pharmacy, radiology, diagnostic laboratory, infectious disease screening and care, substance use disorder screening and treatment. We serve patients with extraordinarily complex medical and social needs, including poverty, food insecurity, homelessness, trauma, and difficulty accessing transportation and employment. We serve all people regardless of their insurance status or ability to pay.

Like many other Community Health Centers across the country, we serve our patients holistically, meaning that we provide healthcare that pays attention to and aims to address all aspects of a person's life, as they all impact their health. We screen, assess and address their care across multiple levels and domains of need addressing everything from food access to disease management. We practice this way because it is our mission to do so, and it is a way to promote wellness for individuals who might not otherwise engage in preventative services. This strategy is beneficial to the patients and restrains costs to the medical system, as the patient's engagement in our integrated primary care teams can reduce unnecessary utilization of higher levels of care.

One recent example of this is the case of a 21-year-old male with multiple medical conditions, including seizure disorder, who was in and out of the hospital due to seizures. Unfortunately, he was not engaging in his medical treatment due to undiagnosed severe depression. After becoming aware of his medical disengagement and his frequent trips to the hospital, his primary care provider at BNHC engaged the integrated behavioral health clinician, who was able to begin to build trust with this traumatized young individual. Together, the primary care provider, behavioral health clinician, and patient began to make slow but steady progress in his participation with his healthcare. The patient has not visited the emergency room since the holistic treatment team has collectively engaged him. Now that he has built trust with this team, he is willing to meet with specialists who can stabilize his medical condition. Given his many needs, the behavioral health team is also working with his family and friends to know how to support his health and wellness. This is a person who was in a revolving door pattern of medical exacerbation to the emergency department—until he was engaged by his primary care provider and an integrated behavioral health clinician. Now, he is stabilized and moving toward illness management and an improved quality of life.

At BNHC, like many other health centers, the integrated model of care is foundational to how we provide primary care services. Our patients are universally screened for health-related social needs (i.e., social drivers of health), as well as risky substance use and depression. Just as we measure vital signs such as blood pressure, temperature, and weight, we ask them about the social conditions that impact their health and wellness; and we have staff on the team who assist with addressing the issues that patients report. This universal screening and team-based approach to access is crucial because it communicates that health-related social needs, substance use and behavioral health concerns are all part of their primary care. It destigmatizes these issues and creates easy access to needed services that improve their health, well-being, and effective participation in their own treatment, in their own lives and in their communities.

Another illustrative example of the benefits of Primary Care-Behavioral Health Integration and universal screening for BH and SUD conditions is the story of Gloria, a 73-year-old woman who had recently moved to our service area and was a newer patient. She completed our standard, universal screening process and was found to have an elevated score on the depression screening tool. Her response on the screening indicated suicidal ideation, and the PCP was planning to complete a Section 12 for the patient, meaning sending her to the hospital for inpatient hospitalization. However, because of the integrated model of care, the PCP reported the result to the integrated BH clinician, who met with the patient and carefully assessed the patient's risk. Rather than hospitalizing the patient, the integrated clinician was able to make a referral to one of our in-house psychiatric providers, who consulted with the PCP to start psychotropic medications. The BHI clinician helped the patient to connect with other resources in the community because the patient had acknowledged that the primary drivers for her current state were loneliness and hopelessness due to multiple losses, including loss of employment.

This patient did not need a hospital. She needed connection. The integrated care team model, which is a cornerstone for how BNHC and so many other CHCs around the country operate, made those connections possible. We strive, train, practice, commit and recommit to seeing the whole person. And in doing so, we are privileged to know the patients and support them through accessing what they need to cope more effectively with the many stressors associated with their lives. Access to effective behavioral health and substance use disorder screening and treatment within the community and through the primary care doorway is an essential strategy for maximizing access in this time of tremendous need.

Increasing Access through Mobile Units and Telehealth Services

Another fundamental way that Community Health Centers operate is that we are innovative and driven to meet the needs of our community. Additionally, we are committed to our communities' health and our patients' care, whether the patient is attending visits or not. We continuously track population health level data to monitor who is in or out of care, whose healthcare metrics (such as blood pressures or A1c's are out of control or have not been checked recently enough) etc. We launch population health text and mail campaigns to outreach and engage patients who are out of care. We mobilize community health and outreach workers to locate and reconnect these patients to their trusted medical home. However, many individuals remain disconnected, and it has worsened throughout the pandemic. We have observed that this has been particularly true for certain vulnerable populations, such as those experiencing homelessness, children, and seniors.

BNHC was fortunate to be awarded a grant in 2020 that yielded our first mobile health unit. The "Community Care in Reach" mobile unit provides services specifically to those experiencing homelessness, as well as people who use drugs. Started in 2021, this mobile unit can provide primary care, some acute care services, peer recovery coaching, and referrals to specialty services—all occurring where the patients are located. According to the CDC, there were over 100,000 drug-related overdose deaths in 2021 alone, which has steadily increased over the last 5 years. The screening, education and interventions provided on this mobile unit have undoubtedly saved lives! Additionally, it offers a patient-centered approach to high-quality, evidence-based care while also serving to contain costs through the reduction of ED utilization for services that are offered on the unit.

In addition to a mental health and substance use crisis in those who use drugs and in individuals experiencing homelessness, we have observed and measured an incredible increase in the behavioral health needs of our pediatric patients during and coming out of the pandemic. BNHC is actively seeking funding to acquire another mobile unit serve the pediatric populations of the city as a school-based service site. The integrated care team would include a full-time Nurse Practitioner, as well as a Behavioral Health Clinician, community health workers and Peer Recovery Coach. While not yet operational, this model (across any willing school system) can bring necessary and easily accessible resources to kids who are falling through the cracks, despite the school, parents' and health centers' best efforts.

On the other end of the age spectrum, I have also professionally observed and have been informed by behavioral health providers across the city of Brockton and the state that there is great concern for the mental health and well-being of many seniors. Having been more socially isolated during COVID (in order to protect themselves), they are now struggling to re-emerge, including struggling to re-engage with their health care providers.

I am privileged to treat a senior struggling with depression, who has said to me that she is deeply lonely, but is scared to leave her home without certain trusted individuals (her adult children). Despite the best efforts to coordinate transportation and engage her family, there are times when she simply does not feel well enough to leave the street on which she lives. She has missed appointments as a result. And like her, there are many others! BNHC is hoping to acquire a mobile unit that can visit senior centers, senior housing sites, the council on aging and potentially other locations (as determined by data) to bring integrated care, including screening and treatment for behavioral health and substance use disorder to their living space. Making care accessible reduces inefficiencies in the system, is cost-effective, and, most importantly, promotes patients' health and well-being.

I am so appreciative that last year this Committee recognized the value of mobile care units when it passed the MOBILE Health Care Act by unanimous consent to make it easier for health centers to finance mobile health units. These mobile units can offer primary or dental care or provide behavioral health services to sparsely populated rural areas or underserved urban populations. While the MOBILE Health Care Act provided the necessary flexibility to health centers to use Federal funding for mobile units, it did not provide any additional New Access Point dollars to take advantage of this flexibility. Additional New Access Point funding is necessary for health centers to take advantage of this unique opportunity. With this funding, health centers, like BNHC, can provide easier access to patients who are not engaging in their integrated primary care homes. This prevents the worsening of their conditions, thus improving their health and well-being while being cost-effective.

In addition to launching mobile clinical units to provide integrated care services to the homeless, at schools, and for seniors, I strongly support permanently extending the telehealth flexibilities, including audio only telehealth care, implemented during the COVID–19 public health emergency. Telehealth has been particularly effective in creating and maintaining access to behavioral health and substance use disorder treatment. This should remain an option to maximize access to services so critically needed by so many. We are experiencing a mental health crisis, and our providers feel it. When 1 in 5 adults and 1 in 2 adolescents live with a mental health illness, these nimble and flexible strategies can save lives, prevent the need for higher levels of care and promote well-being.

Prioritizing Pediatrics

While I spoke about children generally, I would like to call out the critical importance of early childhood mental health. At BNHC, our experienced pediatric providers are deeply disturbed and overwhelmed by the number of children with symptoms of psychological distress. Senior pediatricians who have worked with our patient population for decades, are reporting a particular concern about seeing young children (0–5 years old) exhibiting symptoms that are consistent with Autism Spectrum Disorder but having difficulty accessing diagnostic evaluations due to a limited supply of professionals (psychologists and psychiatrists) trained in these assessment protocols, particularly to serve patients who are uninsured or underinsured.

Fortunately, at BNHC, we have had a robust primary care-behavioral health integration program for years, but we expanded in 2019 with the help of a private grant through the Transforming and Expanding Access to Mental Health Care in Urban Pediatrics (TEAM UP for children) program. TEAM UP is an initiative to build the capacity of 7 Community Health Centers in MA to deliver high-quality, evidence-based, integrated behavioral health care to children and families. The TEAM UP transformation model is rooted in three principles: transforming care, strengthening foundations, and creating a learning community. BNHC has been implementing the TEAM UP model since 2019 and continues to transform to meet the behavioral health needs of its early childhood, pediatric population through integration of behavioral health and social services into primary care. A study of the utilization of services for children who have engaged with TEAM UP sites showed an increase in access to behavioral health services for Medicaid-enrolled children.[1] The mental health needs of our pediatric patients are enormous, and Community Health Centers have innovative and proven strategies to increase access to mental health services. I strongly support investments in health center service expansions, as health centers are well-positioned to meet the needs of our children, who continue to demonstrate the repercussions of the traumatic effects of the last 3 years.

Workforce Development

Nationally and locally, workforce recruitment and retention pose major barriers to maximizing access to services that can address this mental health crisis we are experiencing. According to HRSA estimates based on national benchmarks, nearly one-third of Americans live in a federally designated Mental Health Professional Shortage Area, 7.7 million health center patients are currently going without needed mental health care, and 4.9 million health center patients are going without needed substance use disorder treatment. The models of care to maximize access exist and can be leveraged to meet these needs. However, staffing is critical to addressing this mental health crisis.

In full awareness of our challenge, BNHC has designed and launched a number of grant-funded professional pipeline projects, including one designed for the training, recruitment, and retention of behavioral health clinicians. In this program, BNHC commits to accepting, training, supervising and paying stipends to a cohort of behavioral health students completing their Masters degrees. Additionally, BNHC will pay a recruitment bonus to new hires, and a retention bonus to Behavioral Health Clinicians who have been with the organization for 2 years or more. Our intention is to incentivize training at and

---

[1] Association of Integrating Mental Health into Pediatric Primary Care at federally Qualified Health Centers with Utilization and Follow-Up Care. Jihye Kim, PhD1; R. Christopher Sheldrick, PhD2; Kerrin Gallagher, MPH2; et al.

hopefully also working at BNHC, or another Community Health Center. We would love for this Committee to provide more flexible funding to support a project like ours. These projects encourage training and working at community health centers, thus increasing the supply of trained behavioral health clinicians to meet the needs of this mental health crisis.

According to a survey by the National Association of Community Health Centers, behavioral health staff are in the top three categories for the highest rate of job loss for health centers. Competition from other employers and burnout from the pandemic are the most common reasons for staff departure. Additional Federal funding would help recruitment and retention. Another top priority impacting retention of staff are wellness programs and other interventions for employees to mitigate employment-related stress. I appreciate that last year, the HELP Committee passed the Lorna Breen Act by unanimous consent, which authorized funding for provider burnout. These programs are valuable because our staff are extraordinarily burnt out. As the Deputy CEO of BNHC, and a psychologist, I have the privilege and responsibility of listening to a lot of staff, and many of them have reported that they have ‘‘never felt worse’’.

We genuinely appreciate any support that our staff can receive to remain well in their roles as they continue to work daily to save lives and serve as the healthcare heroes who have been heralded throughout the pandemic. While not fighting COVID, they are fighting to address the effects of COVID including increased overdose deaths and substance use as well as serious mental health concerns.

Conclusion

Health centers like Brockton Neighborhood Health Center need long-term, sustainable, and predictable funding to meet our patients' behavioral health and substance use disorder needs. I recognize the difficult decisions Congress must make to balance funding levels with the need to maintain our Nation's fiscal health. Still, medical inflation has outpaced health centers' funding increases since 2015, leading to a 9.3 percent decrease in actual funding levels. Decades of research show that Federal investments in health centers reduce overall health spending by expanding access to efficient and effective primary care. Patients who access primary care at health centers show positive health outcomes and reduced use of emergency departments and hospital stays.

I appreciate that this budget environment makes additional investments challenging. Still, millions of patients could benefit by expanding access to mental health and substance use disorder care at the health centers where they are already receiving primary care. For example, the National Association of Community Health Centers estimates that an additional investment of $500 million over 5 years would allow health centers to hire more than 2,500 behavioral health specialists and reach more than 5 million additional patients. This level of commitment by Congress would leverage the existing network of care and build on a proven model that saves the health system billions of dollars.

Chairman Markey, Ranking Member Marshall, and Members of the Committee, thank you for allowing me to share the great work my team at BNHC is doing to fight the mental health and substance use disorder crisis in our Country. With this Committee's support, we will continue to find new ways to provide affordable, accessible, and high-quality care to the communities we serve. I look forward to your questions.

Senator MARKEY. Thank you, Dr. Celli, so much. Now, Senator Marshall will introduce our next witness.

Senator MARSHALL. Well, thank you, Mr. Chairman. I am certainly honored to introduce our second witness, Mr. Steven Denny, a fellow Jayhawk and a multi-generational Kansan. Mr. Denny is the deputy director of the Four County Mental Health Center. Their main office is in Independence, Kansas, and they proudly serve five counties now across Southeastern Kansas, including Montgomery County, Wilson, Elk, and Chautauqua.

As I think about that, that is probably an area of about 100 miles by 70 miles, very sparsely populated, and probably—it is the most economically challenged portion of Kansas. In addition to serving the mental health center, Mr. Denny is also the project director of Four Counties Certified Community Behavioral Health Clinic Expansion Grant, provided by the U.S. Substance Abuse and Mental Health Services Administration.

Under this role, Mr. Denny oversees clinical crises and substance use treatment services, as well as seeing patients every day. Thank you so much for agreeing to testify in person to discuss the work being done at Four County.

Mr. Denny, the floor is yours, thank you.

Statement of Steven Denny, Deputy Director, Four County Mental Health Center, Independence, KS

Mr. DENNY. Chairman Markey and Senator Marshall, thank you so much for this opportunity to testify before the Senate HELP Committee this morning. As I mentioned, my name is Steve Denny.

I serve as Deputy Director at Four County Mental Health Center, serving five counties in Southeast Kansas. You will hear me refer to our organization as Four County throughout this testimony. As I mentioned, I am also the Certified Community Behavioral Health Clinic Project Director, also known as CCBHC.

We were the first Kansas organization awarded a SAMHSA CCBHC expansion grant in May 2020. Since then, six additional centers have followed suit in 2021, and by July 1st of 2024, all Kansas community mental health centers will have the same opportunity to become CCBHCs after the passage of Kansas House Bill 2208.

It is a true honor today to speak to you about this exciting opportunity and what it has done for our state and our Nation. The second C in CCBHC stands for community. My community is Montgomery County, Kansas. It is a rural Kansas county located on the Oklahoma border. It contains both industry and agriculture.

My hometown is a place that I swore I would never return to when I went away to college, and I have been back now for 18 years. My father was a lifelong rancher. My children are the sixth generation to live on our family property, our small farm. My community matters to me.

The CCBHC model requires nine core services that are oriented around the unique needs of each community served by CCBHCs. Those nine services are included in my written testimony for further review. This community focus, combined with the comprehensive care, data driven measures, and a continuous focus on quality improvement, is what makes the CCBHC model such a game changer.

I have worked in this field since 2002 as a therapist and a supervisor of multiple populations. During this time, our field has experienced funding cuts, reduction of inpatient resources, and a state hospital crisis that has brought our system to a breaking point.

Many of my colleagues have left the field for less demanding jobs that often pay more. Meanwhile, the needs of our communities continue to grow, leading to this crisis. CCBHCs have served as a lifeline for our system.

Kansas House Bill 2208 provided foundation for our state to apply for the recent CCBHC planning grant to expand this model, with the support of Senator Marshall, for which we are immensely thankful. One shining example of an expanded program into our model is our Veterans Services Program. This provides specialized care coordination for veterans, service members, and their families.

We have seen a 51 percent increase from baseline of veterans served each quarter since project implementation. This crisis also involves our youth. The pandemic was mentioned as a creator of isolation. We found that 36 percent of our adolescent admissions are identified as at risk for suicide or self-harm. 35 percent from the same demographic report that social media is a negative factor in relationship to their mental wellness.

In response, we have started a robust school-based program that serves ten different districts in our area so that we can move our staff beyond the walls of our clinic. We anticipate continued growth in our youth services. In addition, we have created a special program targeting at risk adults for both legal place or legal issues and homelessness.

This program is known as the ACT, or a sort of community treatment program. It provided a crucial relief valve to law enforcement and emergency services. Initial outcome shows that 80 percent of the population has avoided homelessness and 76 percent have avoided new legal incidents based on quarterly tracking data.

In addition, we have developed a special program in partnership with law enforcement. We have four co-responders and 25 iPad devices deployed to our law enforcement partners to increase connection to law enforcement and emergency services. The CCBHC model increases access to care.

Since implementation, our Four County provides 70 percent of the admissions on the same day that individuals seek services. For those who elect to wait, the average wait time is 3 days compared to the national average of 48 days.

They also receive enhanced care coordination and involvement with primary care. If they don't have a primary care provider, we work hard to get them connected. The next big thing in our field is mobile crisis services, which we will need to develop in partnership with a new 9–8–8 crisis hotline.

National data indicates that this CCBHC model reduces ER visits by 68 percent. It also emphasizes care coordination and improved partnership with our local emergency hospitals. In conclusion, I just want to express my sincere support that we should move this model beyond a demonstration project and have it become a staple of our health care system.

Thank you for the opportunity to testify here today on behalf of the people we serve, and for the incredible workforce. Senator Markey, you said, heroes will go—there are so many unsung heroes that do this work, and I am thankful to be in this field. Thank you.

[The prepared statement of Mr. Denny follows:]

Prepared Statement of Steven Denny

Chairman Markey and Senator Marshall, thank you for the opportunity to testify before the Senate HELP Committee this morning. My name is Steve Denny, and I serve as Deputy Director of Four County Mental Health Center, Inc. (FCMHC) located in Southeast Kansas, where I also serve as the Certified Community Behavioral Health Clinic (CCBHC) project director. FCMHC was the first Kansas organization awarded a SAMHSA CCBHC expansion grant in May 20. Six additional Community Mental Health Centers followed suit and were awarded expansion grants in 2021. I have had the privilege of bearing witness to the milestones that created the rapid development of CCBHCs in Kansas. These milestones include the passage of the Kansas House Bill 2208 which established CCBHCs in Kansas and led to the eventual development of a State Plan Amendment to fund these clinics. By July 1st, 2024, our goal is to have all Kansas Community Mental Health Centers become CCBHCs. It is my honor today to speak to the exciting opportunity that the CCBHC model has brought to Kansas and to our Nation.

The second ‘‘C’’ in ‘‘CCBHC’’ represents the word ‘‘community.’’ My community is Montgomery County, Kansas. It is a rural Kansas county located on the Oklahoma border that contains both industry and agriculture and where CCBHCs have saved lives. The CCBHC model requires 9 core services based on the unique needs assessment of the communities served by each clinic. These services include (1) crisis services, screening, (2) diagnosis and risk assessment, (3) psychiatric rehabilitation services, (4) outpatient primary care screening and monitoring, (5) targeted case management, (6) outpatient mental health and substance use services, (7) person and family centered treatment planning, (8) community based mental health care for veterans and (9) peer and family support services. This community focus combined with comprehensive care, data-driven approaches, and a continuous focus on quality is what makes the CCBHC model such a game changer.

I have worked in the field of behavioral health since 2002 as a therapist and supervisor for services to adults diagnosed with severe mental illness, crisis services, substance use treatment services, and adult and child outpatient therapy services. During this time, our field has experienced funding cuts, reduction of inpatient resources that brought us to the breaking point. Many colleagues have left the field for less demanding jobs that pay more. Meanwhile, the behavioral health needs of our communities continue to rise, leading us to a mental health and substance use crisis. Both personally and professionally, I've experienced the impact of suicide involving a variety of demographics, including adults, older adults, veterans and adolescents. One out of every five of FCMHC's crisis assessments are in response to a suicide attempt. In addition, we are facing an unparalleled mental health and substance use provider workforce shortage that has been growing for years and now is at a tipping point.

CCBHCs serve as a lifeline to the people of Kansas. Legislative efforts in Kansas established CCBHCs and provided the foundation for us to apply for the recent CCBHC planning grant to expand this model, with the tremendous support from Senator Marshall, for which we are immensely thankful. CCBHC implementation meant our organization could start and bolster mental health and substance use services based on the community needs. One shining example is FCMHC's Veterans Services program, which provides specialized care coordination for Veterans, service members, and their families. As a result, our organization serves an average of 140 unduplicated veterans each quarter which is a 51 percent increase from baseline all while improving our working relationship with two Veterans Administration facilities with the support of Senator Moran.

Part of the nationwide mental health and substance uses crisis involves our youth. Our children have been isolated with nothing but screens and devices, left alone at times to try and survive without the support of a community that teaches them to not just survive but to thrive. Youth suicide rates in Kansas increased by 63.8 percent in the most recent 15 year period (Kansas Health Institute) Outpacing the national average, which is also rising. 36 percent of adolescent admissions at FCMHC are identified as at risk for suicide or self-harm and 35 percent of the same demographic report that social media is a negative factor in relationship to their mental wellness. In response, we started a robust school-based program along with long standing programs that offer rehabilitation services to youth with more intensive needs. We are currently serving 9 school districts with CCBHC staff embedded in schools. We anticipate that opportunities to serve our youth will increase under the CCBHC model.

In addition, we have created special programs to work with the most ''at risk'' adults who have been diagnosed with mental health and substance use challenges and are often homeless and/or involved with the legal system. This program is known as the Assertive Community Treatment (ACT) model and has provided a crucial relief valve to law enforcement. The initial outcome data shows 80 percent of the population has avoided homeless incidents and 76 percent have avoided new legal incidents. Nationally, 96 percent of CCBHCs are actively engaged in one or more innovative activities in partnership with criminal justice agencies, including 77 percent who—like us—have used their CCBHC status to launch intensive outreach and engagement services to divert people at high risk from further involvement with the criminal justice system.

Of equal importance is the increased access to services in a timely manner while improving care coordination. Since CCBHC implementation, our organization provides 70 percent of admissions on the same day that they seek services. For those who do have to wait, the average wait time is 3 days compared to the national average of 48 days. Individuals in our care receive enhanced care coordination with primary care. 74 percent of our active population has an active primary care provider. When individuals do not have a primary care provider or require additional referrals, care coordinators work hard to close the referral loop. Through data collection, we identified the need to develop a tobacco cessation program. FCMHC currently provides tobacco cessation services to 72 individuals with 47 percent successfully quitting or reducing usage by more than half after starting the program. This is especially encouraging for the long-term cost implications for populations that have co-occurring chronic health conditions.

As we look ahead to CCBHC implementation in Kansas, we need to develop more mobile crisis services in partnership with the national 988 crisis hotline. Mobile crisis services reduce the number of emergency room visits. National data indicates that the CCBHC model reduces emergency room admission percentages by 68 percent. In addition, the CCBHC model emphasizes care coordination agreements between the CCBHC and the hospital. This improves partnerships and helps individuals from falling through the cracks upon discharge to the community.

In conclusion, I wish to express my support that the CCBHC model should move beyond ''demonstration'' status and become a staple of our healthcare system. As Daniel Tsai, the Director of Center for Medicaid and CHIP services at the Center for Medicare and Medicaid Services (CMS) and past Medicaid Director for the State of Massachusetts articulated during the national meeting for the National Council for Mental Well-being just a few weeks ago, the CCBHC model represents a crucial part to the pyramid of health care that we need to ensure high quality access to care for all people across our Nation. We have clearly seen this to be true for Kansas. Thank you for the opportunity to testify on behalf of the countless individuals that the CCBHC system serves and the incredible workforce that provides this care.

Senator MARKEY. Thank you, Mr. Denny, so much. I am going to recognize Senator Tuberville for an introduction of Dr. Taylor. Dr. Taylor is President Elect of the American Society of Addiction Medicine, a triple board certified in general child, adolescent addiction and sports psychiatry. Dr. Taylor also serves as the Medical Director of the NBA.

Senator Tuberville.

Senator TUBERVILLE. Thank you. Thank you, Senator Markey and Senator Marshall, for having this. Just a quick statement, and I note, I am not a Member of this Committee, but I will say this is—the importance of this Committee. I dealt with hundreds of families every year in my former job, and there weren't many families that I would ever run into that didn't have some type of mental health problem in their family.

This is not a crisis. This is a national emergency. I don't think we really understand the problems that we have now. We are going to continue to have it. It is going to get worse if we don't address it, and it is by having hearings like this. I tell people all the time, they say, wait, we can't afford to attack mental health problems. It is too big.

My comment to that is we can't afford not to fund mental health in this country. We have to attack mental health in this country, and we have got to fund it no matter what it takes. So, tough times requires tough leaders. Dr. Taylor, it is my privilege to introduce Stephen Taylor from Birmingham, Alabama.

He is completing his 13th season as the Medical Director of the Player Assistance Anti-Drug Program with the NBA, the National Basketball Players Association. He also serves as the Chief Medical Officer of the Behavioral Health Division of Pathway Health Care, a company that operates 17 outpatient addiction treatment offices spread throughout the South. Additionally, Dr. Taylor is President Elect of the American Society of Addiction Medicine.

Dr. Taylor is uniquely positioned to understand the scope and the extent of the mental health crisis and emergency we are experiencing in this country. This crisis affects children and adults of all ages and all walks of life. He is a perfect witness for today's hearing, a crisis in mental health and emergency substance use disorder care.

He will discuss the work that needs to be done to fix our broken mental health care infrastructure in this country. I am incredibly proud to have someone like Dr. Taylor working on these issues in the great State of Alabama, and I look forward to partnering with him, moving forward, to help keep up these efforts. I am also pleased that this Subcommittee is focusing on this today and hope that the entire HELP Committee can understand the importance of this.

Dr. Taylor, welcome and thank you, Mr. Chair.

Senator MARKEY. Thank you, Senator. You are recognized, whenever you are comfortable, Dr. Taylor. Please begin.

Statement of Stephen Taylor, President Elect, American Society of Addiction Medicine, Birmingham, Al

Dr. TAYLOR. Thank you for that kind introduction, Senator Tuberville. Chairman Markey, Ranking Member Marshall, and esteemed Members of this Subcommittee, thank you for inviting me to participate in today's hearing on closing gaps in access to mental health and substance use disorder care by bringing that care into communities across this Nation.

Today, I am testifying in my capacity as President elect of the American Society of Addiction Medicine, known as ASAM. ASAM is a National Medical Society representing over 7,000 physicians and other clinicians who specialize in the prevention and treatment of addiction and co-occurring conditions.

I would like to begin by recognizing the bipartisan work that Congress has done over the years to help address what is turning out to be the deadliest addiction and overdose crisis in American history. Thank you for your efforts.

Still, at a time of elevated death rates and medical complications associated with synthetic opioids like fentanyl, psycho stimulants like methamphetamine, and the non-opioid veterinary tranquilizer Xylazine, much more work needs to be done to create a sustainable and robust addiction care infrastructure, one that addresses addiction as a preventable and treatable chronic medical disease.

Accordingly, ASAM asks this Subcommittee to focus on three areas that are ripe for policy intervention. First, the addiction specialist physician workforce. ASAM estimates that there are only about 7,000 addiction specialist physicians defined as physicians who are board certified in addiction medicine or addiction psychiatry in this country.

While addiction treatment in the United States is often delivered to patients by multidisciplinary health care teams that work to address patients bio-psychosocial needs, the distinct clinical knowledge and skill set of addiction specialist physicians best situates us to lead those teams.

Addiction specialist physicians can increase our health care team's capacity to prevent and treat more complicated medical cases involving substance use disorder. Addiction specialist led care teams also lead to the greater integration of addiction care into general medical and mental health treatment settings.

Even more importantly, such care models can enable our health care system to increase its capacity to provide addiction treatment in primary care settings, which is especially important in areas where there is a dearth of specialty addiction treatment facilities.

For this and other reasons, Congress created the groundbreaking Substance Use Disorder Treatment and Recovery Loan Repayment Program, or STAR-LRP, in the Support Act of 2018. When individuals pursue a full-time job to provide addiction treatment in high need geographic areas, HRSA's STAR-LRP can help them repay up to $250,000 in their student loans. Demand for this program has been overwhelming.

Therefore, ASAM strongly supports the Substance Use Disorder Treatment and Recovery Loan Repayment Program Reauthorization Act of 2023, which was introduced yesterday in the House on a bipartisan basis and would further strengthen the program while preserving its focus on addiction care workforce.

Additionally, ASAM urges this Congress to pass legislation to encourage teaching health center graduate medical education program applicants to sponsor addiction medicine fellowship programs, and to require all HRSA funded health centers to offer addiction and mental health services.

Second, decriminalization of the prescribing of methadone for the treatment of OUD by addiction specialist physicians for dispensing at pharmacies. While ASAM is grateful for SAMHSA's ongoing efforts to update Federal regulations governing opioid treatment programs known as OTPs, continuing to restrict patient access to methadone for OUD to OTP settings is a public health threat that unnecessarily limits access to this lifesaving medication for those who need it.

Therefore, ASAM strongly supports passage of the bipartisan, bicameral, Modernizing Opioid Treatment Access Act, which would responsibly expand access to methadone treatment for all OUDs by decriminalizing its prescribing by addiction specialist physicians for dispensing at pharmacies.

Third, enforcement of Federal mental health and addiction parity law. It has been well documented that we need better enforcement of Federal mental health and addiction parity law in this country. Under current law, the U.S. Department of Labor lacks the authority to assess civil monetary penalties for violations of Federal parity law already on the books.

This prevents DOL from effectively ending parity violations with respect to group health plans. That is why ASAM strongly supports the soon to be introduced Parity Enforcement Act, which would finally add civil monetary penalty authority to the DOL's oversight.

In conclusion, these policies and resources are imperative to bringing addiction care into communities across this Nation and to saving more lives. Thank you, and I look forward to answering your questions.

[The prepared statement of Dr. Taylor follows:]

Prepared Statement of Stephen Taylor

Chairman Markey, Ranking Member Marshall, and esteemed Members of this Subcommittee, thank you for inviting me to participate in today's critically important hearing on closing gaps in access to mental health and substance use disorder (SUD) care by bringing that care into communities across this Nation. My name is Dr. Stephen Taylor. I am board-certified in addiction medicine, addiction psychiatry, child and adolescent psychiatry, and general psychiatry. I take care of patients with addiction and co-occurring conditions in Birmingham, Alabama where I serve as the Chief Medical Officer of Pathway Healthcare—a company operating 17 outpatient mental health and addiction treatment offices in five southern states. I am also the Medical Director of the Player Assistance and Anti-Drug Program of the National Basketball Association (NBA) and the National Basketball Players Association (NBPA) . Today, I am testifying in my capacity as President-Elect of the American Society of Addiction Medicine, known as ASAM. ASAM is a national medical society representing over 7,000 physicians and other clinicians who specialize in the prevention and treatment of addiction and co-occurring conditions.

I would like to begin by recognizing the bipartisan work that Congress has done over the years to help address—what is turning out to be—the deadliest addiction and overdose crisis in American history. Your efforts have made a positive difference. Thank you.

Still, at a time of elevated death rates and medical complications associated with synthetic opioids like fentanyl, psychostimulants like methamphetamine, and the non-opioid veterinary tranquilizer xylazine, much more work needs to be done to create a sustainable and robust addiction care infrastructure—one that addresses addiction as a preventable and treatable chronic medical disease.

Accordingly, ASAM asks this Subcommittee to focus on the following three areas that are ripe for policy intervention:

1) Prioritization of the recruitment, training, and retention of addiction specialist physicians—defined as physicians who are board certified in addiction medicine or addiction psychiatry;[2]
2) Decriminalization of the prescribing of methadone for the treatment of opioid use disorder (OUD) by addiction specialist physicians (and OTP (defined below) clinicians) for dispensing at pharmacies; methadone is the only full opioid agonist medication that is approved by the Food and Drug Administration (FDA) for the treatment of OUD; and
3) Enforcement of Federal mental health and addiction parity law that is already on the books.

Prioritization of the Addiction Specialist Physician Workforce

Addiction is a chronic medical disease involving complex interactions among brain circuits, genetics, the environment, and an individual's life experiences. People with addiction use substances or engage in behaviors that become compulsive and often continue despite harmful consequences. A lack of knowledge and misinformation about addiction within the medical community

---

[2] ASAM. Public Policy Statement on Recognition and Role of Addiction Specialist Physicians in Health Care in the United States. *https://www.asam.org/advocacy/public-policy-statements/details/public-policy-statements/2022/01/28/public-policy-statement-on-the-recognition-and-role-of-addiction-specialist-physicians-in-health-care-in-the-united-states* (describing the four medical subspecialty certifications that demonstrate and define physician expertise in addiction treatment).

has been a longstanding problem. Therefore, the fact that there remains far too few physicians and other clinicians who specialize in the assessment of substance use disorder (SUD) and the prevention and treatment of the disease of addiction is of grave concern. According to the Substance Abuse and Mental Health Services Administration (SAMHSA), in 2021,

well over 40 million Americans had SUD in the past year.[3] For purposes of comparison, the State of California has nearly 40 million residents. At the same time, deaths continue to persist at record levels from drug overdoses, according to the Centers for Disease Control and Prevention.[4]

Shortfalls exist at all levels of the addiction care workforce, but one of the most grievous is among addiction specialist physicians. ASAM estimates that there are only about 7,000[5] of said physicians in this country—defined as physicians holding board certification in the medical subspecialty of addiction medicine or addiction psychiatry. As of March 2023, there were only 96 ACGME-accredited addiction medicine fellowship programs in the nation 5[6]—far below the recommended goal of 125 fellowships by 2022 set by the President's Commission on Combating Drug Abuse and the Opioid Epidemic over 5 years ago.[7] 6 Our failure to meet this goal should be unacceptable.

---

[3] Substance Abuse and Mental Health Administration. ''Key Substance Use and Mental Health Indicators in the United States: Results from the 2021 National Survey on Drug Use and Health.'' U.S. Department of Health and Human Services Substance Abuse and Mental Health Services Administration, Center for Behavioral Health Statistics and Quality, Populations Survey Branch, no. PEP22–07–01–005 (December 2022). *https://www.samhsa.gov/data/sites/default/files/reports/rpt39443/2021NSDUHFFRRev010323.pdf.*

[4] Ahmad FB, Cisewski JA, Rossen LM, Sutton P. Provisional drug overdose death counts. National Center for Health Statistics. 2023. Designed by LM Rossen, A Lipphardt, FB Ahmad, JM Keralis, and Y Chong: National Center for Health Statistics.

[5] According to an email that ASAM received from the Executive Director of the American Board of Preventive Medicine (ABPM), as of January 2023, there were 4,347 Addiction Medicine Diplomates through ABPM with active status. According to an email that ASAM received from the Executive Director of the American College of Academic Addiction Medicine (ACAAM), as of January 2023, there were 1,312 addiction medicine physicians through the American Board of Addiction Medicine (ABAM). (According to ACAAM's Executive Director, there may be small overlap of people who remain both certified by ABAM and ABPM, but it would not be a significant number.) According to the 2021—2022 ABMS Board Certification Report, as of June 30, 2022, there were 1,398 board-certified addiction psychiatrists in the U.S. (some of whom may be retired). ASAM was unable to confirm the number of AOA board-certified addiction medicine physicians as of the date of this hearing, but estimates a few hundred physicians holding such board certification.

[6] American College of Academic Addiction Medicine. *https://www.acaam.org/fellowship-training.*

[7] THE PRESIDENT'S COMMISSION ON COMBATING DRUG ADDICTION AND THE OPIOID CRISIS. *https://trumpwhitehouse.archives.gov/sites/whitehouse.gov/files/images/Final—Report—Draft—11-15-2017.pdf.*

While addiction treatment in the U.S. is often delivered to patients by multidisciplinary healthcare teams that work to address patients' biopsychosocial needs,[8] the distinct clinical knowledge and skill set of addiction specialist physicians best situate them to lead those teams. Addiction specialist physicians can increase a healthcare team's capacity to prevent and treat more complex medical cases involving substance use disorder. Addiction specialist-led care teams can also lead to the greater integration of addiction care into general medical and mental health treatment settings. Even more importantly, such care models can enable our healthcare system to increase its capacity to provide addiction treatment in primary care settings—which is especially important in areas where there is a dearth of specialty addiction treatment facilities.

Indeed, Congress acknowledged just how severe the overall SUD workforce shortage is—including its addiction specialist shortage—when it created a groundbreaking loan repayment program, known as the Substance Use Disorder Treatment and Recovery Loan Repayment Program, or STAR-LRP, in the SUPPORT for Patients and Communities Act of 2018. When individuals pursue a full-time job to provide SUD treatment in high-need geographic areas, the Health Resources and Services Administration (HRSA)'s STAR-LRP can help them repay up to $250,000 in their student loans. Unsurprisingly, demand for this program has been overwhelming. In Fiscal Year 2021, alone, over 3,000 people applied for the program, but HRSA only had enough funding to serve 8 percent—or 255 of them— at an average award amount of a little over $100,000, which is far below the maximum award amount allowed. Reauthorizing and strengthening STAR-LRP this year, while retaining its laser focus on the SUD workforce, is a top priority for ASAM. That is why ASAM strongly supports passage of the Substance Use Disorder Treatment and Recovery Loan Repayment Program Reauthorization Act of 2023, which is bipartisan legislation in the House that would further strengthen the program while preserving its focus on the addiction care workforce.

In addition, while ASAM urges Congress to ensure that addiction specialist physicians are included across all HRSA Behavioral Health Workforce Development Programs, I also want to highlight that addiction specialist physicians often hold primary board certifications in the primary

[8] Examples of multidisciplinary team models include specialized addiction treatment programs, the Patient Centered Medical Home (PCMH), the "hub-and-spoke" model, the nurse care management model, and the Collaborative Care Model, which exist on a spectrum of integration with general medical treatment.

care specialties recognized by HRSA's Teaching Health Center Graduate Medical Education (THCGME) program. Those primary care specialties include family medicine, internal medicine, pediatrics, and general psychiatry. This multispecialty characteristic of addiction medicine is, therefore, why ASAM recommends that Congress pass legislation that would prioritize (or otherwise incentivize) THCGME program applicants that sponsor addiction medicine fellowship programs. ASAM also strongly supports the President's Budget proposals to (1) make additional investments in addiction and mental health services at health centers and (2) amend section 330 of the Public Health Service Act to require all HRSA-funded health centers to offer addiction and mental health services.[9]

Decriminalization of the Prescribing of Methadone for OUD by Addiction Specialist Physicians for Pharmacy Dispensing

Second, we all know that the long U.S. history of treating addiction in siloed settings separate from the rest of medicine exacerbates the addiction care workforce shortage. SAMHSA estimates that less than four in ten patients with OUD—who are primarily admitted for OUD to publicly funded SUD treatment—receive treatment with medications for OUD.[10] Other studies have shown even worse rates of appropriate medication usage for alcohol use disorder.[11,12] We no longer accept this in other parts of American medicine, and it is not acceptable for caring individuals with addiction.

---

[9] Johnson, Carole. HRSA Administrator. Testimony before the U.S. House of Representatives Committee on Energy and Commerce Subcommittee on Health on ''Examining Existing Federal Programs to Build a Stronger Health Workforce and Improve Primary Care.'' *https:// d1dth6e84htgma.cloudfront.net/Witness—Testimony—Carole—Johnson—HE—Hearing—04—19—23—e3abe98943.pdf'updated—at=2023—04—17T20:18:01. 021Z.* Published April 19, 2023. Accessed April 24, 2023.

[10] Substance Abuse and Mental Health Services Administration, Center for Behavioral Health Statistics and Quality. Treatment Episode Data Set (TEDS): 2020. Admissions to and Discharges from Publicly Funded Substance Use Treatment Facilities. Rockville, MD: Substance Abuse and Mental Health Services Administration, 2022.

[11] Arms L, Johl H, DeMartini J. Improving the utilization of medication-assisted treatment for alcohol use disorder at discharge. BMJ Open Quality 2022;11:e001899. doi: 10.1136/ bmjoq— 2022—001899.

[12] Policymaker Summary: Pharmacotherapy for Adults with Alcohol Use Disorder in Outpatient Settings. Content last reviewed January 2021. Effective Health Care Program, Agency for Healthcare Research and Quality, Rockville, MD. *https://effectivehealthcare.ahrq.gov/ products/alcohol-misuse-drug-therapy/policymaker.*

In 2019, a national report noted that the fragmentation that has occurred as a result of separating OUD treatment settings from other medical care not only creates significant access barriers, but is not supported by evidence.[13] More specifically, while models of integrated methadone treatment of OUD with primary and other medical care sometimes exist in the U.S., they are much more common internationally. A 2017 international meta-analysis showed a significant reduction in all-cause mortality among people treated with methadone for OUD, both by general practitioners and specialty clinics.[14,15] Randomized controlled trials—the gold standard—have demonstrated the safety and efficacy of methadone treatment of stable patients in primary care.[16,17] Safety has also been shown in multiple non-randomized studies, some with 9 to 15 years of follow-up.[18,19,20] Methadone has been available by prescription in Australia since 1970, and in Great Britain since 1968.[21] Moreover, office-based prescribing and pharmacy dispensing of methadone increase the number of individuals with OUD with access to

---

[13] National Academies of Sciences, Engineering, and Medicine. 2019. Medications for opioid use disorder save lives. Washington, DC: The National Academies Press. doi: *https://doi.org/ 10.17226/25310*.

[14] Sordo L, Barrio G, Bravo MJ, et al. Mortality risk during and after opioid substitution treatment: systematic review and meta-analysis of cohort studies. BMJ. 2017;357:j1550.

[15] Samet JH, Botticelli M, Bharel M. Methadone in Primary Care—One Small Step for Congress, One Giant Leap for Addiction Treatment. N Engl J Med. 2018;379(1):7–8. doi:10.1056/ NEJMp1803982.

[16] Fiellin DA, O'Connor PG, Chawarski M, Pakes JP, Pantalon MV, Schottenfeld RS. Methadone maintenance in primary care: a randomized controlled trial. JAMA. 2001 Oct 10;286(14):1724–31. doi: 10.1001/jama.286.14.1724. PMID: 11594897.

[17] Carrieri PM, Michel L, Lions C, et al. Methadone induction in primary care for opioid dependence: a pragmatic randomized trial (ANRS Methaville). PLoS One. 2014;9(11):e112328. Published 2014 Nov 13. doi:10.1371/journal.pone.0112328.

[18] Novick DM, Joseph H, Salsitz EA, et al. Outcomes of treatment of socially rehabilitated methadone maintenance patients in physicians' offices (medical maintenance): follow-up at three and a half to nine and a fourth years. J Gen Intern Med. 1994;9(3):127–130. doi:10.1007/ BF02600025.

[19] Salsitz EA, Joseph H, Frank B, et al. Methadone medical maintenance (MMM): treating chronic opioid dependence in private medical practice—a summary report (1983–1998). Mt Sinai J Med. 2000;67(5–6):388–397.

[20] Schwartz RP, Brooner RK, Montoya ID, Currens M, Hayes M. A 12-year follow-up of a methadone medical maintenance program. Am J Addict. 1999;8(4):293–299. doi:10.1080/ 105504999305695.

[21] Samet JH, Botticelli M, Bharel M. Methadone in Primary Care—One Small Step for Congress, One Giant Leap for Addiction Treatment. N Engl J Med. 2018;379(1):7–8. doi:10.1056/ NEJMp1803982.

methadone treatment, as occurred in Canada following its 1996 implementation of such practices.[22]

Here, in the U.S., methadone was first used for OUD treatment in the 1960's under Investigational New Drug applications issued by the FDA, at a time when providing opioid medications for OUD remained illegal otherwise.[23] In 1972, the FDA determined and approved methadone as safe and effective for treatment of OUD.[24] At the same time, erroneous beliefs that methadone replaced one addiction for another, reports of methadone-related deaths and diversion,[25] and concerns over increasing crime rates[26] created a climate of skepticism and hostility toward methadone-based OUD care. In 1974, Congress granted additional jurisdiction over methadone to the Drug Enforcement Administration (DEA).[27] Both FDA, and subsequently SAMHSA, replaced the usual practice of physician autonomy with strict rules governing the provision of methadone for OUD treatment that—to this day-do not apply when methadone is prescribed for pain and dispensed from a community pharmacy.

These exceptional Federal regulations specified criteria on eligibility, initial methadone dosages, required counseling services, supervised dosing, and restricted methadone treatment to provision within a closed system of regulated clinics, then known as narcotic treatment programs, now known as opioid treatment programs or OTPs.[28] Such detailed regulations surrounding a specific medical practice have led into an orientation toward regulatory

---

[22] Nosyk B, Anglin MD, Brissette S, et al. A Call For Evidence-Based Medical Treatment Of Opioid Dependence In The United States and Canada. Health Affairs. 2013;32(8): 1462—1469. *https://doi.org/10.1377/hlthaff.2012.0846.*

[23] Jaffe JH, O'Keeffe C. From morphine clinics to buprenorphine: regulating opioid agonist treatment of addiction in the United States. Drug Alcohol Depend. 2003 May 21;70(2 Suppl):S3–11. doi: 10.1016/s0376–8716(03)00055–3. PMID: 12738346.

[24] Institute of Medicine (US) Committee on Federal Regulation of Methadone Treatment; Rettig RA, Yarmolinsky A, editors. Federal Regulation of Methadone Treatment. Washington (DC): National Academies Press (US); 1995. Executive Summary. Available from: *https://www.ncbi.nlm.nih.gov/books/NBK232111/.*

[25] Jaffe JH, O'Keeffe C. From morphine clinics to buprenorphine: regulating opioid agonist treatment of addiction in the United States. Drug Alcohol Depend. 2003 May 21;70(2 Suppl):S3–11. doi: 10.1016/s0376–8716(03)00055–3. PMID: 12738346.

[26] Kleber, Herbert D. Methadone Maintenance 4 Decades Later. JAMA. 2008;300(19):2303–2305. free: *https://jamanetwork.com/journals/jama/fullarticle/182898.*

[27] Jaffe JH, O'Keeffe C. From morphine clinics to buprenorphine: regulating opioid agonist treatment of addiction in the United States. Drug Alcohol Depend. 2003 May 21;70(2 Suppl):S3–11. doi: 10.1016/s0376–8716(03)00055–3. PMID: 12738346.

[28] Jaffe JH, O'Keeffe C. From morphine clinics to buprenorphine: regulating opioid agonist treatment of addiction in the United States. Drug Alcohol Depend. 2003 May 21;70(2 Suppl):S3–11. doi: 10.1016/s0376–8716(03)00055–3. PMID: 12738346.

compliance, to the detriment of incentivizing innovation, quality, or individualized patient care. The detailed regulations also have carried along with them a misguided conception of abstinence defined as cessation of methadone pharmacotherapy.[29] Experts have written about how such a highly regulated system of methadone-specific clinics in the U.S. reflects structural racism and contributes to health disparities among people with OUD.[30]

It is progress and good news that outdated Federal OTP regulations will be updated soon to address OUD treatment standards in that setting. Drawing on research, evidence, and experience from the past two decades, thankfully, SAMHSA has indicated forthcoming regulatory updates when it issued a notice of proposed rulemaking in December 2022.[31] 30 However, by continuing to largely restrict access to methadone for OUD to OTPs, the potential for expanded access to methadone treatment for OUD remains severely limited. Despite an expansion of OTPs in the U.S. in certain sectors in recent years, the prevalence of OUD has grown more quickly.[32] Most U.S. counties do not even have an OTP.[33] OTPs have established only a limited number of ''mobile components,'' known as medication vans,[34] and a limited

---

[29] White WL, Mojer-Torres L. Recovery-Oriented Methadone Maintenance. 2010. *http://www.williamwhitepapers.com/pr/dlm—uploads/2010Recovery—orientedMethadoneMaintenance.pdf.* Accessed April 22, 2023.

[30] Miller, NS. Racial disparities in opioid addiction treatment: a primer and research round- up. The Journalist's Resource. 2021. *https://journalistsresource.org/home/systemic-racism-opioid-addiction-treatment/*. Accessed April 22, 2023.

[31] SAMHSA. SAMHSA Proposes Update to Federal Rules to Expand Access to Opioid Use Disorder Treatment and Help Close Gap in Care*https://www.samhsa.gov/newsroom/press-announcements/20221213/update-Federal-rules-expand-access-opioid-use-disorder-treatment*. Published December 13, 2023. Accessed April 24, 2023. In addition, in April 2023, SAMHSA issued newly revised April 2023 Guidance extending methadone take-home flexibilities—effective upon the expiration of the COVID–19 public health emergency and remaining in effect for the period of 1 year from the end of the COVID–19 public health emergency, or until such time that the final rules revising 42 CFR part 8 are published. *https://www.samhsa.gov/medications-substance-use-disorders/statutes-regulations-guidelines/methadone-guidance*.

[32] Substance Abuse and Mental Health Services Administration, National Survey of Substance Abuse Treatment Services (N-SSATS): 2020. Data on Substance Abuse Treatment Facilities. Rockville, MD: Substance Abuse and Mental Health Services Administration, 2021.

[33] Joudrey PJ, Chadi N, Roy P, Morford KL, Bach P, Kimmel S, Wang EA, Calcaterra SL. Pharmacy-based methadone dispensing and drive time to methadone treatment in five states within the United States: A cross-sectional study. Drug Alcohol Depend. 2020 Mar 27;211:107968. doi: 10.1016/j.drugalcdep.2020.107968. Epub ahead of print. PMID: 32268248; PMCID: PMC7529685.

[34] Biden-Harris Administration Expands Treatment to Underserved Communities with Mobile Methadone Van Rule. *https://www.whitehouse.gov/ondcp/briefing-room/2021/06/*

number of satellite medication units in locations such as pharmacies, jails, prisons, federally qualified health centers (FQHCs), and residential treatment facilities, resulting in limited geographic reach,[35] and complex demographic inequities in access to treatment.[36]

For these reasons, ASAM strongly supports passage of the bipartisan and bicameral Modernizing Opioid Treatment Access Act (M-OTAA) (S. 644/H.R. 1359). M-OTAA would responsibly expand the capacity for lifesaving methadone treatment for individuals with OUD through our existing medical infrastructure. Specifically, it would decriminalize[37] OTP clinicians and addiction specialist physicians—the latter representing some of the most educated and experienced physicians using pharmacotherapies for OUD in the nation[38]—who prescribe methadone

---

29/biden-harris-administration-expands-treatmentto-underserved-communities-with-mobile-methadone-van-rule—2021/. Published June 29, 2021. Accessed April 22, 2023.

[35] ''Methadone Barriers Persist, Despite Decades Of Evidence, ''Health Affairs Blog, September 23, 2019. DOI: 10.1377/hblog20190920.981503.

[36] Joudrey, Paul, Gavin Bart, Robert Brooner, Lawrence Brown, Julia Dickson-Gomez, Adam Gordon, Sarah Kawasaki, et al. ''Research Priorities for Expanding Access to Methadone Treatment for Opioid Use Disorder in the United States: A National Institute on Drug Abuse Center for Clinical Trials Network Task Force Report.'' Substance Abuse 42 (July 3, 2021): 245—54. *https://doi.org/10.1080/08897077.2021.1975344.*

[37] Lampe, J.R. (2023). The Controlled Substances Act (CSA): A legal overview for the 118th Congress (CRS Report No. R45948). Congressional Research Service, 9. *https://crsreports.Congress.gov/product/pdf/R/R45948* (stating that a violation of the Controlled Substances Act's registration requirements is a criminal offense if the violation is committed knowingly, and the Department of Justice may bring criminal charges against individual registrants; for example, a first criminal violation of the registration requirements by an individual is punishable by a fine or up to a year in prison).

[38] The American College of Graduate Medical Education (ACGME) sets the program requirements for graduate medical education in addiction medicine and addiction psychiatry. ACGME common core program requirements for addiction medicine fellowships include: pharmacotherapy and psychosocial interventions for SUDs across the age spectrum, (IV.B.1.c.).(1).(k)); the mechanisms of action and effects of use and abuse of alcohol, sedatives, opioids, and other drugs, and the pharmacotherapies and other modalities used to treat these (IV.B.1.c).(1).(m)); the safe prescribing and monitoring of controlled medications to patients with or without SUDs (IV.B.1.c).(1).(n)); at least 3 months of structured inpatient rotations, including inpatient addiction treatment programs, hospital-based rehabilitation programs, medically managed residential programs where the fellow is directly involved with patient assessment and treatment planning, and/or general medical facilities or teaching hospitals where the fellow provides consultation services to other physicians in the Emergency Department for patients admitted with a primary medical, surgical, obstetrical, or psychiatric diagnosis; (IV.C.3.a).(1)); at least 3 months of outpatient experience, including intensive outpatient treatment or ''day treatment'' programs, addiction medicine consult services in an ambulatory care setting, pharmacotherapy, and/or other medical services where the fellow is directly involved with patient assessment, counseling, treatment planning, and coordination with

for OUD that can be dispensed from a community pharmacy. Among other safeguards contained in M-OTAA, these separately registered prescribers would remain subject to SAMHSA's continued regulation and guidance on supply of methadone for unsupervised use.

While it is true there is widespread stakeholder support for SAMHSA's proposals for greater OTP clinician discretion in determining take-home methadone doses for OUD,[39] certain OTP stakeholders have expressed concerns with M-OTAA's provisions that would allow addiction specialist physicians practicing outside of OTPs to prescribe methadone for OUD. These critics often cite the risks of methadone overdose and diversion as the primary reasons for this concern. However, when more closely examined, the totality of that opposition puts more patients with OUD at risk for overdose in a time of an alarming death toll.

For starters, any analysis of M-OTAA must be situated in a contemporary framework for the current crisis. The adulteration of the illegal drug supply with illicitly manufactured fentanyl, fentanyl analogs, and xylazine has created an unprecedented and catastrophic moment in U.S. history. Today, it is a more dangerous time than it has ever been to be an American with OUD. However, patients with OUD who are engaged in addiction treatment are less likely to die than those who remain untreated, and for some patients, methadone is essential to a successful recovery.[40] Methadone can facilitate

---

outpatient services (IV.C.3.a).(2)). *https://www.acgme.org/globalassets/pfassets/programrequirements/404—addictionmedicine— 2022—tcc.pdf.*

[39] Two studies published in January 2023 raise questions about the role of Federal regulatory OTP flexibilities during the COVID public health emergency in increases in methadone-involved overdoses deaths. However, both studies' authors identify significant limitations of their study in demonstrating direct causality. While there remains no direct evidence of causality, ASAM recognizes that granting more flexibilities within the OTP setting must be carried out with caution and with Federal agencies' continual, longitudinal regulations and monitoring for unintended consequences, notwithstanding the widespread support of making such Federal take home policy changes permanent, including among OTP stakeholders. OTP medical directors are not required to be addiction specialist physicians, and not all OTP clinicians are physicians. See Kleinman, Robert A., and Marcos Sanches. ''Methadone-Involved Overdose Deaths in the United States before and during the COVID–19 Pandemic.'' Drug and Alcohol Dependence 242 (January 1, 2023): 109703. *https://doi.org/10.1016/j.drugalcdep.2022.109703*. See also Kaufman, Daniel E., Amy L. Kennalley, Kenneth L. McCall, and Brian J. Piper. ''Examination of Methadone Involved Overdoses during the COVID–19 Pandemic.'' Forensic Science International 344 (January 31, 2023): 111579. *https://doi.org/10.1016/j.forsciint.2023.111579.*

[40] National Academies of Sciences, Board on Health Sciences Policy, Committee on Medication Assisted Treatment for Opioid Use Disorder. The Effectiveness of Medication-Based Treatment for Opioid Use Disorder. National Academies Press (US); 2019. Accessed March 31, 2022. *http://www.ncbi.nlm.nih.gov/books/NBK541393/.*

abstinence from illegal substance use, support recovery, and prevent overdose deaths.[41] Thus, restrictions that continue to limit methadone treatment for OUD to OTPs are a well-recognized vulnerability in the response to the nation's addiction and overdose crisis.[42]

Furthermore, there are underlying complexities in the early trends of diversion of methadone and related overdoses, which were, in large part, associated with historical trends in the acceleration of prescribing opioids for chronic, non-cancer pain.[43], 1A,[44,45] Methadone is unusual among opioid agonists in that the slow accumulation of serum levels during initial dose adjustment may contribute to the risk of fatal methadone overdose,[46] especially if healthcare professionals overestimate a patient's degree of opioid tolerance.[47] And, when methadone is used to treat chronic pain—especially by prescribers lacking training in pain medicine, the frequent dosing regimens tend to play into methadone's pharmacological risks.[48] M-OTAA, however, does not increase methadone prescribing for chronic pain (which happens to remain available through prescription and pharmacy dispensing today). Indeed, historical and contemporary research support a responsible expansion

---

[41] Stone AC, Carroll JJ, Rich JD, Green TC. Methadone maintenance treatment among patients exposed to illicit fentanyl in Rhode Island: Safety, dose, retention, and relapse at 6 months. Drug Alcohol Depend. 2018;192:94–97. doi:10.1016/j.drugalcdep.2018.07.019.

[42] NASEM. Methadone Treatment for Opioid Use Disorder Examining Federal Regulations and Laws A Workshop National Academies. Published 2021. Accessed December 6, 2021. *https://www.nationalacademies.org/event/03—03—2022/methadone-treatment-for-opioid-usedisorder-examining-Federal-regulations-and-laws-a-workshop.*

[43] Paulozzi L, Mack K, Jones CM. Vital Signs: Risk for Overdose from Methadone Used for Pain Relief—United States, 1999—2010. Published July 6, 2012. Accessed December 11, 2021. *https://www.cdc.gov/mmwr/preview/mmwrhtml/mm6126a5.htm.*

[44] Jones CM. Trends in Methadone Distribution for Pain Treatment, Methadone Diversion, and Overdose Deaths—United States, 2002—2014. MMWR Morb Mortal Wkly Rep. 2016;65. doi:10.15585/mmwr.mm6526a2.

[45] DEA. Methadone Diversion, Abuse, and Misuse: Deaths Increasing at Alarming Rate. Published October 16, 2007. Accessed April 22, 2023. *https://www.justice.gov/archive/ndic/pubs25/25930/index.htm—Diversion.*

[46] Clark JD; Understanding Methadone Metabolism: A Foundation for Safer Use. Anesthesiology 2008; 108:351—352 doi: *https://doi.org/10.1097/ALN.0b013e318164937c.*

[47] Center for Substance Abuse Treatment, Methadone-Associated Mortality: Report of a National Assessment, May 8–9, 2003. SAMHSA Publication No. 04–3904. Rockville, MD: Center for Substance Abuse Treatment, Substance Abuse and Mental Health Services Administration, 2004.

[48] FDA. Highlights of Prescribing Information—Methadone.

in access to methadone treatment for OUD, including through office-based practices.[49], 1A[50,51]

To be clear, M-OTAA is not methadone for everyone, prescribed by anyone. It represents a responsible expansion in methadone access for OUD, including through a highly trained, modern-day workforce of expert physicians who can manage this essential treatment for Americans who need it. Inaction on M-OTAA is the risk that this country cannot continue to take.

Enforcement of Existing Federal Mental Health and Addiction Parity Law

Last, despite over a decade since the passage of the Paul Wellstone and Pete Domenici Mental Health Parity and Addiction Equity Act of 2008, such parity of coverage for care remains elusive for millions of Americans suffering with mental health and substance use disorders. A wide disparity in network use and provider payment rates between mental health and addiction treatment, on the one hand, and general medical care on the other, have been well-documented.[52] A recent report to Congress, issued by the U.S. Departments of Labor, Health and Human Services, and the Treasury, suggests that health plans and issuers are not always delivering parity for mental health and substance use disorder benefits to their beneficiaries.[53]

While the reasons for parity elusiveness are many, one sits squarely within your jurisdiction. Under current law, the U.S. Department of Labor (DOL) lacks the authority to assess civil monetary penalties for violations of Federal

---

[49] Salsitz EA, Joseph H, Frank B, et al. Methadone medical maintenance (MMM): treating chronic opioid dependence in private medical practice—a summary report (1983–1998). Mt Sinai J Med N Y. 2000;67(5–6):388–397.

[50] McCarty D, Bougatsos C, Chan B, et al. Office-Based Methadone Treatment for Opioid Use Disorder and Pharmacy Dispensing: A Scoping Review. Am J Psychiatry. 2021;178(9):804–817. doi:10.1176/appi.ajp.2021.20101548.

[51] Novick DM, Salsitz EA, Joseph H, Kreek MJ. Methadone Medical Maintenance: An Early 21stCentury Perspective. J Addict Dis. 2015;34(2–3):226–237. doi:10.1080/10550887.2015.1059225.

[52] Davenport S, Gray T, Melek SP. Addiction and mental health vs. physical health: Widening disparities in network use and provider reimbursement. *https://www.milliman.com/en/insight/addiction-and-mental-health-vs-physical-health-widening-disparities-in-network-use-and-p*. Published November 20, 2019. Accessed May 14, 2023.

[53] USDOL. US DEPARTMENTS OF LABOR, HEALTH AND HUMAN SERVICES, TREASURY ISSUE 2022 MENTAL HEALTH PARITY AND ADDICTION EQUITY ACT REPORT TO CONGRESS. *https://www.dol.gov/newsroom/releases/ebsa/ebsa20220125*. Published January 25, 2022. Accessed May 6, 2023.

parity law already on the books. Without this power, DOL cannot effectively end parity violations with respect to group health plans. That is why ASAM strongly supports passage of the Parity Enforcement Act,[54] which would finally add civil monetary penalty authority to the DOL's oversight, by amending the Employee Retirement Income Security Act (ERISA) to allow the DOL to levy Federal parity violation penalties against covered health insurance issuers, plan sponsors, and plan administrators. According to the same report to Congress noted above, the Employee Benefits Security Administration (EBSA) ''believes that authority for DOL to assess civil monetary penalties for parity violations has the potential to greatly strengthen the protections of MHPAEA [the Paul Wellstone and Pete Domenici Mental Health Parity and Addiction Equity Act of 2008].''[55]

Conclusion

In conclusion, ASAM is actively designing, implementing, and advocating for the policies and resources that will secure a stronger foundation for addiction prevention, treatment, harm reduction, and recovery in this country. The policies and resources I have mentioned today are not inconsequential; they are imperative to saving lives.

We know what to do to treat addiction. We also know that systemic change—a disruption of the status quo, which is currently falling short of our Country's full potential—is exceptionally difficult. But, working together, we must effect change, nonetheless. It is a matter of life or death.

Thank you, and I look forward to answering your questions.

Senator MARKEY. Thank you, doctor, so much. And our final witness is Dr. Warren Ng. Dr. Ng is the President of the American Academy of Child and Adolescent Psychiatry, and a Professor of Psychiatry at Columbia University Medical Center in New York City.

---

[54] The Parity Enforcement Act was introduced by Senator Christopher Murphy during the 117th Congress. *https://www.Congress.gov/bill/117th-congress/senate-bill/4804—qpercent7B percent22search percent22 percent3A percent5B percent22parity+ enforcement+act percent22 percent5D—percent7D&s=1&r=41*. It is expected to be reintroduced during the 118th Congress.

[55] USDOL. US DEPARTMENTS OF LABOR, HEALTH AND HUMAN SERVICES, TREASURY ISSUE 2022 MENTAL HEALTH PARITY AND ADDICTION EQUITY ACT REPORT TO CONGRESS. *https://www.dol.gov/newsroom/releases/ebsa/ ebsa2022 0125*. Published January 25, 2022. Accessed May 6, 2023.

At the American Psychiatric Association, he served on the Council for Children, Adolescents and their Families. Dr. Ng, welcome. Whenever you are ready, please begin.

Statement of Warren Ng, President, American Academy of Child and Adolescent Psychiatry, New York, NY

Dr. NG. Good morning. Thank you, Chairman Markey and Ranking Member Marshall, as well as Members of the Senate HELP Subcommittee.

The members of the American Academy of Child and Adolescent Psychiatry, or AACAP, thanks you for hosting this hearing, as well as your opportunity to share our thoughts on how to bridge the gap to access to care, particularly for the pediatric mental health and substance use treatment.

AACAP represents over 10,000 child and adolescent psychiatrist and trainees, all of whom grasp the gravity of the current situation in the pediatric mental health crisis. Our members work in every child facing system of care in rural and urban communities, as well as hospitals, schools, to families and communities across our Country.

No one in our Nation has been spared the impact of the COVID– 19 pandemic. Child and adolescent psychiatrists with their teams have been on the front lines. That is the reason why in October 2021, the American Academy of Child Analysis and Psychiatry with the American Academy of Pediatrics and the Children's Hospital Association officially declared a national state of emergency for children's mental health.

While there are many factors that contribute to poor access to pediatric mental health care, my testimony today will focus on the impact of the insufficient behavioral health workforce on access to care, as well as some potential solutions.

There has been a silent pandemic of pediatric mental health building for decades. This has largely impacted minoritized groups, including racial, ethnic, as well as gender diverse youth, as well as those who are still living in poverty.

The social disruptions, fear and grief caused by COVID–19 has turned the world upside down for all children, especially those most vulnerable. The escalating rates of pediatric suicide, as well as mental illnesses, compounded by the chronic workforce shortages are well-documented.

We, in collaboration with the Federal and state policymakers, must support immediate, short, and long term strategies. In the short term, to increase access. We can extend the reach of child and adolescent psychiatry workforce by supporting primary care and school-based providers in their settings.

Pediatric mental health care access programs, as well as school based mental health programs, integrated behavioral health, as well as primary care partnership, and tele-psychiatry have all increased access to care.

AACAP is grateful for the recent congressional investments in these models and urges Congress to promote state financing innovations, provider adoption to ensure these models are sustainable. We must meet children where they are at and reduce the barriers to care.

We can also supplement our physician supply by recognizing the invaluable contributions of our international medical graduates. These American trained physician experts are an important part of the mental health care teams, particularly in underserved areas.

Long term strategies to address access counts must include building a strong pipeline of pediatric mental health providers. There are significant workforce shortages even before the pandemic. This was especially true for child and adolescent psychiatrists, whose educational requirements as physician subspecialists are expensive and costly.

Targeted student loan repayment programs and programs set to first student loan payments interest free while training make a difference. Research has shown that these solutions directly influence physician practice choices. The good behavioral health will not attract qualified, highly trained providers, reduce stigma, nor accommodate the growing demand until it is on equal footing with physical health and surgical care.

Poor reimbursement is a disincentive to recruiting medical students into psychiatry and building robust behavioral health services. This contributes to limited in-network psychiatry access, longer wait times, higher expenses for patients who are forced to go out of network to find any care.

Full parity for insurance coverage and reimbursement rates for mental health substance use treatment are critical. AACAP also recommends the Centers for Medicare and Medicaid Services, and other insurance regulators require health plans to use nationally recognized service intensity tools to making medical necessity determinations.

These standardized assessment tools determine the appropriate level of service intensity needed for a particular patient and could assist payers in making appropriate coverage determinations.

Last, we must acknowledge that America is becoming more racially and ethnically diverse and requires a pediatric mental health care system that reflects the communities being served.

The COVID–19 pandemic and preexisting disparities for minoritized youth, including gaps in access to high quality care, truly to bridge this gap in all access to care, we need a workforce that reflects the patients' experiences, language, and background. This leads to better outcomes overcoming stigma, as well as addressing inequities.

We can do this by investing in recruitment, training, and broader distribution of a more diverse representative workforce. AACAP encourages Congress to support programs and improve health equity by providing support for training to racially, ethnically diverse pediatric behavioral health professionals, to scholarship tuition assistance, as well as professional development opportunities.

Thank you again for this opportunity to testify. AACAP is grateful for this opportunity give input into closing the gap in access for lifesaving behavioral health care for children and all Americans. Thank you for taking care of our—being our heroes, as well as our angels in terms of taking care of our children. Thank you.

[The prepared statement of Dr. Ng follows:]

Prepared Statement of Warren Ng

Chairman Markey, Ranking Member Marshall, and Members of the Senate HELP Subcommittee on Primary Health and Retirement Security, the members of the American Academy of Child and Adolescent Psychiatry, AACAP, thank you for hosting this hearing and for the opportunity to share our thoughts on how to bridge the gap in access to pediatric mental health and substance use disorder care. I am Warren Ng, AACAP President, and Director of Outpatient Behavioral Health for New York Presbyterian Hospital in New York City.

AACAP represents over 10,000 child and adolescent psychiatrists and trainees all of whom grasp the gravity of our Nation's pediatric mental health crisis and have been responding. Our members work in every child-facing system of care, in urban and rural communities, from hospitals to schools, and across the lifespan. No one in our Nation has been spared the impact of the COVID–19 pandemic, and child and adolescent psychiatrists and their teams have been on the frontlines. In fact, in October 2021, AACAP along with the

American Academy of Pediatrics and the Childrens' Hospital Association, declared a national state of emergency in children's mental health.[56] While there are many factors that contribute to poor access to pediatric behavioral health care, my testimony today will focus on the impact the insufficient behavioral health workforce has on access to care and potential solutions.

There has been a silent pediatric mental health pandemic building for decades, disproportionately impacting minoritized groups including racial, ethnic, and gender diverse youth, and those living in poverty. The social disruptions, fear and grief caused by the COVID–19 pandemic turned the world upside down for all children, especially those vulnerable to mental illness and substance use disorders. The escalating rates of suicide and mental illness-related morbidity and mortality are well documented. Behavioral health workforce shortages are also chronic and well documented, especially for children. We, in collaboration with our Federal and state policymakers, must support immediate short and long-term strategies.

In the short-term to increase access, we can extend the reach of the child and adolescent psychiatry workforce by supporting primary care and school-based providers in identifying, assessing, and stabilizing pediatric behavioral health disorders and in escalating to specialty behavioral healthcare when the patient's needs require a higher level of care. Pediatric Mental Healthcare Access (PMHCA) consultation programs, school based mental health care, integrated behavioral health and primary care models, and telepsychiatry have all proven to be effective means of connecting patients to behavioral health care. AACAP is grateful for recent congressional investments in these models and urges Congress to promote state financing innovation and provider adoption to ensure these models are sustainable. We must meet children where they are and eliminate additional barriers.

We can also supplement our physician supply by recognizing the invaluable contributions of our international medical graduate (IMG) colleagues. These American trained physician experts are an important part of our mental health care teams, particularly in rural and underserved areas. In fact, recent data shows that 31 percent of child and adolescent psychiatrists are IMGs.[57] We encourage Congress to reauthorize the Conrad 30 Waiver and extend for another 3 years.

---

[56] Pediatricians, CAPs, and Children's Hospitals Declare National Emergency (aacap.org).

[57] Active Physicians Who Are International Medical Graduates (IMGs) by Specialty, 2021—AAMC.

Long-term strategies to address access gaps must include building a strong pipeline of pediatric mental health providers, including child and adolescent psychiatrists. Long before the COVID–19 pandemic, the workforce shortages of pediatric mental health providers were significant. This is especially true for child and adolescent psychiatrists, whose educational requirements as physician subspecialists are extensive and costly. Targeted student loan repayment programs that support pediatric mental health professionals and programs that defer student loan payments, interest-free, while training, help mitigate the barrier of student debt. Research has shown that these solutions directly influence physician practice choices.

The field of behavioral health care will not attract qualified, highly trained providers, reduce stigma, nor accommodate the growing demand for such services until it is on equal footing with physical health and surgical care. In addition to extensive time in training and student debt, poor reimbursement is a disincentive to recruiting medical students into psychiatry and building robust psychiatric services. This contributes to limited in-network psychiatry access, longer wait times, and higher expenses for patients—who are often forced to go out of their insurance networks to find any care. Full parity in insurance coverage and reimbursement rates for mental health and substance use treatment in Medicare and Medicaid would support children's access to high quality and timely mental health care by covering the full range of evidence-based behavioral health care services.

AACAP recommends that the Centers for Medicare & Medicaid Services (CMS) and other insurance regulators require health plans to use nationally recognized service intensity tools developed by professional organizations in making medical necessity determinations. These standardized assessment tools provide determinations of the appropriate level of service intensity needed by a particular patient and could assist payers in making appropriate coverage determinations relating to mental health and substance use services.

Last, we must acknowledge that America is becoming more racially and ethnically diverse and that the current pediatric mental health care system does not sufficiently serve the needs of our communities. The COVID–19 pandemic amplified pre-existing mental health disparities in minoritized children and adolescents, including gaps in access to high quality mental health care. To truly bridge the gap in all children's access to mental health and substance use disorder care, we need a behavioral health workforce that understands and identifies with their patient's experiences, language, and background. We can do this by investing in the recruitment, training, and broader distribution of a more diverse and representative workforce.

Physicians who understand, speak the language, and identify with their patient's life experiences lead to better outcomes and are better equipped to overcome stigma and address inequities. AACAP encourage Congress to support programs that improve health equity by supporting the training of racial and ethnically diverse pediatric behavioral health professionals through scholarship, tuition assistance, and professional development opportunities.

Thank you, again, for the opportunity to testify on this important topic. AACAP appreciates the opportunity to provide input as the Senate HELP Subcommittee on Primary Health and Retirement Security works to close gaps in access to life-saving behavioral healthcare for all Americans who need it, including those who hold our promise for the future, our children.

Senator MARKEY. Thank you. Thank you, Dr. Ng, very much. Now we will turn to questions from the Senators. Dr. Taylor, thank you for raising the Modernizing Opioid Treatment Access Act. Methadone for chronic pain can be prescribed by doctors and picked up at a pharmacy.

But methadone for opioid use disorder, it has a stigma. It is restricted. You talked about SAMHSA and ensuring that we decriminalize methadone as a treatment. Can you talk about why that is such an important step for our Country to take?

Dr. TAYLOR. Absolutely, Senator. As you know that methadone is the only full agonist opioid treatment for opioid medication that is FDA approved for treatment of patients with opioid use disorder.

It seems strange, to say the least, to put it mildly, that I, as an addiction specialist physician, board certified in addiction medicine and addiction psychiatry, would be committing a crime to prescribe a patient methadone in my office who needs methadone for treatment and stabilization of their opioid use disorder.

But someone who has no training in addiction treatment, a doctor who is maybe a general family medicine physician or someone in some other specialty, as long as they have a DEA registration, can prescribe methadone in their office for pain, and can do so and have that patient go pick up that medication in a pharmacy.

That does not make sense, to be honest. And that is a remnant of a really stigmatizing approach to the treatment of people with opioid use disorder. That is really the only way to understand how that came about.

What we are trying to advocate for, and what we hope Congress will pass with the Modernizing Opioid Treatment Access Act, is to make it so that we can be very thoughtful and very careful in our approach to prescribing methadone for treatment of patients with OUD.

That it is addiction specialist physicians, defined as someone who is board certified in addiction medicine or addiction psychiatry, who can prescribe the medication in a patient, in our office, or in one of the other various settings in which addiction specialist physicians work.

Some of those settings are actually even more carefully monitored than OTPs, so called methadone clinics. But can prescribe it to patients and then have those patients pick up that medication in a pharmacy.

It just increases access to care at a time when, as was mentioned, 106,000 patients died, people died last year from overdoses. We have to increase access to care.

Senator MARKEY. Thank you, Dr. Taylor. I wanted unanimous consent to enter into the record two letters from 94 supporting organizations and other clinicians supporting expanding access to methadone and to pass the Modernizing Opioid Treatment Access Act.

Without objection, so ordered.

[The following information can be found on page 42 in Additional Material.]

Senator MARKEY. Social media, its role in creating this teenage, young people mental health crisis in our Country. I would love to hear any of you step up and speak about this, and what you believe the correlation is. Dr. Celli, would you like to take that on?

Dr. CELLI. Sure. This one hits close to home as I have two teenagers and a preteen at home. But I think what we have observed is that social media is—distracts children. It is extraordinarily appealing and gives instant gratification for the desire to connect with somebody.

Now, this was happening prior to the pandemic, but of course, during the pandemic, in a time where children were isolated, had to remain at home in many cases, were not in their school settings, they were not practicing social skills.

It is much the anecdotes that I will hear in the office or from behavioral health clinicians who are seeing teens where I work is that it takes 1 second for a child to put in a friend into some sort of a platform where they can connect with other peers, and instantly your friends come up and they begin to connect.

But these are not actual practiced social skills sort of relationships. And what I think is appealing is that it is so instant, and it can be very engrossing. What is—as a result, the adolescents and children are feeling more isolated.

In fact, I mean, we call these social skills because they are skills they need to be practiced. I think this is impacting how our children are—whether or not they are connecting with their peers and how they are feeling about themselves.

Senator MARKEY. Thank you, doctor, so much. It is unbelievable. One in three teenage girls contemplated suicide last year. One in ten teenage girls attempted suicide last year. One in five LGBTQ youth attempted suicide last year.

Social media is implicated. It is an accessory to this tragedy that we are seeing in our Country, and we have to do something. We need a teenage privacy bill of rights online. We just have to pass one this year. It is urgent. Thank you.

Senator Marshall.

Senator MARSHALL. Thank you again, Chairman. Mr. Denny, I want you to talk just a second about your mobile crisis center. As I travel around the State of Kansas, I think I have been in every hospital, the emergency room is the epicenter of the crisis, and the mental health epidemic has definitely impacted that.

The National Nurses Organization in my office 2 weeks ago, concerned about the violence in the emergency room. There is a right place, there is a tough place to take care of folks with mental health crisis going on, but it is tough in the emergency room.

ER docs are leaving the field. We are not getting new year docs to go into to the field. How have you interacted with your emergency room, and what does your mobile crisis center do?

Mr. DENNY. Well, our mobile crisis services to degree have always been mobile. We are now taking it to 2.0 in terms of being able to respond to anywhere in the community. One strategy is to divert crisis in someone's home or a school or another location, so they do not end up in the emergency room.

That is one of the big strategies that we will employ. Stabilization during a wait for a placement in inpatient hospitalization is an adaptive challenge. And what I mean by that is that there is no technical fix that is going to immediately resolve this issue.

But what we have found, first of all, is partnership on the front end with our emergency rooms, and we serve rural areas, so getting to know and having plans on how we deal with emergency situations are important.

Training for emergency room staff is important, at least some base level behavioral health response training. There are different options out there. And last, one of the things we have developed in Kansas, or are still developing, are the regional crisis centers, which would provide an alternative for someone to go and wait, and be assessed and stabilized, versus an emergency room.

Anytime we can find a different setting to accomplish that purpose that is not as triggering or as difficult as an emergency room, I think the more of that we can do, that is a state program with Federal support, but the more of that we can do, the less of those incidents we will see over time.

But it is a challenge. It is a frustration. It takes partnership between both of our systems to work through those issues.

Senator MARSHALL. Certainly, a patient waiting days in an isolated room in the emergency room is not the solution. And it takes one on one nursing staff, so it takes away resources.

We literally just have a shortage of those inpatient opportunities. Maybe, kind of turn to Dr. Ng, tell us, what is working and what is not working out there in your world? Just take like 1 minute to tell me what you think is cutting edge, and what do you think we have been doing that is not working?

Dr. NG. Thank you very much, Senator Marshall. I think that what is working and what is not working is also acknowledging, I think what Mr. Denny mentioned, is really creating that better continuum of care that goes from community to more intensive treatment, whether or not that is emergency department or inpatient psychiatric units.

I think what is really important to hold center is the fact that person who is experiencing that mental health or emotional crisis is probably scared and frightened and overwhelmed as well.

Being able to center our experience with that person is also understanding that emergency departments are never the place to be when you are in that situation. And how do we humanize that environment, whether or not this an adult or as a child, or a family member.

I think that creating that continuum of care, of escalating intensity of outpatient and community services, that are embedded within communities, partnering with communities to provide the most culturally competent, as well as responsive care is really important.

I think that means that we have to create some innovative programs that are funded and sustainable so that we can provide wraparound care for young people, and their families, and adults within communities.

I think that we are thinking about these intensive outpatient programs, partial hospitalization, wraparound, as well as some of the critical time intervention programs that can sometimes be helpful, but I think the important thing is that they are networked toward a system of care that is a continuum, so that people who are experiencing that care don't have to jump through hoops, but experience it as being surrounded by people who can provide the care they need.

Senator MARSHALL. Yes. Thank you so much. Mr. Chairman, I yield back and maybe we can get some follow-up questions after our colleagues finish.

Senator MARKEY. Absolutely. Senator Baldwin.

Senator BALDWIN. Thank you, Mr. Chairman, Ranking Member, for holding this important Subcommittee hearing, and thank you to all of our witnesses today. I will never forget meeting with three moms in my office who all lost their children to fentanyl overdoses.

Poisonings is the word they used, I think, in part because they believe their children perhaps didn't know that there was fentanyl lacing the illegal pill that they had taken. It is so clear that we have to do more to stop fentanyl from coming into our Country and our communities, and increase prevention and treatment efforts, and make overdose reversal drugs much more widely available.

To do so, we have to use every tool we have to combat this epidemic. I know as Chair of the LHHS Subcommittee of Appropriations, I am committed to fighting for sufficient resources. I am also proud to co-sponsor Bruce's law with my colleague, Senator Murkowski, who has led that important measure.

It would bolster Federal prevention and education efforts surrounding fentanyl. I look at how the opioid epidemic has changed and evolved, if that is the word you want to use, but changed fundamentally just in the last decade or so.

Dr. Taylor, maybe you can describe why the fentanyl phase of this crisis has proven to be so especially challenging for health care providers. How have you experienced this transformation or evolution in our opioid epidemic and in the country?

Dr. TAYLOR. Thank you for that question, Senator Baldwin. So, you hit something right on the head, which is fentanyl represents a third phase of this opioid crisis. Sort of the first phase was the prescription opioid proliferation and the overdose—the overdose death and the addiction epidemic that resulted from that.

Second phase being heroin, as prescription opioids were made more difficult to access and much more expensive, and heroin came in and was much cheaper and much more readily accessible. One of the challenges is that fentanyl is even cheaper than heroin.

As people developed ongoing addiction, marked, of course, with particularly with opioids, with the development of tolerance to whatever dose of drug that they were taking, and withdrawal, which is incredibly unpleasant when someone attempts to abruptly stop using opioids, then the person is driven to find something else that they can take.

Of course, with fentanyl being less expensive and more readily available, it was predictable, if you think about it, that people would then turn to fentanyl. The problem is that it wasn't just pharmaceutical fentanyl.

When you think of fentanyl, it is important to recognize there is pharmaceutical fentanyl, and then there is the illicitly manufactured synthetic product. And then beyond that, there is a number of different synthetic fentanyl analogs that are even more potent than fentanyl.

People are familiar with the word carfentanyl, which is an analog, a synthetic analog of fentanyl that is—has been used to put down elephants. And that is how potent that drug is, and that is the drug that you hear people first responders showing up in situations and just by casual contact with it, ending up with significant levels of it in their system.

Part of the challenge is that as people have continued on with addiction, that may have started from the time they were on prescription opioids, they now are at a point where they are addicted to fentanyl. The other part of the challenge for us as addiction treatment professionals is that because fentanyl and its analogs are so incredibly potent, it is actually much harder to provide treatment for someone who is addicted to fentanyl.

We literally now are scrambling. ASAM just had our annual meeting a couple of weeks back, actually about a month ago in— right here in the D.C. area. And we literally had several conferences with people on the front lines sharing with our general membership what are the strategies for taking someone who is addicted to fentanyl, or even one of the more potent fentanyl analogs, and trying to get that person inducted on to buprenorphine or even methadone.

Because the challenge is that the withdrawal syndrome is so severe when we try to transition a person, that very often people end up not continuing with the treatment and going back out to use fentanyl. And so, we have had to figure out, and we are actively working on, strategies that work to address the severe withdrawal that people go through long enough so that they can transition smoothly to a medication like buprenorphine or methadone.

Which is why we are pushing to make it possible for us to be able to prescribe methadone and have people get it from pharmacies, because for many patients, buprenorphine isn't the medicine that they are going to need for that transition—it is methadone.

That is—and we need to have every tool available in the toolbox to be able to take care of people, particularly because of this extremely complicated, potent drug to which so many people are addicted.

Senator BALDWIN. Thank you. Senator MARKEY. Senator Murkowski.

Senator MURKOWSKI. Thank you, Mr. Chairman. I want to thank my colleague for your support on Bruce's law. I think, Dr. Taylor, this goes exactly to what you are talking about is the intensity of the addiction for those that have been using, whether it was prescription drugs or heroin.

The intensity of the addiction is such that I think people need to understand that we are dealing—we are dealing with something at a higher, more intense level, and what that actually means. And the intensity of fentanyl itself and the lethality.

As we work to educate people, to try to explain that this is not something that you can engage in lightly—you will be poisoned, and you will die. And part of what I am hearing with fentanyl is that the treatment, as you have indicated, is very, very challenged. But, that the likelihood of being poisoned as Sandy Snodgrass' son Bruce was, is out there as a very real reality.

The lethality of fentanyl is something that scares the living daylights out of me. I want to ask, and I am not entirely sure who to address this to, but this week in our largest newspaper in the state was a front-page article about traumatic brain injury and how Alaska has the highest rates of TBI deaths, related deaths in the country.

One out of every four deaths in Alaska under the age of 30 is related to TBI. So, we know that we do a lot of rock climbing and some things that are inherently dangerous, four-wheeling, snow machining. We get all that.

But the reality is, of those deaths, 43 percent were due to suicide. Suicide attempts are more common in individuals that have sustained a brain injury. Almost half of brain injury survivors reporting symptoms of depression.

The question to you all is, what protocols are in place to ensure that those who have sustained a TBI get the mental health that they need, that they get it on the front end? We recognize that this is—this is a pretty tight correlation here.

Are we doing anything with regards to that? If you have got— if you have had a traumatic brain injury, is there follow-up then to help on the mental health side? Dr. Ng.

Dr. NG. Thank you, Senator Murkowski. I think that this is a really incredibly important question to ask around how are we integrating mental health, and behavioral health, and suicide screening throughout all of our health care systems.

It is really understanding that there is no health without mental health, and it is being able to ask those questions, but also work collaboratively with teams.

When we integrate mental health and behavioral health services within medical settings and primary care settings, in specialty pediatric settings, it is really important. It allows us to have that conversation, to ask those questions.

But also, when there are issues related to suicide, that we are able to address it directly and we are not having to refer to someone else. But when you are talking within your trusted medical care team and you are able to provide that level of identification, screening assessment, and referral to treatment, I think that is really key.

Senator MURKOWSKI. Dr. Ng, let me ask about that, because part of our big challenge in Alaska is lack of access to the providers, and particularly pediatric health providers who would be encouraged to practice in rural and medically underserved communities.

Senator Smith and I have a bill, the Mental Health Professionals Workforce Shortage Loan Repayment Act, again, designed to get professionals out into rural areas. But it is a challenge for us in Alaska, I know, but I know that it is also equally challenging in other parts of rural America.

I don't know that we can do enough fast enough, and particularly when we are looking at suicide statistics for young people who are struggling and are just simply not able to get the mental health treatment that they need.

In Alaska, unfortunately, if a young person has been told that we don't have any services that we can provide to you, the care that they receive is outside. And when I say outside, it is not outside of a building, it is outside of the State of Alaska. So, they have to fly to Seattle, if they are lucky. A lot of times the medical help is available in Utah. You are separated from your family, from your support systems. This is not a tenable situation.

I look at what we need to do to grow this workforce, but I also think that—Dr. Ng, you talk about this continuum of care and wraparound services, what more we can do to help parents and families and educators and local community leaders to help be that support in these smaller communities until you can get to the medical professional. I don't know if there is a question in there, but we are really struggling with this at home. Dr. Ng.

Dr. NG. Thank you, Senator. I think that—thank you very much for your leadership and support for S. 462, because I think the workforce shortage issues are really key. But also, being able to fund and support providers to be able to provide those mental health services within the medical setting and within communities is also really key.

Being able to finance some of those strategies, the pediatric mental health care access programs that provides consultation to medical providers, particularly pediatric providers in urgent settings. The other thing is tele sychiatry has been really important to be able to bridge some of those gaps.

I think that partnership with families within communities is key so that we can also encourage tele-psychiatry to be able to be helpful, to bring in key members of the community, as well as family members, to be a partner to that care.

I totally agree that there isn't a quick fix to this because this problem existed well before, but at the same time, the loan repayment, as well as trying to finance integrated behavioral health interventions, as well as leveraging tele-psychiatry and continuing to fund those innovations that have been helpful during the pandemic would be key.

Senator MARKEY. Thank you. Thank you. Senator from Colorado.

Senator HICKENLOOPER. Thank you, Mr. Chair. And thank all of you for being here today, but also for your ongoing work. Clearly, very, very important time to address some of these issues. Peer to peer mental health programs are taking off across school districts around the country.

These programs where trained students offer a listening ear to their peers, they look for concerning signs, help connect students with professional resources appear to add real value. Students often feel more comfortable asking for help from a peer than from an adult, and this step alone can help break the stigma, especially for young people, around going forward and seeking care.

Dr. Ng, why don't I start with you and just say, why do you think so many schools are gravitating—I mean, beyond that trying to work around the stigma, why are they gravitating toward these peer-to-peer programs, and what more can we do to support them?

Dr. NG. Thank you, Senator Hickenlooper. I think that is really a key perspective, is really bringing in the youth voice, as well as the youth involvement, and the youth solutions.

I think that they are incredibly creative, and they are also an incredible resourced for us to continue to partner with, and that is partnering with them at a level that respects the information that they are giving us.

I think it is really important that we honor that and also the diversity among the youth perspectives. And as you heard, the number of adolescent females that are experiencing helplessness and the rates of suicide with regards to the LGBTQ and gender diverse youth, as well as racial or ethnic diversity youth as well.

I think that having the youth voice, and the youth is definitely— they will connect with each other in a way that we are not easily connected to them, and we can also gain from them that wisdom. But the important thing is, is that is not where we stop, that is where we start.

Where we need to end up is actually connecting those youth peers, as well as support services, with other additional help and services along a larger continuum. So being able to reinforce the school based mental health programs embedded within those, as well as crisis response, so that those young people who need more urgent and critical care can be coordinated through that system, through their youth advocates.

Senator HICKENLOOPER. Great. Appreciate it. Mr. Denny, you are from—your approach is from a different ecosystem. Would you agree with that?

Mr. DENNY. Yes, especially in relation to the development of peer services. That is one of the nine required services under CCBHC, person, peer and family support services organization. We have hired our first peer services supervisor and our hope is to continue to develop those services.

One of the exciting things in Kansas too is we have just recently passed a code that would allow us to provide parent peer support services for parents of youth in our services, and I am really excited to see those develop. But it is as it was addressed earlier, there is not always a provider nearby.

Our need to identify across multiple areas, whether it be schools, hospitals, there is a lot of different community-based trainings to help identify people in need and not always rely on a service provider to be there. Because a lot of times when the crisis happens, a behavioral health professional is right around the corner.

Programs for us, such as mental health first aid, psychological first aid, question—for QPR training. There is a lot of different models that help train the community and engage around suicide, particularly in rural areas where we don't always have someone readily available.

We don't have to go to Seattle, but we are two and a half hours away sometimes from a hospital. I totally get the isolation. And what do we do when we are here—kind of out here on our own.

Senator HICKENLOOPER. Great. Thank you. Dr. Celli, I was going to— Colorado hospitals often don't have the resources to provide the care for kids, just as Mr. Denny was describing. Hospital staff are trying to do too much with too little, and again, especially in rural areas.

Your testimony highlighted the outsized importance of community health centers, I think, in this community health programs, but not just—centers and programs.

What do community health centers and certified community behavioral health clinics do to help address these gaps in the behavioral health care system? And how do we—how can we do more, since there are still so many people struggling to access care?

Dr. CELLI. Thank you so much, Senator Hickenlooper, for the question. So, one of the cornerstones of community health centers is that all of the service—all of the services are within the same team.

That team can be very large thousands of staff, but they are all within the same team. And that makes coordination of care, as Dr. Ng was referring to, much easier. You don't have to go through— to another institution. It is one of your colleagues.

That makes access to care much faster, more seamless, and feel like a standard part of your health care, once again, reducing stigma. So, addiction services, mental health services, help for health-related social needs.

Many times, a person is subthreshold diagnostic depression, but then food insecurity or housing insecurity is that one stressor that takes them to a level of being quiet quite ill.

I think that is one of—again, one of the cornerstones of community health centers, that integrated model, and the ability to have all of those services within the same system helps with coordination of care. I did want to highlight for a moment around pediatrics, in particular.

At Brockton Neighborhood Health Center, we have the good fortune of having a program that is called—a grant funded initiative that trains not only the behavioral health providers.

You could have a behavioral health provider who maybe had worked more with adults but is able to get trained in working with children because there is such a gap in services for pediatrics of trained professionals.

This program trains providers on the medical side, medical assistance, nurses, behavioral health clinicians, clinical secretaries, everybody who is on the team, on how to create that space that really engages both the child and the family, and in some cases, other community members as well.

Senator HICKENLOOPER. Yes, I love that approach. I think that is very useful. Thank you all. Dr. Taylor, I have got questions for you as well, and we will put them into the written. I am out of time. I apologize. I yield back to the Chair.

Senator MARKEY. Thank you, Senator, so much. I would just like to follow-up, if I could, on Senator Murkowski's line of questioning of, with so few practitioners, how can telehealth help deliver services?

What is necessary to be able to bridge this gap between Anchorage and Seattle, or Salt Lake City? What are the reimbursement issues? What are the licensing issues so that people can practice across state lines virtually?

What are those new licensing opportunities that are going to have to be put in place if we are going to ensure that we get the resources to where the problem is? Yes, Dr. Ng.

Dr. NG. I will give it a try. I think that there are multiple strategies. I think one of that is the state compacts and being able to provide regional support.

I think that familiarity for the child and adolescent psychiatrist consultant, to know that system of care, to understand that community being served is really key, until the time that you can develop in resources. So, specialists who are actually embedded within, for Senator Murkowski, within the State of Alaska.

Really being able to partner with the local resources, with the community health centers, with the CCBHCs, with that network of care and the educational system is key. Also being able to finance appropriate consultation.

When we are providing that expertise, as child and adolescent psychiatrists and physician experts in mental health, one of the things that we do, we are able to integrate is the health, as well as the mental health, as well as the psychosocial issues.

Being able to integrate all of those in terms a comprehensive treatment plan involving all members, as well as the youth, the family, the community, and the school resources, is really key.

Senator MARKEY. How will that help Senator Murkowski's problem in Alaska? Do you have a recommendation in terms of ensuring that somebody doesn't have to leave Anchorage, can get a topnotch psychiatrist in another state online, so that it can be integrated with perhaps the physical care in Anchorage? What is your recommendation?

Dr. NG. Those wonderful programs, the pediatric mental health care access programs, which really helps to partner child and adolescent psychiatrists with pediatricians, if we are talking about that population.

It is really helping them talk through the care of that young person to develop and acquire some of the skills and the tools necessary to providing that care onsite. And it is really building that capacity for the care.

There are other models, such as the Echo models, that can help extend the clinical expertise locally, whether or not it is with a primary care provider or if it is a provider within the CCBHC, or a community health center, or a private practice provider as well. I think that is the most rapid way of expanding your current short-term strategy, in addition to building some long-term strategies.

Senator MARKEY. Dr. Taylor, I would like to come back to you one more time, and that is on this suboxone, methadone issue, in terms of the help which people need. Can you just put an exclamation point on the need for that law to change?

Dr. TAYLOR. Senator, I have—about a few months ago, I got a message on LinkedIn from a gentleman who was the father of a young man who had been a patient of mine.

The message was thanking me for helping his son and letting me know that his son was just about to graduate from law school. His son had been a patient of mine with a severe opioid use disorder, and I took care of him in my office for several years when he had flunked out of college and was—had gone through the progression, very much like I described previously, of addiction to prescription opioids, and then had moved on to snorting heroin and then injecting heroin, and had really severe addiction to opioids.

I worked with him in the office, and I treated him with buprenorphine, and he did well for periods of time, and then would have a recurrence of his illness. And then I, at one point, had to refer him to a methadone program, an OTP, because I was not able to provide that for him in my office.

During that period of time, I stayed in touch with him, and I tried to liaison with the doctor at the methadone program, who was not necessarily an addiction specialist, but we made the best of it. And then at other periods of time, we then transitioned him back to buprenorphine and I was able to then be the one prescribing and monitoring his medication.

It was a torturous process taking care of that young man because of the fact that he wasn't able to just have me work with him on a consistent basis, prescribing whatever it was that he needed, that I, as an addiction specialist, was more than qualified to prescribe him.

The bottom line—and so he had to come and see me for a while, and then go to the OTP for a while, and then come back into my office for a while, and it was a very difficult treatment course.

I can't guarantee that he would have had a shorter or easier time of it if we had been—if I had been able to prescribe him the methadone the same way I was able to prescribe him buprenorphine, but it certainly would have made more sense for him, and it would have been more convenient for his family.

Thankfully, he is in recovery now. He is doing great. He just graduated from law school. But it shouldn't be necessary for him to go through all of that, and not everyone has the kind of outcome he had.

Senator MARKEY. Senator Marshall.

Senator MARSHALL. Thank you again, Mr. Chairman. Mr. Denny, you have led this prototype of the Certified Community Behavioral Health Clinics. What are the three most important lessons that you would pass on, if we are going to set up something like this up in Alaska or other parts of Kansas? What is the secret recipe, in your opinion—lessons learned?

Mr. DENNY. From the National Council was just letting me know there are two clinics being piloted in Alaska currently, two CCBHC clinics. So that is—the model is off the ground there.

Senator MARSHALL. That is great. And we should ask the Senator Murkowski's staff to follow-up with you and the clinics, and share some lessons learned.

Mr. DENNY. Yes. In terms of setting, it up, it is so important to have an effective community needs assessment and make sure that you are really assessing the needs of each community served. You know, the accessibility conversation, particularly as it relates to telehealth, I always think about rural frontier areas, right.

A lot of our areas that we serve don't necessarily have connectivity. So, making sure that whenever—wherever we offer, those services have the tools and resources, that the right people are at the table. So, an effective needs assessment that truly identifies the unique needs of each community.

The second thing is really developing providers' skill sets and practices that are going to have outcomes. So, the models you choose need to be applicable to the populations you are serving. I think Kansas has done a really good job of choosing evidence-based practices that are really relevant to the needs of Kansans we are serving.

The third thing is, and this is a practical thing, but there is a lot of talented CCBHC clinics throughout our Country. When we were starting, I had people from all over the country reaching out to me saying, try this, try that, consider this, consider that. Here is how you get started on your data.

But the thinking of a data collection strategy that is practical, meaning that you can get started with meaningful outcomes that are going to tell your story, but at the same time, having a plan to how to build and grow that.

You know, in Kansas, in the next 6 months to a year, we will have a data warehouse that will allow us to track outcomes across our entire state population. That will be a really unique opportunity just to begin observing how we are using these clinics to truly impact change.

Senator MARSHALL. Thank you. Dr. Taylor, I know you are a treatment specialist, but I want to go to the prevention side for a second. You know, as a physician, we take family histories.

You say, oh, my goodness, you are at risk for colon cancer, so therefore you need to start your screening at an earlier age. Or you are at risk for diabetes, and your weight is up a little bit this year, and your blood pressure is up we have—how are we doing identifying at risk people, and what other ounces of prevention would you be recommending out there from your experiences?

Dr. TAYLOR. Thanks for that question, Senator Marshall. I am actually also a big-time prevention hawk. Our organization, ASAM, is very much concerned about prevention as well as treatment. We know what the risk factors are for a young person to develop an addiction disorder. We know that addiction is a disease of pediatric onset, in fact.

We know that effective interventions—and when I say—just want to say pediatric onset, we know most of the time when someone develops an addiction disorder, the onset of use and the onset of the disorder is actually in adolescence. So that is what I mean by pediatric onset.

But we know that there are effective evidence-based interventions, prevention and prevention interventions that work at the community-based level. They often involve building social skills, teaching adolescents social skills, and many of these are school based programs. We know that if—the No. 1 risk factor for a young person to develop an addiction is to have a parent who has or has had an addiction disorder.

One of the most effective things you can do is to provide effective treatment for parents who have an addiction disorder, get them stabilized, so that their children are not subject to the ACES, the adverse childhood experiences, that a child of a person with an addiction is at risk for, and then target those young people, knowing that they are at increased risk, with early intervention.

I have done that on the individual level in my office, but also organizations can do that. And I am involved in community-based organizations in Birmingham, one specifically called the Addiction Prevention Coalition that actually does a lot of programing in and around Birmingham, specifically designed to target young people in schools with mental health first aid, with peer programs like Senator Hickenlooper had described.

That is something that is doable. We at ASAM support the implementation of those programs. The key is to fund ones that are evidence based and to actually de-emphasize and not continue to fund those that have been shown to not be effective.

Senator MARSHALL. Well, thanks so much. Again, I want to thank all the witnesses. I think you can tell this is a very thoughtful Subcommittee, and your testimony is very valuable, and we hope that there is follow-up at the staff level. And you all certainly made us think about several issues, and I appreciate you being here. Thank you.

Senator MARKEY. Thank you, Senator Marshall. Thanks to our great panel here today. This is obviously a period where there is a devastating behavioral health crisis that threatens every community in this country, and disproportionately impact communities of color and low income and other marginalized communities.

Thanks to these experts here today and so many people across the country, we have the opportunity to build on what has already been done to create a society where everyone has a fair and just opportunity to attain their highest level of health, and I look forward to continuing to work with each of you to do that.

We have to discuss how we can get more resources into the hands of all of the practitioners, all the families out there. A vision without funding is a hallucination. You need—if you get the tools, you will be able to help families.

I ask unanimous consent to enter into the record statements from various stakeholders outlining priorities for closing the gaps in access to mental health and substance use disorder care.

[The following information can be found on pages 64 through 77 in Additional Material.]

Senator MARKEY. For any Senators who wish to ask additional questions for the record, they will be due in 10 business days, on June 1st at 5.00 p.m.

The Committee stands adjourned.

Additional Material

May 16, 2023

Hon. KEVIN MCCARTHY, Speaker,
Hon. HAKEEM JEFFRIES, Minority Leader

Hon. CHUCK SCHUMER, Majority Leader,
Hon. MITCH MCCONNELL, Minority Leader,
Hon. MCMORRIS RODGERS, Chair,
Hon. FRANK PALLONE, Ranking Member,
Hon. JIM JORDAN, Chair,
Hon. JERROLD NADLER, Ranking Member,
U.S. House of Representatives House of Representative Washington, D.C. 20515.
Hon. BERNIE SANDERS, Chair,
Hon. BILL CASSIDY, Ranking Member,
U.S. Senate Committee on Health, Education, Labor, and Pensions, Washington, DC. 20510.

Dear Speaker Mccarthy, Majority Leader Schumer, Minority Leader Jeffries, Minority Leader Mcconnell, Chair Mcmorris Rodgers, Ranking Member Pallone, Chair Jordan, Ranking Member Nadler, Chair Sanders, and Ranking Member Cassidy:

The undersigned organizations, representing a broad base of stakeholders, write today to endorse S. 644/H.R. 1359—the Modernizing Opioid Treatment Access Act (the ''M-OTAA''). This bipartisan, bicameral legislation would responsibly expand access to methadone treatment for opioid use disorder (OUD) in medical settings and areas where it is not available now. There is a shortage of methadone treatment for OUD that contributes to racial, gender, and geographic inequities in access to such treatment in the U.S.—especially in rural areas—despite an increasing number of opioid treatment programs (OTPs) in the for-profit sector in recent years.[58] Therefore, imminent passage of the M-OTAA is critical to saving lives, helping families, and strengthening American communities.

Only three medications have been approved by the Food and Drug Administration to treat OUD: methadone, buprenorphine, and naltrexone. OUD is associated with a 20fold greater risk of early death due to overdose, infectious disease, trauma, and suicide.[59] Methadone is the most well-studied

[58] Joudrey, Paul, Gavin Bart, Robert Brooner, Lawrence Brown, Julia Dickson-Gomez, Adam Gordon, Sarah Kawasaki, et al. ''Research Priorities for Expanding Access to Methadone Treatment for Opioid Use Disorder in the United States: A National Institute on Drug Abuse Center for Clinical Trials Network Task Force Report.'' Substance Abuse 42 (July 3, 2021): 245—54. https://doi.org/10.1080/08897077.2021.1975344.

[59] Schuckit MA. Treatment of Opioid-Use Disorders. N Engl J Med. 2016;375(4):357–368. doi:10.1056/NEJMra1604339.

pharmacotherapy for OUD, with the longest track record.[60] According to myriad experts, methadone is safe and effective for patients when indicated, dispensed, and consumed properly.[61] But federal law largely limits its availability for OUD to OTPs and prevents the broader use of this medication to address fentanyl's deadly role in driving the rise of, and disparities in, drug overdose deaths in America.

The M-OTAA would allow OTP clinicians and board-certified physicians in addiction medicine or addiction psychiatry to prescribe methadone for OUD treatment that can be picked up from pharmacies, subject to the Substance Abuse and Mental Health Services Administration rules or guidance on supply of methadone for unsupervised use. This legislation would capitalize on the existing addiction expert workforce and pharmacy infrastructure to integrate methadone treatment for OUD with the rest of general healthcare. In doing so, the M-OTAA would help increase innovation in the OTP industry and narrow gaps in access to methadone for OUD for those who need it.

Our organizations are unified in our support of the M-OTAA and our strong belief that it will help turn the tide on the addiction crisis facing our Nation.

Sincerely,

1) American Society of Addiction Medicine
2) American Association of Psychiatric Pharmacists
3) American College of Academic Addiction Medicine
4) American College of Osteopathic Emergency Physicians
5) American College of Medical Toxicology
6) American College of Physicians
7) American for Multidisciplinary Education and Research in Substance Use and Addiction, Inc. (AMERSA)
8) American Medical Association
9) American Osteopathic Academy of Addiction Medicine
10) American Pharmacists Association

---

[60] Substance Abuse and Mental Health Administration. Medications for Opioid Use Disorder: For Healthcare and Addiction Professionals, Policymakers, Patients, and Families. Treatment Improvement Protocol (TIP) Series, No. 63. Chapter 3B: Methadone.; 2018. Accessed March 31, 2022. *http://www.ncbi.nlm.nih.gov/books/NBK535269/*.

[61] Baxter LES, Campbell A, DeShields M, et al. Safe Methadone Induction and Stabilization: Report of an Expert Panel. J Addict Med. 2013;7(6):377–386. doi:10.1097/01.ADM.0000435321.39251.d7.

11) American Psychological Association
12) AIDS Foundation Chicago (AFC)
13) AIDS UNITED
14) Alabama Society of Addiction Medicine
15) A New PATH (Parents for Addiction Treatment & Healing)
16) Anxiety and Depression Association of America
17) Any Positive Change, Inc.
18) Arkansas Society of Addiction Medicine
19) Association for Behavioral Health and Wellness
20) Being Alive
21) Big Cities Health Coalition
22) Broken No More
23) CADA of Northwest Louisiana
24) California Society of Addiction Medicine
25) Center for Adolescent Behavioral Health Research, Boston Children's Hospital
26) Center for Housing & Health
27) Clinical Social Work Association
28) Collaborative Family Healthcare Association
29) Community Outreach Prevention and Education Network
30) Coolidge Consulting
31) DAP HEALTH
32) Drug Policy Alliance
33) Faces & Voices of Recovery
34) Florida Society of Addiction Medicine
35) The Grand Rapids Red Project
36) Grayken Center for Addiction at Boston Medical Center
37) Harm Reduction Action Center
38) Hawai'i Health & Harm Reduction Center
39) Hawai'i Society of Addiction Medicine
40) Hep Free Hawai'i
41) Honoring Individual Power and Strength (HIPS)
42) Illinois Society of Addiction Medicine
43) Indiana Recovery Alliance
44) Inseparable
45) International Society for Psychiatric Nurses
46) The Kennedy Forum
47) Landmark Recovery
48) Legal Action Center

49) Louisiana Society of Addiction Medicine
50) Massachusetts Association of Behavioral Health Systems
51) Massachusetts Association for Mental Health, Inc.
52) Massachusetts Society of Addiction Medicine
53) Mental Health America
54) Michigan Society of Addiction Medicine
55) Midwest Society of Addiction Medicine
56) Minnesota Society of Addiction Medicine
57) National Alliance for Medication Assisted Recovery (NAMA Recovery)
58) National Association of Pediatric Nurse Practitioners
59) National Alliance on Mental Illness
60) National Association of Addiction Treatment Providers
61) National Association of Social Workers
62) National Board for Certified Counselors
63) National Council on Alcoholism and Drug Dependence
64) National Harm Reduction Coalition
65) National Health Care for the Homeless Council
66) National League for Nursing
67) National Safety Council (NSC)
68) National Survivors Union
69) New Bedford Community Health
70) New York Society of Addiction Medicine
71) Northern New England Society of Addiction Medicine
72) Oklahoma Society of Addiction Medicine
73) Oregon Society of Addiction Medicine
74) Overdose Crisis Response Fund
75) Partnership to End Addiction
76) Pennsylvania Harm Reduction Network
77) The Porchlight Collective SAP
78) Public Justice Center
79) RI International
80) Rural Organizing
81) San Francisco AIDS Foundation
82) Shatterproof
83) The Sheet Metal and Air Conditioning Contractors National Association (SMACNA)
84) SMART RECOVERY
85) South Shore Health

86) Southwest Recovery Alliance
87) Students for Sensible Drug Policy
88) Tennessee Justice Center
89) Tennessee Society of Addiction Medicine
90) Today I Matter, Inc.
91) Vital Strategies
92) Washington Society of Addiction Medicine
93) Wisconsin Society of Addiction Medicine
94) Young People in Recovery

March 30, 2023

U.S. Committee on Energy and Commerce, 2125 Rayburn House Office Building, Washington, DC 20515.

U.S. Senate Committee on Health, Education, Labor, and Pensions, Subcommittee on Primary Health and Retirement Security, 428 Dirksen Senate Office Building, Washington, DC. 20510.

Dear United States Senators and Representatives:

We write from the frontlines of our Nation's addiction and overdose crisis, as board-certified physicians in addiction medicine or addiction psychiatry, some of whom work in opioid treatment programs (OTPs). As you help lead us out of this public health emergency, we humbly ask that you consider this message with the seriousness it deserves. Our aim is to inform recent discourse on the delivery of high-quality and effective treatment for people with opioid use disorder (OUD) with methadone, and provide critical clarifications to complex issues that have arisen in the context of that discussion on Capitol Hill.

Currently, Federal law limits the availability of methadone for OUD to heavily regulated OTPs at both the Federal and state level, a structure that has implications for access to, and quality of, care. During the COVID–19 pandemic, public health recommendations for social distancing compelled the Federal Government to reform Federal regulations governing methadone treatment for OUD at OTPs. As a result, a natural experiment occurred,[62] and our Nation learned that the Federal Government could move quickly and

[62] Krawczyk, Noa, Bianca D. Rivera, Emily Levin, and Bridget C. E. Dooling. "Synthesising Evidence of the Effects of COVID–19 Regulatory Changes on Methadone Treatment for Opioid Use Disorder: Implications for Policy." The Lancet Public Health 8, no. 3 (March 1, 2023): e238—46. *https://doi.org/10.1016/S2468–2667(23)00023–3.*

responsibly to protect patients' health and safety, while ensuring that they receive the addiction care they need. Thus, as you consider next steps to tackle our Nation's addiction and overdose crisis, we urge you to support swift passage of the bipartisan and bicameral Modernizing Opioid Treatment Access Act (S. 644/H.R. 1359) (the ''M-OTAA'').

The Modernizing Opioid Treatment Access Act

The M-OTAA would modernize Federal law governing the delivery of OUD treatment with methadone—law which has largely remained unchanged since 1974, despite the scientific and medical consensus, dating as far back as 1995, calling for the Federal Government to regulate methadone for OUD more in alignment with other Schedule II Food and Drug Administration (FDA)-approved medications.[63] Notably, existing Federal law predates the establishment and recognition by the American Board of Medical Specialties of the medical subspecialties of addiction medicine and addiction psychiatry. This explains one reason for the prescriptive Federal laws enacted in the 1970's that were to govern methadone treatment for OUD in a practice environment without recognized addiction specialist physicians. In brief, the M- OTAA would authorize the Drug Enforcement Administration (DEA) to issue special registrations for physicians who are board-certified in addiction medicine and/or addiction psychiatry, as well as OTP prescribing clinicians, who could then use their clinical expertise in prescribing methadone for OUD

[63] In 1995, experts at the Institute of Medicine (IOM) wrote, ''In light of these considerations, the committee urges reassessment of the appropriate balance between the risks of methadone and its benefits. The current regulations foster situations where addicts cannot obtain a treatment program tailored to their individual circumstances, physicians are unable to exercise professional judgment in treating individual patients, programs are isolated from mainstream medical care (thus depriving patients of important ancillary services), and significant economic costs are incurred in assuring compliance with regulatory requirements—costs that are shared by programs, insurers, patients, and taxpayers. We have concluded that there is no compelling medical reason for regulating methadone differently from all other medications approved by FDA, including schedule II controlled substances. Nevertheless, the committee is not recommending abolition of the methadone regulations. The regulations serve important functions, not the least of which is to maintain community support for methadone treatment programs by assuring that the programs maintain standards and are subject to outside review.'' See Institute of Medicine (US) Committee on Federal Regulation of Methadone Treatment; Rettig RA, Yarmolinsky A, editors. Federal Regulation of Methadone Treatment. Washington (DC): National Academies Press (US); 1995. Available from: *https://www.ncbi.nlm.nih.gov/books/NBK232108/—doi—10.17226/ 4899.*

treatment that could be dispensed by community pharmacies, subject to SAMHSA rules or guidance on supply of methadone for unsupervised use.

Areas of Concern: Patient and Public Safety, the Current Quandary in Outpatient Treatment with Buprenorphine, and High-Quality and Effective OUD Treatment and Persistent Stigma

Methadone is a lifesaving medication that also has risks that we take very seriously. It can be a challenge to balance the risk of adverse individual and community-related impacts associated with the inappropriate provision, and diversion, of the medication against the well-established individual and public health benefits of properly treating certain patients with OUD with methadone. Our aim with this letter is to provide salient information on three relevant areas of concern: 1) the safety of patients with OUD who may be treated with methadone, and more broadly, of the public, 2) the current quandary in outpatient treatment with buprenorphine (a partial agonist) for patients with OUD who are increasingly using fentanyl or other high potency synthetic opioids, and 3) what constitutes high-quality and effective treatment for patients with OUD and the persistent stigma that surrounds those patients.

Patient and Public Safety

Evidence gathered over the last several decades illustrates that, for many people with OUD, treatment with methadone is critical to preventing overdose and promoting remission and recovery.[64] In addition, because methadone is also a very effective analgesic and has a long half-life, it is also sometimes used to treat chronic pain in pain management practice.

---

[64] National Academies of Sciences, Engineering, Health and Medicine Division, Board on Health Sciences Policy, Committee on Medication-Assisted Treatment for Opioid Use Disorder, Michelle Mancher, and Alan I. Leshner. The Effectiveness of Medication-Based Treatment for Opioid Use Disorder. Medications for Opioid Use Disorder Save Lives. National Academies Press (US), 2019. https://www.ncbi.nlm.nih.gov/books/NBK541393/.

Decades Ago, Methadone-Involved Overdoses Correlated with Its Use in the Treatment of Pain

As an opioid analgesic for pain, methadone was swept up in the confluence of factors that lead to the inappropriate prescribing of opioids for pain treatment in the 1990's and 2000's.[65] The scientific and medical consensus after examining these trends concluded that there was a strong, positive correlation between rates of methadone prescription for use in pain treatment and methadone diversion and overdose deaths.[66] Methadone for use in pain treatment and its involvement in overdoses, however, drastically declined as public health and law enforcement agencies took measured steps to limit its injudicious use for pain, while still making it available via prescription and pharmacy dispensing when clinically appropriate for pain treatment.[67]

New Studies Have Been Used Opportunistically, And Their Nuances Have Not Been Explained

With that said, we share concerns expressed by others of methadone becoming a potential contributor of more overdoses and deaths if careful policy changes are not enacted. For example, there was an increase in methadone-involved overdose deaths in 2020; however, evidence shows such increase was likely associated with the synthetic opioid-driven spike in drug overdose deaths that year.[68] Unfortunately, some advocates use that increase opportunistically to convey a fatalistic approach that risks paralyzing lawmakers and preventing any progress. Further, those same advocates may even mention two other studies published in January 2023 that raise questions about the role of Federal regulatory OTP flexibilities during the COVID PHE—which allowed for more unsupervised use of methadone in the treatment of OUD within OTP settings—to increases in methadone-involved

---

[65] Paulozzi, Leonard, Karen Mack, and Christopher M. Jones. ''Vital Signs: Risk for Overdose from Methadone Used for Pain Relief—United States, 1999—2010,'' July 6, 2012. https://www.cdc.gov/mmwr/preview/mmwrhtml/mm6126a5.htm. ''Examination of Methadone Involved Overdoses during the COVID–19 Pandemic.'' Forensic Science International 344 (January 31, 2023): 111579. https://doi.org/10.1016/j.forsciint.2023.111579.

[66] Jones, Christopher M., Grant T. Baldwin, Teresa Manocchio, Jessica O. White, and Karin A. Mack. ''Trends in Methadone Distribution for Pain Treatment, Methadone Diversion, and Overdose Deaths—United States, 2002—2014.'' Morbidity and Mortality Weekly Report 65, no. 26 (2016): 667—71.

[67] Id.

[68] Jones, Christopher M., Wilson M. Compton, Beth Han, Grant Baldwin, and Nora D. Volkow. ''Methadone-Involved Overdose Deaths in the US Before and After Federal Policy Changes Expanding Take-Home Methadone Doses From Opioid Treatment Programs.'' JAMA Psychiatry 79, no. 9 (September 1, 2022): 932—34. *https://doi.org/10.1001/jamapsychiatry.2022.1776.*

overdoses deaths. Specifically, one such study found an increase in methadone-involved overdose deaths in the year after March 2020 compared with prior trends, both with and without co-involvement of synthetic opioids;[69] the other found an increase of methadone-involved overdose deaths by 48.1 percent in 2020 relative to 2019.[70]

Neither of those two studies, however, includes or examines additional, provisional overdose death data after March 2021, when the rate of methadone-involved overdose deaths stabilized and declined. The authors' failure to include this data may bias the models in their studies. Indeed, the relative rate of methadone-involved overdose deaths has declined by 9.5 percent between August 2021 and August 2022,[71] while overdose deaths related to a lack of access to medications for OUD increased in the same period.[72] In addition, there is no direct evidence of causality that links any change in Federal OTP take-home policies to an increase in methadone-involved overdose deaths, as is noted in one study.[73] Nor do the authors in the other study wish to add to misconceptions about the safety of methadone for OUD, as stated by those authors themselves.[74] If anything, these two studies demonstrate that modernizing treatment with methadone for OUD—within

---

[69] This study examines absolute counts rather than relative rate increases in methadone-involved overdose deaths. Relative rates are in proportion to the whole, while absolute counts are not, and the use of absolute counts rather than relative rates limits the usefulness of this analysis. See Kleinman, Robert A., and Marcos Sanches. ''Methadone-Involved Overdose Deaths in the United States before and during the COVID–19 Pandemic.'' Drug and Alcohol Dependence 242 (January 1, 2023): 109703. *https://doi.org/10.1016/j.drugalcdep.2022.109703.*

[70] This study points out that the rate of methadone-involved overdose deaths in 2020 was much lower than its peak in 2006–2008, and that these methadone-involved overdose deaths have been largely attributed to methadone prescribed for pain. See Kaufman, Daniel E., Amy L. Kennalley, Kenneth L. McCall, and Brian J. Piper.

[71] See statistical examination of provisional overdose death data from the CDC's National Center for Health Statistics Vital Statistics System. Volkow, Nora, D. Presentation to the American Society of Addiction Medicine Advocacy Conference, ''National Institute of Drug Abuse: What Radical Change Means,'' March 6, 2023.

[72] Kariisa, Mbabazi. ''Vital Signs: Drug Overdose Deaths, by Selected Sociodemographic and Social Determinants of Health Characteristics—25 States and the District of Columbia, 2019— 2020.'' MMWR. Morbidity and Mortality Weekly Report 71 (2022). *https://doi.org/10.15585/ mmwr.mm7129e2.*

[73] ''This study is observational and does not allow for a causal attribution of the increase in methadone-involved overdose deaths to any specific factor,'' and ''this study cannot distinguish whether individuals who die from methadone-involved overdoses receive methadone through OTPs, as prescriptions for pain, or through other sources, including diverted methadone.'' See Kaufman, et al., (2023).

[74] ''We hope that these findings will not add to further misconceptions about the safety of methadone relative to other less widely prescribed Schedule II opioids,'' see Kleinman, et al., (2023).

the OTP setting—must be carried out with caution and with Federal agencies' continual, longitudinal regulations and monitoring for unintended consequences, notwithstanding the widespread support of making such Federal take home policy changes permanent by OTP organizations and associations. By way of contrast, our experience and training as addiction specialist physicians, coupled with the thoughtful guardrails in the M-OTAA, enables us to lead models of methadone treatment for OUD responsibly and safely, while we manage risks to patient and public health. In the absence of continued DEA and SAMHSA Federal regulations, oversight, and monitoring of OTPs on several fronts, however, these two studies do illustrate why we cannot say the same yet for all clinicians within the OTP setting. While some OTP medical directors are board-certified addiction specialist physicians, the Federal Government does not require them to be so credentialed; thus, some are not.

Recently Published Systematic Review Finds No Increased Risk of Methadone Overdose from Federal Regulatory Flexibilities That Allowed For More Unsupervised Use of Methadone

We also draw your attention to a review that synthesized peer-reviewed research between March 2020 and September 2022 on the effect of the Federal regulatory flexibilities on OTPs' operations, the perspectives of patients and providers, and health outcomes of patients at OTPs, including for methadone-involved overdoses, which found no evidence of increased risk of methadone overdose.[75] We do understand from this review, on the other hand, that many OTPs limited their uptake of the Federal regulatory flexibilities and did not universally provide the maximum ceiling of doses allowed for take home methadone, driven in part due potential consequences to patients, concerns about reduced OTP revenue, and uncertainty about when this temporary regulatory flexibility would end.[76]

---

[75] The systematic review of 29 peer-reviewed studies published between March 1, 2020, and September 6, 2022, includes six studies that assessed the association between pandemic flexibilities and overdose risk, which used OTP records or state-level mortality data, national poison-control or mortality data, or qualitative data. See Krawczyk, Noa.

[76] Findings include three studies of OTP providers, three surveys of OTP patients, and one multi-State survey of 170 OTP providers. Krawczyk, Noa, Bianca D. Rivera, Emily Levin, and Bridget C. E. Dooling. ''Synthesising Evidence of the Effects of COVID–19 Regulatory Changes on Methadone Treatment for Opioid Use Disorder: Implications for Policy.'' The Lancet Public Health 8, no. 3 (March 1, 2023): e238—46. *https://doi.org/10.1016/S2468–2667(23)00023–3.*

One Explanation for the Spike in Methadone-Involved Overdoses Is The Increase of Synthetic Opioids in the Non-Pharmaceutical Drug Supply

As previously noted, a plausible explanation for changes in trends in methadone-involved overdose deaths in 2020 is the dominating role that fentanyl and other high potency synthetic opioids have been playing in our non-pharmaceutical drug supply. For example, another recent analysis found an increase in overdose deaths, with and without methadone, in March 2020. Then, overdose deaths not involving methadone continued to increase by approximately 69 deaths per month, while methadone-involved overdose deaths remained stable. In terms of the implementation of the Federal regulatory flexibilities for unsupervised use of methadone at OTPs, in the period before this policy change, and after it, there were similar rates of decline in the percentage of methadone-involved overdose deaths.[77] This study therefore suggests, in light of this data, that in the early months of the COVID–19 pandemic, the spike in drug overdose deaths overall in March 2020 was associated with the increase in synthetic opioids in the drug supply among people who were being treated with methadone from an OTP, not due to methadone risks associated with Federal regulatory flexibilities for OTPs.

Multiple Factors Explain Methadone Being Preferentially Listed on Overdose Death Certificates

Finally, it is important for lawmakers to understand that methadone's long halflife is an additional, confounding variable that can result in the preferential listing of methadone on death certificates, during a period when overdose deaths frequently involve multiple substances. Novel psychoactive substances permeate the non-pharmaceutical drug supply as well, for which drug overdose deaths are not routinely assessed. Moreover, the decentralization of authority in death certification policy and procedure also creates substantial differences in how overdose deaths are characterized and reported, and there is a high error rate in death certificates for overdose deaths.[78]

---

[77] In January 2019, 4.5 percent of overdose deaths involved methadone, and 3.2 percent of overdose deaths involved methadone by August 2021. See Jones, et al., (2023).

[78] Peppin, John F., John J. Coleman, Antonella Paladini, Giustino Varrassi, John F. Peppin, John J. Coleman, Antonella Paladini, and Giustino Varrassi. ''What Your Death Certificate Says About You May Be Wrong: A Narrative Review on CDC's Efforts to Quantify Prescription Opioid Overdose Deaths.'' Cureus 13, no. 9 (September 16, 2021). *https://doi.org/10.7759/cureus.18012.*

The Current Quandary in Outpatient Treatment with Buprenorphine for Patients with OUD Involving Fentanyl or Other High Potency Synthetic Opioids

Under the Code of Federal Regulations Title 21 1306.07(b), the DEA permits an exception to methadone dispensing requirements for DEA-registered physicians outside of OTPs to provide emergency treatment for patients with methadone for OUD for 1 day, and to carry out such treatment for no more than 3 days, while planning for the patients' referral to treatment.[79] Last March 2022, the DEA started allowing certain DEA-registered physicians to dispense a 3-day supply of methadone at one time, so long as the exception is requested.[80] While this change is theoretically helpful, it does not help us face a terrible quandary when we attempt to initiate buprenorphine treatment with patients with OUD involving illegal fentanyl or other high potency synthetic opioids.

Federal Law Currently Prevents the Use of Methadone for the Treatment of Patients Via a ''Low Dose Buprenorphine with Opioid Continuation'' Initiation Process

Patients who use fentanyl in the unregulated drug supply, which increasingly has unpredictable and hazardous novel contaminants, have significant challenges with initiation of buprenorphine (a partial agonist), another highly effective medication for OUD treatment. Under current law, however, it is illegal to prescribe full opioid agonists such as hydromorphone, oxycodone, or morphine for OUD during buprenorphine initiation and titration. Thus, we are sometimes left with a dangerous alternative, which is to advise patients that use of opioids from the unregulated supply should be continued while undergoing buprenorphine initiation via a low dose buprenorphine with opioid continuation initiation process. Access to methadone would be a safe full agonist alternative to use for individuals who are undergoing a low dose buprenorphine with opioid continuation initiation process, and the M-OTAA could allow this to be safely done under expert physician guidance.

---

79 ''21 CFR 1306.07—Administering or Dispensing of Narcotic Drugs.'' Accessed March 16, 2023. *https://www.ecfr.gov/current/title–21/chapter-II/part–1306/subject-group-ECFR1eb5bb3a23fddd0/section–1306.07.*

80 ''DEA's Commitment to Expanding Access to Medication-Assisted Treatment.'' Accessed March 16, 2023. *https://www.dea.gov/press-releases/2022/03/23/deas-commitment-expanding- access-medication-assisted-treatment.*

Restrictions on Methadone for OUD Limit Treatment Options for Patients with OUD Who Do Not Stabilize on Buprenorphine

In addition, methadone is an excellent alternative medication treatment recommended for patients with OUD who do not stabilize on buprenorphine. However, unless it's being dispensed from an OTP, we can only dispense methadone to those patients for up to 3 days. This limitation restricts our being able to offer this critically important medication to those patients, even when they face insurmountable geographical, financial, transportation, or other barriers to continue their treatment at OTPs. In these medical scenarios, the absurdity of antiquated Federal laws that govern methadone for OUD treatment is extremely clear. When the laws are applied to an ever and rapidly changing unregulated drug supply, the laws' out-of-date nature is obvious and distressing.

High-Quality and Effective OUD Treatment and Persistent Stigma

High-Quality and Effective Treatment for OUD Does Not Make Engagement in Psychosocial Counseling a Condition of Receiving Medication

Patients with OUD who are treated with medications for OUD have over 50 percent lower overdose rates.[81] For this reason and to fulfill our medical mission to save lives, our first, most immediate goal is to reach more people with moderate to severe OUD with this life-saving medication.[82] Patients who receive medication for OUD, including methadone, have better rates of retention in treatment; behavioral therapies, alone, do not increase patient retention in treatment.[83] While psycho-social treatment and other services are an important component of quality care and beneficial to many people with

---

[81] National Academies of Sciences, Engineering, Health and Medicine Division, Board on Health Sciences Policy, Committee on Medication-Assisted Treatment for Opioid Use Disorder, Michelle Mancher, and Alan I. Leshner. The Effectiveness of Medication-Based Treatment for Opioid Use Disorder. Medications for Opioid Use Disorder Save Lives. National Academies Press (US), 2019. *https://www.ncbi.nlm.nih.gov/books/NBK541393/.*

[82] NYU Langone News. ''Almost 90 Percent of People with Opioid Use Disorder Not Receiving Lifesaving Medication.'' Accessed March 10, 2023. *https://nyulangone. org/news/almost–90-per-cent-people-opioid-use-disorder-not-receiving-lifesaving-medi cation.*

[83] Timko, Christine, Nicole R Schultz, Michael A Cucciare, Lisa Vittorio, and Christina Garrison-Diehn. ''Retention in Medication-Assisted Treatment for Opiate Dependence: A Systematic Review.'' Journal of Addictive Diseases 35, no. 1 (2016): 22—35. *https://doi.org/10.1080/10550887.2016.1100960.*

OUD,[84] the scientific and medical consensus is that psychosocial treatment should be made available to patients in treatment for OUD, but a patient's willingness to engage in such treatment should not be a condition of the patient receiving medication.[85]

High-Quality and Effective Treatment for OUD Is Patient-Centered

In an office-based practice of addiction medicine or addiction psychiatry, an expert physician may counsel patients with OUD who are willing to engage in psychosocial treatment as part of the physician's medical management; a multidisciplinary team member in the practice may provide more intensive counseling for patients with OUD, or the practice may refer some of those patients to another practice for even more psychosocial treatment. While we are grateful for SAMHSA's recently proposed modifications to 42 CFR Part 8 which, if finalized, should significantly improve the quality of treatment services at OTPs, by making it less ''program centered'' and more ''patient centered''—like expertled office-based practices—patients with OUD need more options for their care, and more OTPs need to face high-quality competition as an incentive to continue to improve their services.

Existing Stereotypes Lend Themselves to Prescriptive, Rigid Models of Methadone Treatment for OUD

Finally, we know that patients with OUD face persistent stigma, including stereotypes that they are non-compliant, out-of-control, unwilling to change risk behaviors, and do not have strong communities.[86] We are extremely concerned that these stereotypes lend themselves to prescriptive, rigid approaches to methadone treatment for OUD. The existing, siloed

---

[84] Dugosh, Karen, Amanda Abraham, Brittany Seymour, Keli McLoyd, Mady Chalk, and David Festinger. ''A Systematic Review on the Use of Psychosocial Interventions in Conjunction With Medications for the Treatment of Opioid Addiction.'' Journal of Addiction Medicine 10, no. 2 (March 2016): 91—101. *https://doi.org/10.1097/ADM.0000000000000193.*

[85] See National Academies of Sciences, Engineering, Health and Medicine Division, Board on Health Sciences Policy, Committee on Medication-Assisted Treatment for Opioid Use Disorder, Michelle Mancher, and Alan I. Leshner. The Effectiveness of Medication-Based Treatment for Opioid Use Disorder. Medications for Opioid Use Disorder Save Lives. National Academies Press (US), 2019. *https://www.ncbi.nlm.nih.gov/books/NBK541393/,* and see American Society of Addiction Medicine. ''National Practice Guideline for the Treatment of Opioid Use Disorder: 2020 Focused Update,'' 2020. *https://sitefinitystorage.blob.core.windows.net/sitefinity-production-blobs/docs/default-source/guidelines/npg-jam-supplement.pdf'sfvrsn=a00a52c2—2.*

[86] Earnshaw, Valerie, Laramie Smith, and Michael Copenhaver. ''Drug Addiction Stigma in the Context of Methadone Maintenance Therapy: An Investigation into Understudied Sources of Stigma.'' International Journal of Mental Health and Addiction 11, no. 1 (February 1, 2013): 110—22. *https://doi.org/10.1007/s11469–012–9402–5.*

infrastructure for methadone treatment for OUD in the U.S. has compounded such stigma, and despite methadone's strong evidence as a life-saving medication, there is neither broad acceptance of methadone as a treatment intervention by the public, nor by healthcare providers, including some addiction providers. [87]

The Integration of Methadone Treatment with Other Medical Care Will Improve the Quality of OUD Care

The separateness of methadone treatment for OUD—which results in methadone dispensed from OTPs, rather than pharmacies, being nearly universally excluded from prescription drug monitoring programs—has rather served to focus OTP services on the administration of one medication for one medical indication.[88] In contrast, the modernization of methadone treatment for OUD, as contemplated by the M-OTAA, will give Americans with addiction involving polysubstance use more conveniently located, comprehensive treatment options that can treat and manage their uncontrolled use of any substance, as well as other chronic, often comorbid diseases with OUD, such as depression, diabetes, bipolar disorder, and hypertension.[89] These additional options are urgently needed, so that we may safely integrate treatment with methadone for OUD with the rest of general healthcare, and continue to improve the treatment of OUD with methadone in this country.

We stand ready to discuss this information further with you at any time. We are hopeful that we can work together to save as many lives as possible. We look forward to hearing from you.

Sincerely,
Ruth A. Potee, M.D., FASAM**,
Medical Director, Franklin County House of Corrections,
Director of Addiction Services, Behavioral Health Network.

---

[87] Madden, Erin Fanning. ''Intervention Stigma: How Medication-Assisted Treatment Marginalizes Patients and Providers.'' Social Science & Medicine (1982) 232 (July 2019): 324—31. *https://doi.org/10.1016/j.socscimed.2019.05.027.*

[88] See Olsen, Yngvild, and Joshua M. Sharfstein. ''Confronting the Stigma of Opioid Use Disorder—and Its Treatment.'' JAMA 311, no. 14 (April 9, 2014): 1393—94. *https://doi.org/ 10.1001/jama.2014.2147,* and National Association of State Alcohol and Drug Abuse Directors, and American Association for the Treatment of Opioid Dependence. ''TECHNICAL BRIEF: CENSUS OF OPIOID TREATMENT PROGRAMS—NASADAD,'' December 5, 2022. *ttps://nasadad.org/2022/12/technical-brief-census-of-opioid-treatment-programs/.*

[89] Olsen, Yngvild, and Joshua M. Sharfstein. ''Confronting the Stigma of Opioid Use Disorder—and Its Treatment.'' JAMA 311, no. 14 (April 9, 2014): 1393—94. *https://doi.org/ 10.1001/jama.2014.2147.*

The views expressed are those of the authors and do not necessarily represent the views of their institutions.

One asterisk (*) indicates an individual has past work experience at an opioid treatment program (OTP); two asterisks (**) indicates the individual currently works at an OTP.

MELISSA WEIMER, DO, MCR, DFASAM
Yale New Haven Hospital, Yale University
JESSICA R. GRAY, MD, FASAM
Massachusetts General Hospital
WILLIAM F. HANING, III, M.D., FASAM, DFAPA
President, American Society of Addiction Medicine Professor of Psychiatry, John A. Burns School of Medicine, University of Hawai'i
Nina Vidmer
Executive Director, American Osteopathic Academy of Addiction Medicine
BRIAN HURLEY, MD, MBA, DFASAM
President-Elect, American Society of Addiction Medicine Medical Director, Substance Abuse Prevention and Control at Los Angeles County
Department of Public Health
STEPHEN M. TAYLOR, MD, MPH, DFAPA, DFASAM
Vice-Chair, Legislative Advocacy Committee, American Society of Addiction
Medicine Pathway Healthcare, LLC
Suneel M. Agerwala, MD*
Yale School of Medicine
Dinah Applewhite, MD
Massachusetts General Hospital
MICHAEL S. ARGENYI, MD, MPH, MSW*
University of Iowa Hospitals & Clinics
Mahreen Arshad, MD, MPH
Addiction Medicine, Obesity Medicine, Internal Medicine
Julia Arnsten, MD
Montefiore Medical Center
Lance Austein, MD, FACP
Monogram Medical, PC
Sarah Axelrath, MD*
Stout Street Health Center Colorado Coalition for the Homeless

Sarah Bagley, MD, MSc
Addiction Consult Service, Boston Medical Center
Jessica Barnes Calihan, MD
Adolescent Substance Use & Addiction Program, Boston Children's Hospital
Raymond Bertino, MD
President, Illinois Society of Addiction Medicine Clinical Professor of Radiology and Surgery, University of Illinois College of
Medicine, Peoria
BENJAMIN BEARNOT, MD, MPH, FASAM
Charlestown Health Center, Massachusetts General Hospital
Annemarie Bonawitz-Dodi, MD, FASAM**
Lexington Center for Recovery
Joseph F. Boyle, MD*
Addiction Consult Service, Faster Paths To Treatment, Boston Medical Center
Jeffrey Brent, MD, PhD
University of Colorado, School of Medicine
EMILY BRUNNER, MD, DFASAM
Gateway Recovery Center
Bradley M. Buchheit, MD, MS
Oregon Health & Sciences University
Michael A Carnevale, DO*
Peacehealth Medical Group
Carolyn Chan, MD*
Yale Hospital and Cornell Scott Hill Health Center (FQHC)
Yale School of Medicine
EDWIN C. CHAPMAN, MD, FASAM*
Edwin C. Chapman, MD, PC
Avik Chatterjee, MD, MPH
Addiction Consult Service, Boston Medical Center
Cynthia Chatterjee, MD, MA, FASAM
San Mateo County Health (Retired)
PAUL CHENG, MD, MPH, MROCC, FASAM
The Clinic
Judy S. Chertok, MD
Penn Family Care, University of Pennsylvania
Samantha Chirunomula, MD*
Department of Medicine, Division of Infectious Diseases

University of Illinois-Chicago
SETH A. CLARK, MD, MPH, FASAM**
Addiction Medicine Consult Service, Rhode Island Hospital
Lifespan Recovery Center
Shawn Cohen, MD*
Yale School of Medicine
D. TYLER COYLE, MD, MS**
University of Colorado School of Medicine
Paul Christine, MD, PhD*
Boston Medical Center
Fabiola A. Arbelo Cruz, MD*
Connecticut Mental Health Center, Yale School of Medicine
Paula Cook, MD**
Moab Regional Recovery
Ashley Coughlin, MD*
Addiction Psychiatrist and Director of Intensive Outpatient Psychiatric Services
Lawrence and Memorial Hospital Northeast Medical Group Yale New Haven Health
Phoebe Cushman, MD, MS
Boston University School of Public Health
Catherine DeGood, DO**
CODAC Behavioral Healthcare, Butler Behavioral Health
MICHAEL DELMAN, MD, FACP, FACG, DFASAM**
Medical Director, Seafield Center
Regina DiGiovanna, MD, FASAM*
Wellness Center-AMEX
Dora Dixie, MD**
Family Guidance; The Women's Treatment Center; Symetria Recovery
FRANK DOWLING, MD, FASAM, DLFAPA
Long Island Behavioral Medicine, PC
Honora Englander, MD
Principal Investigator and Director, Improving Addiction Care Team (IMPACT)
Oregon Health & Science University
Mark Eisenberg, MD
Massachusetts General Hospital Boston Health Care for the Homeless
Caitlin Farrell, DO, MPH
Boston Medical Center

ALLEN FEIN, MD, FASAM
Stonybrook Community Medical Group
Casey Ferguson, MD*
CODA, Inc.
Central City Concern
Bridget Foley, DO
Director, Office-Based Addiction Treatment (OBAT), Tufts Medical Center
MARTIN FRIED, MD, FACP
Wexner Medical Center, Ohio State University
PETER D. FRIEDMANN, MD, MPH, DFASAM, FACP
Chief Research Officer, Baystate Health Office of Research, University of Massachusetts Chan Medical School-Baystate
Jennifer Frush, MD, MTS
Boston Medical Center Emergency Department
Jennifer L. Fyler, MD**
Greenfield Opioid Treatment Program, New View Residential Treatment Program,
Behavioral Health Group
Hiroko Furo, MD, PhD*
University of Texas Health Science Center-San Antonio
Evan Gale, MD
Associate Medical Director, Addiction Consult Team
Massachusetts General Hospital
JOSEPH GARBELY, DO, DFASAM**
Brookdale Premier Addiction Recovery
HEIDI GINTER, MD, FASAM**
Recovery Centers of America
MELODY GLENN, MD, MFA, FASAM*
Director, Addiction Medicine Consult Team Banner—University Medical Center, University of Arizona
David Goodman-Meza, MD, MAS**
Division of Infectious Diseases, David Geffen School of Medicine, UCLA
ANDREA GOUGH-GOLDMAN, MD, MPH, FASAM**
Oregon Health & Science University
Paul Grekin, MD**
Evergreen Treatment Services
Lucinda Grovenburg, MD Scott Hadland, MD, MPH, MS, FASAM

Massachusetts General Hospital; Harvard Medical School
JOHN HARDY, MD, FASAM
John Hardy MD LLC, AMG Physicians LLC, Transformations Wellness Center
Miriam Harris, MD, MSc**
Boston Medical Center Health Care Resource Centers, Boston Methadone Treatment Program
Nzinga Harrison, MD, FASAM
Chief Medical Officer, Eleanor Health
LEAH HARVEY, MD, MPH
Infectious Disease and Addiction Medicine Physician, Boston Medical Center
BENJAMIN HAYES, MD, MS, MPH
Montefiore Medical Center
Andrew A. Herring, MD
Systemwide Medical Director, Substance Use Disorder Treatment, Alameda Health System
JANET J. HO, MD, MPH, FASAM
Addiction Consult Service, University of California-San Francisco
LYNDA KARIG HOHMANN, MD, PHD, MBA, FAAFP, FASAM
(Retired)
RANDOLPH P. HOLMES, MD, DFASAM
Los Angeles Centers for Alcohol and Drug Abuse (LACADA)
Stephen Holtsford, MD, FASAM
Recovery Centers of America; Lighthouse Recovery, Inc.; BrightHeart Health
STANLEY T. HOOVER, MD, FASAM
Dan Hoover, MD
Oregon Health & Sciences University Addiction Medicine ECHO Director
Connie Hsaio, MD**
APT Foundation; Connecticut Mental Health Center
Cornell Scott—Hill Health Center, Yale School of Medicine
Ilana Hull, MD, MSc
University of Pittsburgh Medical Center
Michael Incze, MD, MEd
Department of Internal Medicine, Primary Care, University of Utah
CHRISTINA E. JONES, MD, FASAM*
Behavioral Health Group; Community Connections

Ayana Jordan, MD, PhD*

Sunset Terrace Family Health Center New York University Grossman School of Medicine

Joseph Joyner, MD, MPH*

Chelsea Health Care Center, Massachusetts General Hospital

Kimberly A. Kabernagel, DO, FASAM**

Medical Director, Marworth Treatment Center, Geisinger Health

DAVID KAN, MD, DFASAM*

Bright Health Volunteer Clinical Professor, University of California-San Francisco

PETER KASSIS, MD, FASAM**

BayMark, Health Care Resource Centers

Ghulam Karim Khan, MD*

Clinical Research Fellow, Infectious Disease and Addiction Medicine, Boston

Medical Center

Laura Gaeta Kehoe, MD**

Massachusetts General Hospital

Andrea Kermack, MD**

Wellness Center—Port Morris, Montefiore Medical Center

Stefan G. Kertesz, MD, MSc

Professor of Medicine, Heersink UAB School of Medicine

Laila Khalid, MD, MPH

Montefiore Medical Center

Simeon Kimmel, MD, MA*

Assistant Professor of Medicine at Chobanian and Avedisian School of Medicine Attending Physician, General Internal Medicine and Infectious Diseases; Boston Medical Center

Rachel King, MD*

South End Community Health Center

Boston Medical Center

Miriam S. Komaromy, MD

Medical Director, Grayken Center for Addiction, Boston Medical Center

Juleigh Kowinski Konchak, MD, MPH, FASAM

Attending Physician, Behavioral Health, Department of Family and Community

Medicine Cook County Health

JARED W. KLEIN, MD, MPH*

Harborview Medical Center, University of Washington School of Medicine

Elizabeth E. Krans, MD, MSc

University of Pittsburgh Medical Center

ARI KRIEGSMAN, MD, FASAM*

Medical Director, Addiction Consult Service, Mercy Medical Center

Sunny Kung, MD

Merrimack Valley Bridge Clinic

JORDANA LAKS, MD, MPH*

Boston Medical Center

JAMES R. LATRONICA, DO, FASAM**

University of Pittsburgh Medical Center; University of Pittsburgh School of Medicine

DAVID LAWRENCE, MD, FASAM**

Medical Director, Veterans Affairs Greater Los Angeles Health System

Diana Lee, MD*

Addiction Medicine and Primary Care Physician, New York University Grossman School of Medicine

SKY LEE, MD, AAHIVS

Board Certified in Family & Addiction Medicine

XIMENA A. LEVANDER, MD, MCR*

Addiction Medicine Clinician and Researcher Oregon Health & Science University

SHARON LEVY, MD, MPH, FASAM

Director, Adolescent Substance Use and Addiction Program, Boston Children's

Hospital Associate Professor in Pediatrics, Harvard Medical School

MOXIE LOEFFLER, DO, MPH, FASAM**

Lane County Treatment Center Oregon Society of Addiction Medicine

Sara Lorenz Taki, MD**

Medical Director, Greenwich House Methadone Maintenance Treatment Program

Margaret Lowenstein, MD, MSHP*

University of Pennsylvania

TIFFANY LU, MD, MS, FASAM*

Montefiore Medical Center

Cynthia Sue Marske, DO**

Benton County Health Services

Marlene Martin, MD

University of California-San Francisco; San Francisco General Hospital

STEPHEN MARTIN, MD, EDM, FASAM, FAAFP

Barre Family Health Center, University of Massachusetts Memorial Health

Boulder Care

Mariya Masyukova, MD, MS

Attending Physician, Montefiore Medical Center; Assistant Professor, Albert

Einstein College of Medicine

MARY G. MCMASTERS, MD, DFASAM* NICKY MEHTANI, MD, MPH*

San Francisco Department of Public Health University of California-San Francisco

Sarah Messmer, MD*

Mobile MAR Program, University of Illinois-Chicago College of Medicine

Jennifer Michaels, MD

The Brien Center, Berkshire Medical Center

KENNETH MORFORD, MD, FASAM**

APT Foundation, Yale New Haven Hospital, Yale School of Medicine

Katherine Mullins, MD, AAHIVS*

New York University—Langone Health

Rayek Nafiz, MD*

Penn Medicine

ANNE N. NAFZIGER, MD, PHD, FASAM, FCP, FACP**

Conifer Park, Inc.

CHRISTINE NEEB, MD, FASAM**

University of Illinois Health Mile Square Health Center; Stonybrook Center

AARON NEWCOMB, DO, FASAM

Shawnee Health Services

MARK X. NORLEANS, MD, PHD, FASAM

Addiction Care of Excellence

Sherry Nykiel, MD*

Justus Mental Health; Key Recovery and Life Skills Center Delaware Division of Medicaid and Medical Assistance

Nicole O'Connor, MD

Beth Israel Deaconess Medical Center

Linda Peng, MD*

Hillsboro Medical Center, Oregon Health & Sciences University
Alyssa Peterkin, MD
Hospital, Outpatient Bridge Clinic, Boston Medical Center
Charles Peterson, MD**
Medical Director, New Season Opioid Treatment Program
ARWEN PODESTA, MD, DFASAM
Podesta Wellness, LLC
CARA POLAND, MD, MED, FACP, DFASAM
Michigan State University
SMITA PRASAD, MD, MBA, MPH, FASAM
Longbranch Healthcare Tulane Addition Medicine Fellowship Program
JOSIAH D. RICH, MD, MPH*
Professor of Medicine and Epidemiology, Brown University The Miriam and Rhode Island Hospitals, Rhode Island Department of Corrections
ELISE K. RICHMAN, MD, FASAM
Montefiore Behavioral Health Center
EOWYN RIEKE, MD, MPH, FASAM
Fora Health
Daniel Rosa, MD**
Senior Medical Director, Acacia Network
A. KENISON ROY, III, MD**
Behavioral Health Group, New Orleans
LIPI ROY, MD, MPH, FASAM
Housing Works
Kenneth Saffier, MD, FASAM
Contra Costa Health Services
KELLEY SAIA, MD, F-ACOG, D-ABAM*
Project RESPECT, Substance Use Disorder in Pregnancy Treatment Center
Boston Medical Center
ELIZABETH M. SALISBURY-AFSHAR, MD, MPH, FAAFP, DFASAM, FACPM
Associate Professor, Department of Family Medicine and Community Health
University of Wisconsin-Madison
JASLEEN SALWAN, MD, MPH, FASAM*
Montgomery Family Medicine Associates
JEFFREY H. SAMET, MD, MA, MPH, FASAM
John Noble Professor of Medicine and Professor of Public Health, Boston

University Primary Care, Inpatient Medicine Service, and Addiction Consult Service, Boston

Medical Center

MARIO SAN BARTOLOME, MD, MBA, MRO, FASAM

KCS Health Center

RANDY SEEWALD, MBBS, MD, FASAM, HMDC**

Lexington Center for Recovery

JEFFREY SELZER, MD, DFASM, DLFAPA*

Medical Director, Committee for Physicians Health

CHRISTOPHER W. SHANAHAN, MD, MPH, FASAM, FACP**

Frontage Road Methadone Clinic, Boston Public Health Commission

DEAN SINGER, DO, FASAM*

Bridge Primary, Clinical and Support Options (CSO)

Deepika E. Slawek, MD, MS

Montefiore Medical Center

MARCELA SMID, MD, MA, MS

University of Utah School of Medicine

Eleasa Sokolski, MD*

Oregon Health & Science University

MIA D. SORCINELLI SMITH, MD, FASAM, FAAFP**

Greater Lawrence Family Health Center

Spectrum Health Systems Massachusetts Behavioral Health Partnership

Peter Smith, MD, MSc

Boston Medical Center

Natalie Stahl, MD, MPH*

Greater Lawrence Family Health Center

PAUL J. STEIER, D.O., FASAM, FAOAAM

G Street Integrated Health; Serenity Lane; Centro Latino Americano; South Lane

Mental Health

STEPHANIE STEWART, MD, MPHS, FASAM, MRO**

University of Colorado School of Medicine

JOSHUA ST. LOUIS, MD, MPH, FASAM*

Greater Lawrence Family Health Center

Sarah Bronwyn Stuart, MD*

Syracuse Recovery

LESLIE SUEN, MD, MAS*

San Francisco General Hospital University of California-San Francisco

Mohsin Syed, MD

Slocum-Dickson Medical Group
Ashish Thakrar, MD*
University of Pennsylvania Health System Philadelphia Veterans Affairs
Jessica L. Taylor, MD
Medical Director, Faster Paths to Treatment
Boston Medical Center
CARLOS F. TIRADO, MD, MPH*
Travis County Integral Care, CARMAHealth PLLC
Kristine Torres-Lockhart, MD, FASAM*
Port Morris Wellness Center—Opioid Treatment Center
Montefiore Medical Center
JOSEPH M. VALDEZ MD, MPH, FASAM
Outpatient Addiction Medicine Clinic, Geisinger Center of Excellence
SARAH E. WAKEMAN, MD, FASAM
Medical Director, Massachusetts General Hospital Substance Use Disorder
Initiative Harvard Medical School
William Joseph Walsh, III, MD
Weber Recovery Center
NALAN WARD, MD, FASAM**
Massachusetts General Hospital; Harvard Medical School
CAROLYN WARNER-GREER, MS, MD, FACOG, FASAM**
The Bowen Center
ANDREA WEBER, MD, MME, FACP, FASAM
University of Iowa Addiction and Recovery Collaborative
JOHN WEEMS, MD, FASAM*
CommunityCare federally Qualified Health Centers
DANIEL WEINER, DO, FASAM
Rogue Community Health
ZOE M. WEINSTEIN, MD, MS, FASAM**
Boston Medical Center
Annalee Wells, DO
Lynn Community Health Center
Arthur Robin Williams, MD, MBE*
Assistant Professor of Clinical Psychiatry, Columbia University Director, American Academy of Addiction Psychiatry Area II (New York)
JAN WIDERMAN, DO, FAAP, FASAM, FAOAAM
Medically Assisted Recovery Services, PC
TRICIA WRIGHT, MD, FS, FACOG, DFASAM

San Francisco General Hospital University of California-San Francisco
JEFFERY T. YOUNG, MD, FASAM
Hazelden Betty Ford Foundation
Amy Yule, MD*
Medical Director, Addiction Recovery Management Service, Massachusetts General
Hospital Psychiatrist, Boston Medical Center

Additional Signatories:
ROHIT ABRAHAM, MD, MPH, MAT
Boston Medical Center
Marielle Baldwin, MD, MPH
Assistant Professor of Family Medicine, Chobanian and Avedisian School of Medicine, Boston University
Rebecca Barron, MD, MPH
Emergency Medicine, University of Massachusetts Chan—Baystate
Angela R. Bazzi, PhD, MPH Corinne A. Beaugard, MSW
Grayken Center for Addiction, Boston University School of Social Work
ROBERT S. BEIL, MD, AAHIVM
Montefiore Medical Center
Judana Bennett, PMHNP-BC
Massachusetts General Hospital
Cari Benbasset-Miller, MD
Cambridge Health Alliance—Revere
Edward Bernstein, MD
Professor Emeritus, Department of Emergency Medicine, Boston University School of Medicine
Anne Berrigan, LICSW
Boston Medical Center
Alexandra Bessaoud, BSN, RN
Center for Infectious Disease, Boston Medical Center
Samantha Blakemore, MPH
Boston Medical Center
JAMES BLUM, MD, MPP
Boston Medical Center
KIMBERLY BRANDT, MS, FNP-BC*
CODA, Inc.
Bari Brodsky, MD
North Shore Community Health, Cambridge Health Alliance

Ebony Caldwell, MD, MPH**
APT Foundation; Cornell Scott Hill Health Center
Sandra Cagle, NP
Ascension Macomb Oakland Hospital
Mordechai Caplan, Medical Student Brittney Carney, DNP, FNP-BC*
Boston Children's Hospital
Layla Cavitt**
Comprehensive Psychiatric Centers—Miami
Deborah Chassler, MSW
Senior Academic Researcher, Boston University
Benjamin J. Church, DO
Emergency Medicine, Baystate Health
Kaitlyn Clausell, MS4
Albert Einstein College of Medicine
Camille Clifford
Massachusetts HEALing Communities Study, School of Public Health, Boston University
ALEX CLOSE, MD, EM, PGY–2
Bridget Coffey, MSN
Missouri Institute of Mental Health, University of Missouri-St. Louis
Gerald Coste, MD
Cambridge Health Alliance
PATRICIA CREMINS, MA, PA-C, AAHIVS
Chanelle Diaz, MD, MPH
Montefiore Medical Center
Frank DiRenno, MD
Montefiore Medical Center
Catherine Donlon, MD, PGY–1
Cambridge Health Alliance
ASHLEY DEUTSCH, MD, FACEP, FAAEM**
Emergency Medicine, University of Massachusetts Chan School of Medicine
Tala Elia, MD
Emergency Medicine, University of Massachusetts Chan School of Medicine
Anthony English, PA-C
Springfield and Holyoke OTPs, Behavioral Health Network
Liz Evans, PhD

Public Health Researcher Health Promotion and Policy Department, University of Massachusetts

Patrick Felton, MD

Baystate Medical Center

Sean Fogler, MD

Elevyst

NICOLE FORDEY, LCSW, LISAC, LICSW, CCTP*

Monument

Eduardo Garza, MD Pgy–5 Chief Resident FM/Psych

Boston Medical Center

Angela G. Giovanniello, PharmD, L.Ac Amanda Gebel, Overdose Prevention Specialist

Missouri Institute of Mental Health, University of Missouri-St. Louis

MAT GOEBEL, MD, MAS

Baystate Medical Center, Baystate Noble Hospital

Andrea Gordon, MD

Cambridge Health Alliance

Robert M. Grossberg, MD

Montefiore Medical Center

Valerie Gruber, PhD

Clinical Psychologist, Addiction Counselor

Jonathan Hanson, MD, MPH

Resident Physician, Boston Medical Center

Jacqueline Harris, PA-C

Baystate Springfield ED

Iman Hassan, MD, MS

Albert Einstein College of Medicine

ERICA HEIMAN, MD, MS**

Yale Fellow in Addiction Medicine

Kevin T. Hinchey, MD

Matthew Holm, MD Montefiore Medical Center

Jamie Lee Horton

Baystate Medical Center

Sandra Honter-Williams, MBM**

Rapid Access Program, Grayken Center for Addiction, Boston Medical Center

Beth Hribar, MPP** Andrew Hyatt, MD

Cambridge Health Alliance

Fazeelah Ibrahim**

Addiction Medicine Fellow
J. Aaron Johnson, PhD
Professor and Director, Institute of Public and Preventive Health
Augusta University
Michelle R. Johnson, MD
Cambridge Health Alliance
Jennifer Jones, MD Paul Joudrey, MD, MPH*
University of Pittsburgh Medical Center—Shadyside, Mercy IMREP
Darline Justal, NP**
Boston Medical Center
Matthew Kahari, MD**
Geisinger Medical Center
CAROL B. KELLY, MD, FACP
Montefiore Comprehensive Family Care Center
Mark E. Klee, PharmD
Baystate Medical Center, Baystate Health
Sarah Kleinschmidt, MD
Emergency Department
Sarah Kosakowski, MPH
Boston Medical Center
COLLEEN T. LABELLE, MSN, RN-BC, CARN
Boston University
Shilpa Lad
Moses Campus, Montefiore Medical Center
HUNG LE, SPRM, CARN-AP**
Boston Medical Center
Hansel Lugo
Recovery Coach, Boston Medical Center
Casa Esperanza, Bridgewell, Lynn Community Health Center
YinPhyu Lwin
Interfaith Methadone Maintenance Treatment Program
Kirsten Meisinger, MD, MHCDS
Union Square Family Health Center, Cambridge Health Alliance
Harvard Center for Primary Care
CARLA MERLOS, MSN, PMHNP-BC**
Boston Medical Center
Dave Morgan, RPh
Stephen Murray, MPH, NRP
Boston Medical Center

Nicole O'Connor, MD
Beth Israel Deaconess Medical Center
ADELE OJEDA, RN, CARN*
University of Massachusetts Barre Family Health Center
Chiedozie Ojimba
Montefiore Methadone Clinic Interfaith Medical Center Methadone Clinic
Donald Otis
Missouri Institute of Mental Health, University of Missouri-St. Louis
Danielle C. Ompad, PhD
Drug Use Researcher, Professor of Epidemiology New York University School of Global Public Health
Linda Neville, BS
Boston Medical Center
VIRAJ PATEL, MD, MPH
Montefiore Medical Center
LISA PETERSON, LMHC, LCDP, LCDS, MAC**
Chief Operating Officer, VICTA
Sriya Podila, MS1
University of Massachusetts Chan School of Medicine
DANIEL POMERANTZ, MD, MPH, FACP
Montefiore Medical Center
Talia Puzantian, PharmD**
Keck Graduate Institute School of Pharmacy and Health Sciences
San Francisco General Hospital
Heidi Quist, PA-C
Chronic Pain Wellness Center at the Phoenix VA
Gabriela Reed, MD
Addiction Medicine Fellow, Boston Medical Center
DANIEL RESNICK, MBA, OMS-III* DAWN RICE BSN, RN2**
Montefiore's Family Health Center
JOHN ROBERTS, DNP, ANP-BC
Gavin Foundation Acute Treatment Services
Jonathan Ross, MD, MS
Community Health Center, Montefiore Medical Center
Victor Roy*
National Clinician Scholars Program, Yale University VA Homeless Patient Aligned Care Team
Jay Schiff

Co-Founder & CEO, Addinex Technologies, Inc.
Elizabeth Schoenfeld, MD, MS
Vice Chair for Research, Department of Emergency Medicine, UMass Chan-Baystate
Gail Groves Scott, MPH
Director of Research and Advocacy, Health Policy Network, LLC
Ruchi Shah, DO
Family Medicine Residency, Grayken Addiction Medicine Fellow, 2023, Boston
Medical Center
Lauren Shapiro, MD
Montefiore Medical Center; Family Care Center
Anjali Sharma MD, MS
Montefiore Medical Center
Jennifer Sharpe Potter, PhD, MPH
University of Texas Health-San Antonio
MARC SHI, MD, AAHIVS
Montefiore Medical Center
Joseph Sills, MD
Emergency Medicine, University of Massachusetts Chan School of Medicine
ROSEMARY E. SMENTKOWSKI, MSN, RN, PMHNP-BC, CARN
New Hope Integrated Behavioral Health Care
Rachel Smith, BS
Medical Student, Boston University
Mark Spencer, MD Kathleen Sylvester, FNP**
Greenfield OTP, Behavioral Health Services
Mary Tomanovich, MA
Grayken Center for Addiction, Boston Medical Center
Sheila P. Vakharia, PhD, MSW
Drug Policy Alliance
Kyle Vance
Missouri Institute of Mental Health, University of Missouri-St. Louis
Alicia S. Ventura, MPH
Boston Medical Center
Nadia Villarroel, MD Durane Walker, MD
Baystate Medical Center
RYAN WALKER, MD, MPH
Greater Lawrence Family Health Center

Kris Warren
Grayken Center for Addiction, Boston Medical Center
Karrin Weisenthal, MD
Addiction Medicine Fellow, Boston Medical Center
Libby Wetterer, MD
American Academy of Family Physicians
Alexa Wilder, MPH
Grayken Center for Addiction, Boston Medical Center
DAWN WILLIAMSON RN, DNP, PMHCNS-BC, CARN-AP
Massachusetts General Hospital
Rachel Winograd, PhD*
Clinical Psychologist and Associate Professor Missouri Institute of Mental Health, University of Missouri-St. Louis
Emily Zametkin, MD
Baystate Medical Center

American Academy of Family Physicians

May 17, 2023.
Senator ED MARKEY, Chairman
Senator ROGER MARSHALL, Ranking Member
U.S. Senate Committee on Health, Education, Labor, and Pensions, Subcommittee on Primary Health and Retirement Security,
428 Dirksen Senate Office Building, Washington, DC. 20510.

Dear Chairman Markey and Ranking Member Marshall:

On behalf of the American Academy of Family Physicians (AAFP), representing more than 129,600 family physicians and medical students across the country, I write to applaud the Subcommittee's focus on mental health and substance use disorder with today's hearing titled "A Crisis in Mental Health and Substance Use Disorder Care: Closing Gaps in Access by Bringing Care and Prevention to Communities."

Family physicians provide comprehensive mental health services and are a major source for mental health care in the U.S. Nearly 40 percent of all visits for depression, anxiety, or cases defined as "any mental illness" were with primary care physicians, and primary care physicians are more likely to be the source of physical and mental health care for patients with lower socioeconomic status and for those with comorbidities.[90] Family physicians also play a crucial role in safe pain management prescribing practices, screening patients for opioid use disorder (OUD), and prescribing and maintaining treatment of medications for OUD (MOUD). Primary care physicians are often the first point of care for patients and can provide necessary referrals or coordinate care with psychiatric and other mental health professionals when needed.

Unfortunately, access to mental health care and substance use disorder (SUD) treatment remains a significant challenge for many patients across the country, particularly those from underserved communities or marginalized populations. A study published this month found that Black patients lacked equal access to OUD treatment and were far less likely to be prescribed buprenorphine, to live near a prescriber, and to remain in treatment 6 months after first being prescribed it when compared to white patients.[91]

The AAFP shares your commitment to advancing policies that will improve access to mental health and SUD care for all communities across the country. We long advocated for elimination of the X-waiver and applaud Congress for doing so as part of the Consolidated Appropriations Act of 2023. Removing these burdensome requirements for physicians to prescribe MOUD will greatly improve patient access to evidence-based, lifesaving treatment. To build upon this momentum, we urge Congress to consider the following policy recommendations.

Support Integration of Behavioral Health and Primary Care

Given the dire shortage of behavioral health clinicians, especially in many rural and underserved communities, equipping primary care clinicians to provide frontline mental health and substance abuse disorder treatment is essential for ensuring patients have timely access to care. Integrated behavioral health has shown significant cost-savings for payers and physicians, as well as more equitable access to mental health services for traditionally underserved populations.[92] Unfortunately, while many primary

---

[90] Jetty, A., Petterson, S., Westfall, J. M., & Jabbarpour, Y. (2021). Assessing Primary Care Contributions to Behavioral Health: A Cross-sectional Study Using Medical Expenditure Panel Survey: *https://Doi.Org/10.1177/21501327211023871.*

[91] Black patients with opioid addiction lack equal access to treatment (statnews.com).

[92] SY, L.-T., J, E., D, C., & PY, C. (2018). A Systematic Review of Interventions to Improve Initiation of Mental Health Care Among Racial-Ethnic Minority Groups. Psychiatric

care physicians want to integrate behavioral health services in their practices, they face burdensome startup costs and payment and reporting challenges that prevent integration.

The AAFP has continuously advocated for additional Federal investments to initiate and sustain BHI in primary care practices. We applaud Congress for including a provision in the most recent year-end omnibus to authorize grants to support the uptake and adoption of integrated care services, including the Collaborative Care Model (CoCM). We strongly encourage Congress to build upon this by implementing additional legislation to support BHI.

Specifically, the AAFP urges the reintroduction and passage of the bipartisan Improving Access to Behavioral Health Integration Act. This bill makes necessary changes to existing Federal programs to ensure primary care practices can integrate behavioral health care services by providing grant funding that covers the steep startup costs. This initial financial support is critical to improving access to integrated services and ensuring patients and payers can achieve the long-term cost savings that behavioral health integration often provides.

We also urge Congress to pass the Better Mental Health Care for Americans Act (S. 923), which would establish a Medicare add-on code for office visits provided by primary care physicians who have integrated behavioral health into their practice. This enhanced payment recognizes the unaccounted resources required to provide integrated behavioral health care and ensures that primary care practices can sustain it. Additionally, it would establish a Medicaid demonstration program to ensure that all children covered by Medicaid have access to integrated behavioral health care in primary care, schools, or other critical settings. This program would provide infrastructure, technical assistance, and sustainable financing to support expanding access to integrated mental health care for children.

Additionally, to improve access to integrated telmental and behavioral health care in primary care settings, the AAFP encourages Congress to establish a new program for adults that mirrors HRSA's Pediatric Mental Health Care Access Program (PMHCA). This program, recently reauthorized in 2022, promotes behavioral health integration into pediatric primary care by using telehealth, and has a proven track record of increasing mental and behavioral health needs despite ongoing workforce shortages by meeting children and adolescents where they are. Given the well-documented shortage

---

Services (Washington, DC.), 69(6), 628—647. *https://doi.org/10.1176/APPI.PS.—201700382.*

of mental and behavioral health clinicians and the growing demand for specialized care, a HRSA-funded program that provides primary care clinicians with virtual access to specialists could increase timely access to care for adult patients.

Telehealth

The COVID–19 public health emergency (PHE) transformed access to mental and behavioral health care via telehealth, making it possible for many patients to be connected to appropriate clinicians and treatment that had otherwise been unavailable to them due to financial, geographic, coverage, or other barriers. As PHE flexibilities end, we strongly urge that Congress implements policies to minimize disruptions in access to tele-mental and behavioral health care.

The AAFP has consistently advocated to Congress to permanently remove the in-person requirement for tele-mental health services for Medicare beneficiaries. Evidence has shown that telehealth is an effective modality for providing mental and behavioral health services.[93] Meanwhile, family physicians report that persistent behavioral health workforce shortages create significant barriers to care for their patients. Arbitrarily requiring an in-person visit prior to coverage of telemental health services will unnecessarily restrict access to behavioral health care.

As acknowledged in the AAFP's recent comments to the Drug Enforcement Administration (DEA), the in-person connection between a physician and patient can provide a valuable touchpoint for patients receiving MOUD and other OUD treatment services. However, existing shortages of clinicians prescribing buprenorphine for OUD, as well as numerous other barriers faced by patients with OUD, will prevent many patients from being able to obtain an in-person visit, particularly within the DEA's proposed 30-day timeframe. To that end, we strongly urge against requiring an in-person exam for prescribers of buprenorphine for treatment of OUD, given evidence in support of telehealth, limited access to OUD treatment prescribers, and relatively lower rates of buprenorphine diversion.

While an in-person evaluation may be necessary for other primary care treatment, data shows that buprenorphine prescribing is particularly well-

---

[93] Pew Trust. (2021, December 14). State Policy Changes Could Increase Access to Opioid Treatment via Telehealth—The Pew Charitable Trusts. *https://www.pewtrusts.org/en/research-andanalysis/issuebriefs/2021/12/state-policy-changes-could-increase-access-to-opioid-treatment-via-telehealth.*

suited for virtual- only visits. Telehealth initiation of and continued treatment with buprenorphine has shown greater treatment retention, reduced illicit opioid use, improved access to treatment, greater patient satisfaction, and reduced healthcare costs.[94]

Nearly 160 million individuals live in a mental health professional shortage area, and many more have mental health professionals in their area that do not accept the patient's insurance or require unfeasible cost sharing.[95] Nearly 99 million individuals live in a primary care health professional shortage area and would be unable or challenged to receive MOUD without telehealth and audio-only visits.[96] This difficulty in access to care for patients is compounded by transportation, time, and child-care challenges, as well as trauma and stigmatization from past experiences with the health care system. All of which makes virtual visits critically important for initiating and maintaining OUD treatment.

Close the Medicaid Coverage Gap

The AAFP supports efforts to provide coverage for low-income individuals in states that decided to forgo the Affordable Care Act's Medicaid Expansion. Closing the Medicaid expansion coverage gap would grant over 2 million uninsured Americans access to health coverage and would be a critical step in improving access to mental and behavioral health care, as well as addressing existing disparities in access. Data has shown that 60 percent of those in the Medicaid coverage gap are people of color, and more than 1 in 4 are estimated to have a behavioral health condition.[97] Family physicians have repeatedly called upon states to expand Medicaid to avoid coverage gaps, and in the

---

[94] Vakkalanka, J.P., Lund, B.C., Ward, M.M. et al. Telehealth Utilization Is Associated with Lower Risk of Discontinuation of Buprenorphine: a Retrospective Cohort Study of US Veterans. J GEN INTERN MED 37, 1610—1618 (2022). *https://doi.org/10.1007/s11606—021—06969—1.*

[95] Bureau of Health Workforce, Health Resources and Services Administration (HRSA), U.S. Department of Health & Human Services, Designated Health Professional Shortage Areas Statistics: Designated HPSA Quarterly Summary, as of September 30, 2022 available at *https:// data.hrsa.gov/topics/healthworkforce/shortage-areas.*

[96] Ibid.

[97] Sullivan J, Pearsall M, and A Bailey. ''To Improve Behavioral Health, Start by Closing the Medicaid Coverage Gap,'' Center on Budget and Policy Priorities. October 4, 2021. Accessed online: *https://www.cbpp.org/research/health/to-improve-behavioral-health-start-by-closing-the-Medicaid-coverage-gap#—ftn3.*

absence of state action, we support alternative options to cover individuals who would otherwise be eligible.

Improved Access for Justice-Involved Populations

Individuals who have been incarcerated have significant health care needs and face multiple barriers to obtaining health insurance and access to care. These challenges affect not only the formerly incarcerated individuals, but also their families and communities, many of which are disadvantaged, and experience health inequities born out of complex social determinants of health.

It is estimated that nearly half (47 percent) of individuals who are incarcerated meet the Diagnostic and Statistical Manual (DSM)-IV criteria for substance use disorder in the 12 months prior to admission to prison.[98] Unfortunately, only 12 to 15 percent of individuals who have a substance use disorder receive drug treatment while incarcerated.[99] For this reason, individuals who have chronic addictions have a higher risk of going through withdrawal while in custody and then overdosing when they return to the community.[100,101]

The AAFP advocates for individuals who are incarcerated or detained to have access to comprehensive medical services, including mental health care and substance use disorder treatment. We support the funding and implementation of successful re-entry models and other evidence-based programs to assist those who have recently been incarcerated. Access to evidence-based treatments for SUD should be provided by correctional health facilities while individuals are still incarcerated, and connections to housing, employment, comprehensive primary care, and substance use and mental health support should be made to best support their health outcomes and transition back into the community.

---

[98] Maruschak L, Bronson J, and M Apler. ''Survey of Prison Inmates, 2016: Alcohol and Drug Use and Treatment Reported by Prisoners,'' U.S. Department of Justice Office of Justice Programs Bureau of Justice Statistics. July 2021. Accessed online: *https://bjs.ojp.gov/sites/g/files/ xyckuh236/files/media/document/adutrpspi16st.pdf.*

[99] Ibid.

[100] Fu JJ, Zaller ND, Yokell MA, et al. Forced withdrawal from methadone maintenance therapy in criminal justice settings: a critical treatment barrier in the United States. J Subst Abuse Treat. 2013;44(5):502–505.

[101] Magura S, Lee JD, Hershberger J, et al. Buprenorphine and methadone maintenance in jail and post-release: a randomized clinical trial. Drug Alcohol Depend. 2009;99(1–3):222–230.

To that end, the AAFP urges Congress to pass the Reentry Act (S. 1165/ H.R. 2400), which allows Medicaid coverage for incarcerated individuals to automatically begin 30 days prior to their release. This will facilitate better care continuity as part of community reentry, including for those with SUD and mental health needs.

Thank you for the opportunity to offer these recommendations. The AAFP looks forward to continuing to work with you to advance policies that improve patient access to mental health and substance use disorder care. Should you have any questions, please contact Natalie Williams, Senior Manager of Legislative Affairs at nwilliams2@aafp.org.

Sincerely,

Sterling N. Ransone, Jr.,
Board Chair, American Academy of Family Physicians.

American College of Emergency Physicians, May 17, 2023

Senator ED MARKEY, Chairman
Senator ROGER MARSHALL, Ranking Member
U.S. Senate Committee on Health, Education, Labor, and Pensions, Subcommittee on Primary Health and Retirement Security,
428 Dirksen Senate Office Building, Washington, DC. 20510.

Dear Chairman Markey and Ranking Member Marshall:

On behalf of the American College of Emergency Physicians (ACEP) and our nearly 40,000 members, thank you for holding today's hearing, entitled, ''A Crisis in Mental Health and Substance Use Disorder Care: Closing Gaps in Access by Bringing Care and Prevention to Communities.'' We appreciate the opportunity to share some of our experiences on the frontlines of our Nation's mental health and substance use disorder (SUD) crises, and we look forward to continuing to work with you to improve access to the lifesaving care and treatment that our patients need and deserve.

As the health care safety net, the emergency department (ED) is often the first— and sometimes only—point of contact for individuals experiencing mental health crises or other behavioral health challenges, such as substance use disorder (SUD) or overdose. While the ED is the critical frontline safety net and the most appropriate setting for acute unscheduled care for individuals suffering from a mental health crisis, it is not ideal for long-term treatment of mental and behavioral health needs. However, due to the fragmented nature of the mental health care infrastructure in the U.S., persistent lack of sufficient resources, and longstanding shortages of mental and behavioral health professionals, far too many Americans have limited options for the longer-term follow-up treatment they need and deserve. These challenges contribute to long ED wait times and aggravate "boarding" issues, a scenario where patients are kept in the ED for extended periods of time due to a lack of available inpatient beds or space in other facilities where they could be transferred. Overcrowding and boarding are not failures of the ED; rather, they are symptoms of larger systemic issues that must be addressed to eliminate bottlenecks in health care delivery and reduce the burden on the already-strained health care safety net.

Once again, ACEP is grateful for the Committee's attention to the mental and behavioral health challenges affecting millions of Americans. As you continue to examine this pressing public health issue, we urge you to consider several key issues. These include strengthening the mental/behavioral health workforce; increasing integration, coordination, and access to care; ensuring parity; furthering the use of telehealth; and improving access to behavioral health care for children and young people. We also continue strongly urge the Committee to include physician and provider mental health and burnout as necessary considerations in comprehensive mental health policy initiatives, especially in light of the significant mental health toll the COVID–19 pandemic and its lingering effects have taken on frontline health care providers. Improving and providing for the mental health and well-being of the health care workforce is a unique challenge, but one that is absolutely essential to ensure that patients have access to the full continuum of high-quality health care. Additionally, we hope you will examine the many innovative solutions that emergency physicians throughout the country have developed and successfully implemented to reduce emergency psychiatric patient boarding.

Emergency Department Boarding

Patient "boarding" occurs when a patient continues to occupy an ED bed even after being seen and treated by a physician, while waiting to be admitted to an inpatient bed in the hospital, or transferred to psychiatric, skilled nursing, or other specialty facility. As our health care system becomes increasingly strained, these patients must stay in the ED for days or even weeks on end waiting for a bed to become available so they can be admitted or transferred. Patients being boarded in the ED limits the ability of ED staff to provide timely and quality care to all patients, forcing other newly arriving patients with equally important emergency conditions to wait in the ED waiting room for care, with wait times as long as eight or even 12 hours rapidly becoming a new norm, and patients even dying during these waits as staff struggle to keep up with an unsupportable volume of sick patients to care for.

Boarding has become its own public health emergency. Our nation's safety net is on the verge of breaking beyond repair; EDs are gridlocked and overwhelmed with patients waiting—waiting to be seen, waiting for admission into an inpatient bed in the hospital, waiting to be transferred to psychiatric, skilled nursing, or other specialized facilities that have little to no available beds, or, waiting to simply return to their nursing home. And this breaking point is entirely outside of the control of highly skilled emergency physicians, nurses, and other ED staff doing their best to keep everyone attended to and alive.

Any emergency patient can find themselves boarded, regardless of their condition, age, insurance coverage, income, or geographic area. Even patients sick enough to need intensive care may board for hours in ED stretchers not set up for the extra monitoring they need. Those in mental health crises, often children or adolescents, board for months in chaotic EDs while waiting for a psychiatric inpatient bed to open anywhere. But boarding does not just affect those waiting to receive care elsewhere. When ED beds are already filled with boarded patients, other patients are decompensating and, in some cases, dying while in ED waiting rooms during their tenth, eleventh, or even twelfth hour of waiting to be seen by a physician.

> ''At peak times which occur up to 5 days per week we have more patients boarding than we have staffed beds. High numbers have include last week when our 22 bed emergency department had 35 boarders and an additional 20 patients in the waiting room. In addition, we have patients who unfortunately have died in our waiting room while awaiting treatment. These deaths were entirely due to boarding. Our boarding numbers have unfortunately skyrocketed in the wake of COVID as a consequence of increasing surgical volumes and decreasing inpatient nurse staffing.''——anonymous emergency physician

To illustrate the stark reality of this crisis, ACEP asked its members to share examples of the life-threatening impacts of ED boarding. The stories paint a picture of an emergency care system already near collapse. While the causes of ED boarding are multifactorial, unprecedented and rising staffing shortages throughout the health care system have recently brought this issue to a crisis point, further spiraling the stress and burnout driving the current exodus of excellent physicians, nurses, paramedics, and other health care professionals.

We need a health care system that can accurately track available beds and other relevant data in real-time, appropriate metrics to measure ED throughput and boarding, contingency plans and ‘‘load balancing’’ plans for boarding/crowding scenarios, and fewer regulatory or other ‘‘red tape’’ burdens that delay necessary care. Recognizing all EDs are different and there is no one-size-fits-all solution to this multifactorial problem, ACEP is in the process of developing a broad range of potential legislative and regulatory solutions that will alleviate the burdens and overall strain on EDs caused by patient boarding. As we finalize these recommendations and policy solutions, we will share more broadly with you and your staff in the coming weeks. Further, we strongly urge Congress to direct its attention to this critical issue and work with us and other stakeholders through roundtables, hearings, and legislation to provide both short-and long-term solutions to this public health crisis.

Violence Against Emergency Physicians and Health Care Workers

Violence in the emergency department is a serious and growing concern, causing significant stress to emergency department staff and to patients who seek treatment in the emergency department (ED). According to a survey conducted by ACEP in 2022, two-thirds of emergency physicians report being assaulted in the past year alone, while more than one-third of respondents say they have been assaulted more than once. Nearly 85 percent of emergency physicians say the rate of ED violence has increased within the last year.

Beyond the immediate physical impacts and injuries, the risk of violence increases the difficulty of recruiting and retaining qualified health care professionals and contributes to greater levels of physician burnout. In fact, 87 percent of emergency physicians report a loss of productivity from the physician or staff as a result, and 85 percent of emergency physicians report emotional trauma and an increase in anxiety because of ED violence. Most importantly, patients with medical emergencies deserve high-quality care in a place free of physical dangers from other patients or individuals, and care from staff that is not distracted by individuals with behavioral or substance-induced violent behavior.

And unlike the significantly more visible violence against airline employees and other travelers that has become more ubiquitous over the last several years, violence against health care workers often is not seen or addressed because of inadequate reporting and tracking of violent incidents, and other systemic barriers that do not hold violent individuals accountable for their actions. As a result of the inability to prosecute those who are arrested, many health care workers are discouraged from even pressing charges and being forced to accept that it's ''just part of the job.'' Violence is not accepted in any other workplace, and it must not be accepted especially in a setting focused on improving the health and well-being of individuals.

There are many factors contributing to the increase in ED and hospital violence, we recognize there is no one-size-fits-all solution to this issue either. In fact, one of the challenges is that the types of violence one ED typically experiences can be significantly different from another ED, even in the same town. Therefore, ensuring there are adequate resources to help identify best practices and outfitting facilities with resources appropriate to their specific needs is imperative. Overall, employers and hospitals should develop workplace violence prevention and response procedures that address the needs of their particular facilities, staff, contractors, and communities, as those needs and resources may vary significantly.

ACEP supports multi-pronged legislative efforts to address various aspects of health care workplace violence prevention, including the ''Workplace Violence Prevention for Health Care and Social Service Workers Act,'' (H.R. 2663/S. 1176), introduced by Sen. Tammy Baldwin (D-WI) (and by Reps. Joe Courtney (D-CT), Don Bacon (R-NE), and others in the House); as well as the ''Safety From Violence for Healthcare Employees (SAVE) Act,'' (H.R. 2584) introduced by Reps. Larry Bucshon (R-IN) and Madeline Dean (D-PA). The Workplace Violence Prevention for Health Care and Social Service Workers Act would ensure that health care workplaces implement violence prevention plans and techniques and are prepared to respond to acts of violence, while the SAVE Act would establish Federal legal penalties for individuals who knowingly and intentionally assault or intimidate health care workers and provide grants to help hospitals and medical facilities establish and improve workplace safety, security, and violence prevention efforts.

Access to Mental Health Care

The emergency department is not only a safety net for those with physical care needs, but also for individuals suffering from a mental health crisis or acute psychiatric emergency. However, it is not ideal for long-term treatment of mental and behavioral health needs. Due to the fragmented nature of the mental health care infrastructure in the U.S., persistent lack of sufficient resources, and longstanding shortages of mental and behavioral health professionals, far too many Americans have limited options for the longer-term follow-up treatment they need and deserve. These challenges also contribute to the long ED wait times and aggravate ED boarding issues detailed above. In fact, ED boarding challenges disproportionately affect patients with behavioral health needs who wait on average three times longer than medical patients because of these significant gaps in our health care system.

Improving coordination of care across the health care continuum must be one of the highest priorities for any mental health reform effort. The ED serves as the critical health care safety net not only for acute injuries, but for psychiatric emergencies as well. However, most EDs are not ideal facilities to provide longer-term care for patients experiencing a mental health crisis—they are often hectic, noisy, and particularly disruptive for behavioral health patients.

Across the country, communities have adopted innovative alternative models to improve emergency psychiatric care and reduce psychiatric patient boarding. These include Behavioral Health Emergency Rooms (BHERs), separate areas of the ED that specialize in caring for patients experiencing a behavioral health crisis; Emergency Psychiatric Assessment Treatment and Healing (EmPath) Units, a separate, hospital-based setting solely for psychiatric emergencies with the safe, calming, homelike environment of a community mental health crisis clinic but with the ED's ability to care for any patient presenting for treatment; and Psychiatric Emergency Service (PES) models, a ''hub-and-spoke'' model with a dedicated psychiatric ED serving as a central hub with bidirectional spokes going out to a wide variety of mental, behavioral, and physical care, as well as social services.

- *Behavioral Health Emergency Rooms (BHERs).* BHERs are separate areas of the ED that specialize in proactive rapid-assessment, stabilization, and treatment of patients in experiencing a behavioral health crisis. Care is delivered via a multidisciplinary team of emergency physicians, psychiatrists, psychiatric nurses, and social workers. This service is operational 24 hours a day, 7 days a week, 365 days a year. These dedicated spaces provide patients with a safer, private, and more peaceful setting in which to deescalate and receive specialized care. By initiating proactive assessments in a BHER, 40–50 percent of patients can be safely discharged home, reducing ED boarding time. Additionally, optimizing transition of care through Integrated Outpatient Care clinics ensures ongoing high-quality medical and behavioral health care follow-up with convenient and comprehensive treatment options for patients.
- *EmPath (Emergency Psychiatric Assessment Treatment and Healing) Units.* The EmPath unit is a separate, hospital-based setting solely for psychiatric emergencies with the safe, calming, homelike environment of a community mental health crisis clinic with the ED's ability to take care of any patient who presents for treatment. This unit accepts all suitable patients regardless of the severity of their illness, legal status, dangerousness, substance use intoxication or withdrawal, or co-morbid medical problems, as these patients are typically excluded from community programs and thus would likely experience boarding in an ED in the traditional medical system.
- EmPath units provide immediate access to individualized care from a comprehensive mental health care team of psychiatrists, psychologists, mental health nurses, social workers, and other licensed mental health care professionals. This team partners directly with patients and their families to address the immediate mental crisis and to develop a longer-term care plan through appropriate follow-up services. In some instances, EmPath Units have reduced regional ED boarding by 80 percent, and have also reduced the need for—and incidence of—coercive measures (such as physical restraints), episodes of agitation, and psychiatric hospitalization.
- *Psychiatric Emergency Service (PES). The PES model is a multipronged approach for emergency psychiatric patients treated in the ED based on increased availability of psychiatrists and dedicated case managers who focus on psychiatric patients.* This model is

referred to as a ''hub-and-spoke'' model with a dedicated psychiatric ED serving as a central hub with bidirectional spokes going out to a wide variety of mental, behavioral, and physical care, as well as social services. Recognizing that psychiatric patients have vastly different needs and circumstances affecting their overall health, this model helps address the patient's immediate mental health needs and swiftly directs them to the most appropriate follow-up services, which helps alleviate the overall load on the mental health care system. These two-way spokes may also serve to reconnect patients with the psychiatric ED should they require acute stabilization while receiving follow-up services, potentially avoiding an inpatient hospitalization and ensuring the patient receives the most appropriate care and treatment throughout the mental health care continuum.

These innovative approaches have helped communities improve coordination of emergency psychiatric care and they can serve as models for other communities to implement and build upon. However, what is clear from experience is that the ultimate success of any model hinges on the availability of resources, whether monetary, staffing, or access to follow-up services and patient access to long-term mental and behavioral health care. One of the persistent challenges in emergency medicine is that ''one emergency department is one emergency department''—i.e., the needs of each community and the resources available to local EDs, hospitals, and other facilities vary widely, and a model that is successful in one community may not be the best fit for another community.

For example, in 2017, Oregon implemented a dedicated psychiatric ED model in Portland based closely on the Alameda Model (California), but the transition has been marked by challenges for both the dedicated psychiatric ED and surrounding facilities. The dedicated psychiatric ED that was intended to reduce the burden on individual EDs is frequently at capacity or overcrowded, but emergency physicians at other facilities have noted that they are still seeing the same number of acute psychiatric patients in their own EDs. Additionally, the dedicated psychiatric ED has struggled to transfer patients to long-term follow-up treatment at Oregon State Hospital, contributing to long wait times, crowding, and poor outcomes for patients. Despite these challenges, stakeholders have been working to address the short-comings of the system and adapt the model to better meet the needs of the Portland community, but the experience has highlighted that new care models are not necessarily ''plug-and-play'' and do not guarantee immediate results.

To ensure that communities can implement models that best fit their needs, ACEP supports the bipartisan ''Improving Mental Health Access from the Emergency Department Act'' (S. 1346), led by Senators Shelley Moore Capito (R-WV) and Maggie Hassan (D-NH). This legislation would provide critical funding to help communities implement and expand programs to expedite transition to post-emergency care through expanded coordination with regional service providers, assessment, peer navigators, bed availability tracking and management, transfer protocol development, networking infrastructure development, and transportation services; increase the supply of inpatient psychiatric beds and alternative care settings; and, expand approaches to providing psychiatric care in the ED, including telepsychiatry, peak period crisis clinics, or dedicated psychiatric emergency service units. During the 117th Congress, this legislation (H.R. 1205) was passed by the House of Representatives in a voice vote but was not considered by the Senate. We urge Congress to consider and pass this important legislation.

Another longstanding barrier to providing adequate mental health treatment services is the Medicaid Institutions for Mental Disease (IMD) exclusion that prohibits the Federal Government from providing Medicaid reimbursement to states for care provided to most patients in an inpatient psychiatric or SUD facility with more than 16 beds. Though this longstanding policy was intended to reduce the number of people committed to long-term psychiatric treatment facilities without receiving appropriate care, it has perpetuated the problem of disparate treatment of mental health and has stood as a major barrier in the effort to provide necessary non-hospital in-patient psychiatric care options.

As a limited workaround, states have been able to apply for Section 1115 Medicaid waivers to receive matching Federal funds for short-term residential treatment services in an IMD. Congress also recently took steps to address some of the challenges posed by the IMD exclusion in the Substance Use-Disorder Prevention that Promotes Opioid Recovery and Treatment for Patients and Communities (SUPPORT) Act (P.L. 115–271), creating a limited new exception to allow states to provide Medicaid coverage for beneficiaries with at least one SUD in certain IMDs.

The IMD exclusion may also threaten the ability of communities to provide a continuum of crisis stabilization services that includes call centers, mobile crisis units, and crisis stabilization programs. Crisis stabilization programs are a resource distinct from traditional residential treatment facilities for mental health and SUD treatment. These provide individuals with additional immediate-access treatment options, helping them avoid settings detrimental to their condition such as jails, homeless shelters, or the streets. Unfortunately, the IMD exclusion was established before crisis stabilization beds were developed, and the 16-bed limitation for facilities severely restricts the ability of these services to meet the needs of communities with vulnerable Medicaid populations and high demand for such services. We agree with legislators' bipartisan efforts urging CMS to ensure Medicaid reimbursement for crisis stabilization beds and to ensure these programs are not adversely affected by the IMD exclusion.

ACEP has long advocated for full repeal of the IMD exclusion and strongly urges Congress to rescind this harmful policy either as a standalone effort or as a cornerstone of any comprehensive mental health reform legislation Ensuring Parity Between Behavioral and Physical Health Care Limited access to appropriate coverage, narrow provider networks, lack of Federal enforcement mechanisms for parity law violations, and low reimbursement for mental health services remain barriers to achieving parity between mental and physical health care.

In recent years, Congress has taken important steps to improve parity between mental and physical health care by requiring insurers to provide the same level of coverage for mental health and substance use disorder treatment as they do for physical care. But despite Federal law, there is no mechanism for the Federal Government to enforce compliance against plans that continue to violate parity requirements and discriminate against patients with mental health conditions or SUD. ACEP supports providing the Department of Labor (DOL) with the ability to issue civil monetary penalties (CMPs) for violations of the ''Mental Health Parity and Addiction Equity Act'' (MHPAEA; P.L. 110–343) by group health plan sponsors, plan administrators, or issuers. ACEP supports legislative efforts to give the DOL the authority to issue CMPs.

Without enforcement penalties and more explicit parity requirements, we will continue to see insurers attempting to find their way around the law and limit the coverage available to beneficiaries experiencing mental health crisis. As a recent example, Optum in Maryland issued a policy several years ago establishing that only certain provider types (specialty mental health providers) are eligible to bill when the only diagnosis is a psychiatric issue, including homicidal ideation and suicidal ideation, precluding payment for an ED physician's evaluation and management services. This policy ignores the significant challenges emergency physicians are experiencing in seeing and treating mental health needs in the ED and has disproportionate impacts on hospitals with high Medicaid populations. Though Optum ultimately issued an updated provider alert that resolved this matter, it was not without significant confusion and substantial delays that affected patient care.

We also believe this is yet another example of insurers attempting to disregard the Prudent Layperson Standard (PLP), a longstanding and critical policy that protects patients from retroactive denials of insurance coverage for emergency department visits that are ultimately determined to be non-emergent. Patients who believe they are experiencing a medical emergency should not be discouraged from seeking treatment out of fear that their ED visit will not be covered by their insurer.

Ensuring parity for behavioral health care also requires appropriate treatment of substance use and opioid use disorders (SUD/OUD). Individuals with SUD/OUD often seek care in the emergency department, and one of the most effective means emergency physicians have to aid these patients is by using buprenorphine as part of a medications for opioid use disorder (MOUD) protocol. As one of three drugs approved by the U.S. Food & Drug Administration (FDA) for the treatment of opioid dependence, buprenorphine is a very safe and efficacious medication. Strong enough to reduce withdrawal symptoms and cravings but not enough to cause euphoria, it can allow individuals with OUD to more effectively engage in treatment as they pursue recovery. But despite the passage of the MAT Act and subsequent removal of the X-waiver, significant barriers to the use of buprenorphine persist, including limited access to the treatment due to Drug Enforcement Administration (DEA) set quantity limits, which flag pharmacy and hospital purchases of these required SUD/ OUD treatments as suspicious orders. In fact, both prescribers and patients across the Nation are still experiencing difficulty in obtaining buprenorphine prescriptions. According to a recent study that surveyed more than 5,000 pharmacies, less than half stocked buprenorphine.[102] Additionally, a separate survey found that one-fifth of pharmacies were not willing to fill buprenorphine prescriptions.[103] A survey of addiction treatment providers also revealed that 84 percent of their patients

---

[102] Hill, L. G., Loera, L. J., Torrez, S. B., Puzantian, T., Evoy, K. E., Ventricelli, D. J., Eukel, H. N., Peckham, A. M., Chen, C., Ganetsky, V. S., Yeung, M. S., Zagorski, C. M., & Reveles, K. R. (2022). Availability of buprenorphine/naloxone films and naloxone nasal spray in community pharmacies in 11 U.S. states. Drug and alcohol dependence, 237, 109518. *https://doi.org/ 10.1016/j.drugalcdep.2022.109518.*

[103] Kazerouni, N. J., Irwin, A. N., Levander, X. A., Geddes, J., Johnston, K., Gostanian, C. J., Mayfield, B. S., Montgomery, B. T., Graalum, D. C., &; Hartung, D. M. (2021). Pharmacy-related buprenorphine access barriers: An audit of pharmacies in counties with a high opioid overdose burden. Drug and Alcohol Dependence, 224. *https://doi.org/10.1016/ j.drugalcdep.2021.108729.*

experienced a delay in accessing their buprenorphine, which can be life-threatening for those undergoing treatment for opioid use disorder.[104] We urge Congress to ensure that health insurance plans appropriately cover SUD/OUD treatments, and further to ensure that patients are not are not hindered by unnecessary Federal barriers on their path to recovery through arbitrary limitations on the medications they need.

Improving Access to Behavioral Health Care for Children and Young People

The full effects of the COVID–19 pandemic are not limited to the staggering toll on American lives or the long-term physical health challenges from which many recovering patients still suffer. We are still collectively struggling to comprehend the true scope of the pandemic's impact on the mental health and well-being of millions of Americans, particularly on children and younger Americans.

As the recent U.S. Department of Education report, ''Supporting Child and Student Social, Emotional, Behavioral, and Mental Health Needs'' notes, children have experienced isolation, bereavement, depression, worry, and other issues throughout the pandemic, leading to reports of anxiety, mood, and eating disorders, as well as increased self-harm behavior and suicidal ideation at nearly twice the rate of adults.

Pediatric ED visits related to mental health significantly increased during the pandemic—a 24 percent increase for children 5–11 years of age, and 31 percent for children 12–17. These stressors affect children's development and ability to learn in both the immediate and long-term with lasting consequences should their mental health needs not be adequately addressed.

Adding to these long-term considerations are the mental health stresses associated with the loss of a caregiver. According to a recent pre-publication study in the October 2021 issue of the American Academy of Pediatrics journal, Pediatrics, more than 140,000 U.S. children under the age of 18 lost a primary or secondary caregiver due to COVID–19 between April 1, 2020 and

[104] American Society of Addiction Medicine. (2022). Reducing Barriers to Lifesaving Treatment: Report on the Findings from ASAM's Pharmacy Access Survey. *https://sitefinitystorage.blob.core.windows.net/sitefinity-production-blobs/docs/default-source/advocacy/reports/asam-pharmacy-access-survey-report-final11.7.22.pdf'sfvrsn=6da97680—3.*

June 30, 2021.[105] 4 The consequences of the pandemic's disproportionate impact on racial and ethnic minorities, exacerbated by longstanding systemic inequalities, manifest here as well given that children of racial and ethnic minorities account for 65 percent of children who lost a primary caregiver (compared to 39 percent of the total population). The authors note the significant long-term impacts that orphanhood and caregiver loss have on the health and well-being of children, ranging from mental health problems and increased risks of suicide violence, sexual abuse, and exploitation, to disruptions in family circumstances such as housing instability and lack of nurturing support. Especially given the Committee's considerable attention to gaps in equity and longstanding disparities in health care, we urge you to examine the far-reaching effects of pandemic on historically underserved populations and we stand ready to work with you to provide the perspective and experience of emergency physicians to help develop effective and durable policy solutions.

Our health care system is not currently well-equipped to address the long-term effects of the significant trauma so many young Americans have experienced over the course of the last year. Given the substantial strains on the health care and social safety nets that existed long before the pandemic hit, it is clear that EDs, child welfare systems, the child and adolescent mental health workforce, and other related services will need considerable investments and significantly expanded resources in order to appropriately address this unprecedented challenge. As policymakers and stakeholders evaluate suggestions to improve mental and behavioral health access, these proposals and any new treatment models must be considered through the lens of pediatric care in order to prioritize the most vulnerable of the vulnerable.

Once again, thank you for the opportunity to provide our comments and suggestions on how to improve access to mental health and substance use disorder care for our patients and their families. We look forward to working with you on these important efforts. Should you have any questions or require any further information, please do not hesitate to contact Ryan McBride, ACEP's Congressional Affairs Director, at rmcbride@acep.org.

Sincerely,
Christopher S. Kang, M.D., FACEP,
ACEP President.

---

105 COVID–19-Associated Orphanhood and Caregiver Death in the United States *(aappublications.org)*.

American Therapeutic Recreation Association, May 17, 2023

Senator ED MARKEY, Chairman,
Senator ROGER MARSHALL, Ranking Member,
U.S. Senate Committee on Health, Education, Labor, and Pensions, Subcommittee on Primary Health and Retirement Security,
428 Dirksen Senate Office Building, Washington, DC. 20510.

Dear Chairman Markey and Ranking Member Marshall:
On behalf of the American Therapeutic Recreation Association (ATRA), we appreciate the opportunity to submit this testimony for the record regarding the Committee's hearing on A Crisis in Mental Health and Substance Use Disorder Care: Closing Gaps in Access by Bringing Care and Prevention to Communities. As providers that comprise a part of the mental healthcare workforce with a particular focus on community response, we look forward to working with you to develop solutions to address America's mental health and substance use crisis.

ATRA is committed to advancing access to recreational therapy and ensuring that individuals are able to receive care that suits their interests and needs and supports the development of functional skills for daily living and stress release. ATRA is the largest professional association representing recreational therapy. Recreational therapists are nationally certified, and where applicable, state-licensed to provide evidence-based treatment services for individuals with a range of disabling conditions across the lifespan. Recreational therapy is active treatment, medically necessary, and can be prescribed by a physician as part of a client's plan of care.[106]

ATRA has watched with interest and concern as new data has highlighted the mental health crisis that America is currently experiencing. As recreational therapists, we are trained to use a variety of interventions to help clients address mental health challenges, as well as other areas like physical health and emotional/social well-being. Therefore, we recognize the critical need to ensure that resources are in place to address this mental health emergency to ensure that people are able to successfully manage the stress and anxiety of everyday life.

---

[106] Kemeny B, Fawber H, Finegan J, Marcinko D. Recreational therapy: Implications for life care planning. J life care Plan. 2020;18(4):35–58.

In mental health care, recreational therapists support clients with cognitive, social, leisure, and physical interventions, as well as stress management techniques, to improve a client's overall health. Recreation therapy (RT) for mental health incorporates activities including music, sports, dance, art, and outdoor activities to help a client find strategies that work for them to manage stress and ensure they have a healthy outcome for managing their mental health. RT also uses meaningful engagement in life activities or leisure as a means to increase coping and therefore reduce depression and anxiety. This type of therapy can be particularly helpful and attractive to individuals, including adolescents, as an alternative, non-pharmacological outlet.

RT's focus their work on community engagement and specifically work with individuals in their communities and homes to provide opportunities to participate in life activities including leisure, recreation, and play. The primary purpose of recreational therapy is to establish and maintain tools and skills to be successful in their community and home environment.

The Important Role that Recreational Therapists Play

Recreational Therapy (RT) embraces a definition of "health" which includes not only the absence of "illness," but extends to the enhancement of physical, cognitive, emotional, social, and leisure development so individuals may participate fully and independently in chosen life pursuits. Recreational therapists address assessed client needs related to behavior, cognition, function, pain management, physical activity level, socialization, recreation, and leisure.[107] Recreational therapists have the competencies to assess and implement interventions necessary to promote improved mental health, quality of life, and prevent secondary conditions[108,109] by reducing depression, stress, and anxiety in their clients and helping build confidence to socialize in their community. Recreational therapists work in a variety of settings that promote youth and adolescent mental health including community mental

---

[107] Commission on Accreditation of Rehabilitation Facilities. 2020 Medical Rehabilitation Standards Manual. 2020.

[108] Hawkins B, Kemeny B, Porter H. Recreational therapy competencies, Part 2: Findings from the ATRA competencies study. Ther Recreation J. 2020;54(4). doi:10.18666/trj–2020-v54-i4–10238.

[109] Kinney J. Analysis of services performed by recreational therapists. Ther Recreation J. 2020;54(3):227–243. doi:10.18666/trj–2020-v54-i3–10248.

health centers, public and alternative schools, co-occurring disorder programs, day hospitals for outpatient treatment, inpatient psychiatric hospitals, inclusive recreation programs, residential living facilities, nature-based recreation programs, and addiction recovery centers.

In the United States, recreational therapists at a minimum must have a bachelor's degree in recreational therapy or a related field.[110] Anatomy and physiology, assessment, salient characteristics of illness and disabilities, medical terminology, the therapeutic process, and 560 hours of fieldwork are required courses.[111] The Certified Therapeutic Recreation Specialist (CTRS) is the required certification for recreational therapists by NCTRC and shows that the recreational therapist has passed an all-encompassing national certification exam demonstrating extensive knowledge and skill-based training in core therapy skills (assessment, planning, implementation, documentation, and evaluation), a team-oriented approach to care delivery, and training in group processes. The CTRS credential is required for practice as a recreational therapist in Veterans Affairs[112] and designated as the accepted certification for recreational therapists by the Centers for Medicare and Medicaid Services Federal guidelines for skilled nursing facilities. Ethical conduct is mandated by the professional organization, the American Therapeutic Recreation Association (ATRA)'s code of ethics, and quality indicators of RT practice are supported by the ATRA Standards of Practice.

Research has shown the effectiveness of recreational therapy services for mental health outcomes. Through recreational therapy interventions, youth with mental health challenges saw increases in health-related quality of life,[113] positive changes in their perceived self-esteem,[114] and decreases in feelings of social isolation and loneliness.[115] Through outdoor adventure interventions,

---

[110] National Council for Therapeutic Recreation Certification. The CTRS is the qualified provider of Recreational Therapy Services. 2020.

[111] Bureau of Labor Statistics U.S. Department of Labor. Occupational Outlook Handbook, Recreational Therapists. 2020.

[112] U.S. Department of Veterans Affairs. VA Handbook 5005, Part II, Appendix G60. The Recreation and Creative Arts Therapist.

[113] Bennett JR, Negley SK, Wells MS, Connolly P. Addressing well-being in early and middle childhood: recreation therapy interventions aimed to develop skills that create a healthy life. Spec Issue Strengths-based Pract—Part 1. 2016;50(1):unpaginated. *http://js.sagamorepub.com/trj/article/view/6782.*

[114] Concepcion H. Video game therapy as an intervention for children with disabilities. Ther Recreation J. 2017;(3):221–228.

[115] Luchies LB, Barbour AL, Anderson SR. Children's Healing Center involvement reduces social isolation and loneliness among immunocompromised children and their family members. Am J Recreat Ther. 2019;18(3):37–47.

recreational therapists also helped some young people with substance abuse disorder and post-traumatic stress disorder to learn effective strategies for their personal recovery.[116]

To better explain the role of RT, we have provided some examples of recreational therapy services specific to adolescents with mental health conditions:

- A recreational therapist in Virginia works at a residential treatment center for adolescents with mental health diagnoses. Utilizing stress management interventions like guided imagery, progressive muscle relaxation, Tai Chi, and yoga, recreational therapy services help adolescents reach goals like decreasing symptoms of depression and anxiety while increasing self-confidence and personal grounding.
- Another recreational therapist works in a school in New Mexico with high school students with intellectual and developmental disabilities (IDD) who are experiencing increased anxiety during COVID–19. Recreational therapy services help the students cope with feelings of fear, worry, and hopelessness through after-school, group therapy sessions for teaching emotional identification, coping skills, and adjustment strategies to navigate their ever-changing daily schedules.
- Last, a recreation therapist in Colorado utilizes nature-based, adventure therapy interventions for adolescents with mental health diagnoses. Goals of improving adolescents' self-confidence, problem-solving skills, and sense of community are achieved through outcomes-based, recreational therapy modalities that include kayaking, rock climbing, high and low ropes courses, and wilderness hiking.

Conclusion

ATRA is supportive of Congress' work to address the mental health crisis and appreciates the opportunity to provide written testimony. As Congress continues to consider legislative opportunities to address the mental health crisis, we ask that recreational therapists be included in any legislative

---

116 Leighton J, Lopez KJ, Johnson CW. ''There is Always Progress to Be Made:'' Reflective Narratives on Outdoor Therapeutic Recreation for Mental Health Support. Ther Recreation J. 2021;55(2):185–203.

language to support efforts to reduce stress, anxiety, and depression among youth, adolescents and adults. We welcome the opportunity to speak with you more about what RT is, and how it can help in responding to the mental health emergency.

Please do not hesitate to contact the American Therapeutic Recreation Association (ATRA) directly Brent Wolfe, ATRA Executive Director, at brent@atra-online.com.

Sincerely,
Brent Wolfe,
on behalf of ATRA.

Senator ED MARKEY, Chairman,
Children's Hospital Association,
May 17, 2023.

Senator ROGER MARSHALL, Ranking Member,

U.S. Senate Committee on Health, Education, Labor, and Pensions, Subcommittee on Primary Health and Retirement Security, 428 Dirksen Senate Office Building, Washington, DC. 20510.

Dear Chairman Markey and Ranking Member Marshall:

On behalf of the nation's children's hospitals and the children and families we serve, thank you for holding this hearing, ''A Crisis in Mental Health and Substance Abuse Disorder Care: Closing Gaps in Access by Bringing Care and Prevention to Communities.'' We appreciate your leadership on this issue and look forward to working together to ensure that Federal programs are tailored to meet the unique needs of children, adolescents and the pediatric provider community proudly committed to serving them. We appreciate the work Congress has done to date to address the national children's mental health crisis; however, more Federal support and attention is urgently needed to meaningfully impact the troubling trajectory for our Nation's children.

Children's Hospital Association represents more than 220 children's hospitals nationwide, dedicated to the health and well-being of our Nation's children through innovations in the quality, cost, and delivery of care. Children's hospitals serve as a vital safety net for all children across the country regardless of insurance status, including those that are uninsured, underinsured and enrolled in Medicaid, the single largest payer of mental health services for children. As essential providers dedicated to providing the highest quality pediatric care, children's hospitals look forward to working with you to address the crisis in mental health facing America's children.

Prior to the pandemic, trends in child and adolescent mental health were worrying, as mental health symptoms increased among children, and many did not receive needed care. The stressors of the pandemic on families and children have worsened these trends significantly. Concerning evidence of the crisis:

- 1 in 5 children and adolescents experience a mental health condition in a given year.[117]
- In 2021, 29 percent of teens reported experiencing poor mental health, while 4 in 10 reported feeling persistent sadness or hopelessness. Teen girls were twice as likely (57 percent) to report persistent sadness.[118]
- 1 in 5 high school students contemplated suicide and 1 in 10 attempted suicide one or more times.[119]
- Suicide is the second leading cause of death for youth and young adults between the ages of 10 and 24.[120]

An increased demand for mental health services across the continuum of care for children, but particularly for children in crisis, has stressed already inadequate and under-resourced systems, leaving far too many children waiting for needed mental and behavioral health care, frequently ''boarding'' in emergency departments until an appropriate placement becomes available. As compared to pre-pandemic, 84 percent of hospitals report boarding more children and youth and 75 percent report longer boarding stays.[121] As we emerge from the public health emergency, the troubling trends continue with large numbers of children and youth languishing in hospital emergency departments waiting for access to needed care.

---

117 ''*What is Children's Mental Health?*'' Centers for Disease Control and Prevention, April 2019.

118 ''*Youth Risk Behavior Survey Data Summary & Trends Report,*'' Centers for Disease Control and Prevention, February 2023.

119 ''*Youth Risk Behavior Survey Data Summary & Trends Report,*'' Centers for Disease Control and Prevention, February 2023.

120 ''*Facts about Suicide,*'' Centers for Disease Control and Prevention.

121 Leyenaar J, Freyleue S, Bordonga A, et al., "Frequency and Duration of Boarding for Pediatric Mental Health Conditions at Acute Care Hospitals in the US," JAMA: Vol 326, No. 22, 2021.

This crisis in boarding is also reflection of inadequacies within our Nation's pediatric mental health system, which is fragmented and insufficiently supported, too often resulting in delayed care. For many children, their mental health conditions can be managed with less intensive treatment, such as outpatient therapy and medication management through primary care, yet children's mental health conditions often go unidentified and untreated. Nearly 60 percent of children and youth with major depression are not receiving care and it is common for several years to pass between when symptoms first appear and treatment begins.[122] To prevent the children's mental health crisis from continuing we need to do a better job of providing access to needed services across the continuum of care, beginning as early as possible and ideally before children reach a point of crisis.

As you consider changes to existing programs and contemplate new initiatives, it is critical to examine how these changes affect the pediatric population. The importance of investing in services and supports that promote timely access to necessary pediatric mental health care cannot be overstated. Current Federal programs are essential and yet remain insufficient to meet the severity of this compounding national crisis in children's mental health. We look forward to partnering with you as you work to implement programmatic improvements and address the continued mental, emotional, and behavioral health needs of children across the country.

As the Senate HELP Committee moves forward, we urge you to prioritize:

- Creating new programs and investments meeting the needs of children and youth.
- Refining existing programs and increasing support to ensure that they are intentionally designed to meet the unique needs of children and adolescents and ensure access to services as early as possible.
- Increasing and targeting investments to support the recruitment, training, retention, and professional development of a diverse clinical and nonclinical pediatric workforce.

New Tailored Investments to Meaningfully Address the Crisis

Within HHS, there are several programs that focus on mental health broadly and some that focus on children specifically. These are important programs

---

[122] *''The State of Mental Health in America,''* Mental Health America, 2023.

that play a role in meeting children's needs, but more is desperately needed. There are a number of programs that aim to improve children's access to evidence-based treatment for mental health conditions, yet they do not go far enough to address the widespread and unmet needs of children. Both the creation of new initiatives and enhancements to existing programs will be needed to adequately address the growing crisis in child and adolescent mental health.

At the core of a strong pediatric mental health care delivery system is a strong, interconnected network of pediatric health providers and supportive services that are available to deliver high-quality, developmentally appropriate mental and behavioral health care. Building a strong system of care starts with ensuring that children are able to access services in the settings where they are such as: early learning and childcare settings, schools, their pediatrician's office, community settings and emergency departments. A truly comprehensive approach must include the full continuum of clinical and non-clinical health services and supports that encompass promotion and prevention, early intervention and treatment. In too many communities, there are few local options for children in need of mental health treatment and investment is urgently needed to scale up services and support for the pediatric population.

Given the workforce shortages within pediatric mental health professions, the importance of innovative approaches to utilizing our current workforce, such as through integrated care, and support for enhanced care coordination are paramount. When children's and adolescents' mental health needs are significant enough to require services outside of schools and community-based outpatient settings, it is critical that they are delivered in appropriate settings designed for them and staffed by professionals with pediatric expertise. Children's hospitals have seen a growing demand for inpatient psychiatric care, as well as step down levels of care including partial hospitalization, day hospitals and intensive outpatient services. Unfortunately, there are too few of these services designed specifically for children, adolescents, and young adults, which results in significant delays in care and contributes to mental health boarding.

While investing in upstream mental health promotion, prevention, early identification and intervention for children is critical, including to prevent conditions from worsening to the point of crisis, we also need to ensure that there are appropriate treatment options across the full continuum of care for children and adolescents who need them. We urge Congress to provide resources to support efforts to scale up inpatient care capacity, including costs associated with the conversion of general beds to accommodate mental health patients, as well as to support the development of intermediate levels of care such as partial hospitalization, day programs, intensive outpatient services and crisis response and stabilization services which are designed to support families and divert children from emergency departments.

To better support the continuum of care, we strongly support legislation introduced last year by Sens. Casey and Cassidy entitled, Health Care Capacity for Pediatric Mental Health Act of 2022. The bill focused on children and would improve access to community-based services and supports, support training to enhance the workforce and invest in mental health infrastructure. Similar bipartisan legislation has been introduced in the House this year, H.R. 2412, the Helping Children Cope Act, which would provide grants to children's hospitals and other providers to increase their capacity to provide pediatric mental health services such as those described above. We would like to see policies like these enacted this year to address the serious gaps children and youth experience when attempting to access mental health services. We understand it is challenging to create new programs and dedicate spending but the level of the crisis and longstanding impacts for children and families and our Nation warrant the new dedicated investments.

Refining Existing Programs to Better Work for Children and Youth the Community Mental Health Services Block Grant

The Community Mental Health Services Block Grant, frequently called the Mental Health Block Grant, supports state mental health agencies to provide comprehensive community mental health services and investments in evidence-based prevention for adults with severe mental illness or children with serious emotional disturbances (SED). The parameters of the funding as currently written focus on children with SED, making it difficult to spread funds to broader activities, such as evidence-based prevention efforts or mental health services for children whose needs do not reach the threshold of a serious emotional disturbance or have not yet been diagnosed. We strongly support a set-aside within this block grant for prevention and early intervention, to ensure that these Federal dollars can be used by states to expand early intervention and prevention services, especially with children and teens. A similar provision was included in the Mental Health Reform

Reauthorization Act of 2022, led by Senators Cassidy and Murphy last Congress, and received bipartisan support.

Support for Children's Mental Health Workforce. Congress must address the urgent need to relieve pressure on the existing pediatric mental health workforce, as well as invest in its long-term expansion across disciplines to meet the ongoing and growing mental health needs of our children. Pediatric mental health workforce shortages are persistent and projected to increase over time. Nationally, there are approximately 10,500[123] practicing child and adolescent psychiatrists and only 5.4 clinical child and adolescent psychologists per 100,000 children 18 years of age and younger, far fewer than needed to meet the existing and increasing demand.[124] Shortages also exist for other vital pediatric mental health specialties critical to improving early identification and intervention for children with mental health needs. Additionally, racial and ethnic minority providers are under-represented across many mental health professions, which can be an added burden on racial and ethnic minority communities who already face inequitable access to care. More dedicated support for a larger and more diverse pediatric workforce is critical to addressing children's mental health needs now and into the future.

Congress can take several immediate steps to address the current and ongoing mental health workforce shortage.

Loan forgiveness for pediatric mental health providers. Existing loan forgiveness programs can be difficult for pediatric specialty providers to access. We support robust funding for the Pediatric Subspecialty Loan Repayment Program, which would provide loan forgiveness for pediatric subspecialists, including mental health providers practicing in underserved areas. While we were glad to see the program received increased funding in fiscal year 2023, we strongly encourage a larger investment of at least $30 million, to support the pediatric subspecialty workforce and improve longstanding shortages. Additionally, we support S. 462, the Mental Health Professionals Workforce Shortage Loan Repayment Program Act, a bipartisan bill which would extend loan repayment to mental health providers across a wider array of mental health professional fields, who serve in areas with shortages of mental health professionals. We look forward to working with you to identify realistic and effective immediate solutions to support and retain a diverse national pediatric mental health workforce.

---

123 Workforce Maps by State (aacap.org), American Academy of Child and Adolescent Psychiatry.

124 "Supply of Child and Adolescent Behavioral Health Providers." University of Michigan Behavioral Health Workforce Research Center. July, 2020.

Children's Hospitals Graduate Medical Education (CHGME) program. Pediatricians build strong relationships with families and can play a critical role in identifying children with mental and behavioral health needs earlier, before more serious issues emerge. The CHGME program supports the training of more than half of the nation's pediatric physician workforce and is essential to the continued access of children to needed pediatric specialists, including developmental pediatricians and child adolescent psychiatrists. However, CHGME represents only 2 percent of the total Federal spending on GME. These funding shortfalls must be financed by children's hospitals' child-patient care operations and are a key contributor to the overall pediatric workforce shortage. We appreciated the fiscal year 2023 funding level but would encourage Congress to consider a higher overall appropriations level for fiscal year 2024 to reduce the growing and unsustainable gap between other federally funded training programs and CHGME and a bipartisan reauthorization of the program this year supporting the existing goals to secure the future pediatric physician workforce.

Project AWARE. SAMHSA's Project AWARE—Advancing Wellness and Resiliency in Education, supports partnerships between State Mental Health Agencies and State Educational Agencies to expand programs which improve mental wellness and mental health awareness in schools. The program provides funding to develop school-based mental health programs and training for school-based professionals. Given the increased need for early intervention services, and the effectiveness of the existing program we support the Mental Health Services for Students Act, led by Senator Tina Smith and Rep. Grace Napolitano in the 117th Congress. This legislation would provide competitive grants for local education agencies to bring in onsite mental health professionals, improving children's access to mental health services at schools across the country. School partnerships with local mental health providers, including children's hospitals, facilitate early identification and intervention to improve mental health outcomes for school-aged children and teens.

Pediatric Mental Health Care Access Grants. The Pediatric Mental Health Care Access program is administered through HRSA with the goal of improving access to quality health care services through supporting the development of pediatric mental health care telehealth access programs or support existing programs. We were pleased to see the program reauthorized in the Bipartisan Safer Communities Act last year and we look forward to seeing how the program's expansion into more sites, including emergency departments and schools, progresses. Integrated care, including through telehealth consultation supported by this program, can improve identification of mental and behavioral health needs in children and streamline connections to care. While this program provides critical support to pediatricians, enabling them to treat some mental health conditions within primary care, we know that greater investment is needed in pediatric care integration. Integrating mental health with primary care, including through colocation of mental health providers, has been shown to substantially expand access to mental health professionals and increase children's utilization of behavioral health services.

Thank you again for your commitment to improving the mental and behavioral health care delivery system for children and adults. Children's hospitals and their affiliated providers stand ready to partner with you as you continue your work. Children need your help now.

With questions or for more information on Children's Hospital Association's mental health policy recommendations, please contact Vice President of Policy, Aimee Ossman, or Director of Federal Affairs, Cynthia Whitney.

[Whereupon, at 11:17 a.m., the hearing was adjourned.]

Chapter 2

Mental Health and Substance Use Disorders: Responding to the Growing Crisis*

Committee on Health, Education, Labor, and Pensions

Tuesday, February 1, 2022
U.S. Senate, Committee on Health, Education, Labor, and Pensions,
Washington, DC.

The Committee met, pursuant to notice, at 10:04 a.m., in room G50, Dirksen Senate Office Building, Hon. Patty Murray, Chair of the Committee, presiding.

Present: Senators Murray [presiding], Casey, Murphy, Kaine, Hassan, Smith, Rosen, Burr, Collins, Cassidy, Murkowski, Braun, Marshall, Scott, Tuberville, and Moran.

Opening Statement of Senator Murray

The CHAIR. Good morning. The Senate Health, Education, Labor and Pensions Committee will please come to order. Today we are holding a hearing on our Nation's growing mental health and substance use disorder crisis.

---

* This is an edited, reformatted and augmented version of Hearing of the Committee on Health, Education, Labor, And Pensions United States Senate, One Hundred Seventeenth Congress, Second Session, Publication No. S. HRG. 117–387, dated February 1, 2022.

In: Mental Health and Substance Use Disorders: A Growing Crisis
Editor: Darren D. Stewart
ISBN: 979-8-89530-699-4

I will have an opening statement followed by Senator Murkowski, she is standing in for Ranking Member Burr for this hearing, and then we will introduce our witnesses. I believe the Ranking Member will join us a little later as well. After the witnesses give their testimony, Senators will each have 5 minutes for a round of questions.

While we were unable to have the hearing fully opened to the public or media for in-person attendance, live video is available on our Committee website at help.senate.gov. And if you are in need of accommodations, including closed captioning, you can reach out to the Committee or the Office of Congressional Accessibility Services.

We continue to see a high number of new COVID cases, so we are having this hearing in a larger hearing room where we can be socially distanced, limiting the number of people who are in the hearing room, accommodating both some of our Committee Members and our witnesses through video as we have done previously, and taking additional measures such as wearing masks.

As always, I appreciate the work from the staff of the Sergeant- at-Arms, the Architect of the Capitol, and our Committee Clerk and staff to make this hearing as safe as possible. Thank you to all of you. Even before the COVID–19 pandemic, our Nation was facing mental health and substance use disorder challenges on multiple fronts. Millions of people experienced depression, anxiety, and other mental health disorders.

Drug overdoses were on the rise, and our health workforce was stretched far too thin. In 2018, mental health issues were responsible for 56 million doctor office visits and 5 million emergency room visits. In 2019, suicide was the second leading cause of death among adolescents. From 1999 to 2019, the rate of overdose deaths more than tripled, and then COVID–19 hit and made things worse.

Our Nation lost over 100,000 people to drug overdoses in a single year, and overdose deaths, especially deaths involving fentanyl, skyrocketed in my home State during this pandemic. Nationwide, we are also seeing a concerning rise in methamphetamine and cocaine use as well. Across the country, people are stressed, and this pandemic has been especially traumatic for children.

Our schools, teachers, and education leaders are seeing this every day. Our educators are on the front lines trying to help so many students experiencing mental health challenges, often without the support of trained mental health professionals. We have seen sharp increases in kids' visits to the emergency room for mental health crises, thoughts of suicide, and suicide attempts, especially among girls. And as of last December, over a 167,000 children have had their world shattered after losing a parent or caregiver to

COVID–19, some have even lost both parents. And we know marginalized students are facing the worst of these challenges, deepening inequities they already face. We also know educators and caregivers are facing their own mental health challenges from the strain of this pandemic as well.

We need to continue helping our students and educators and ensuring schools have the support, training, and resources they need. But right now, our mental health and substance use disorder workforce is stretched too thin to meet the needs of our kids, let alone our communities at large. And if we just keep stretching without taking action, something is going to break.

For example, nearly half of psychologists reported feeling burnt out last year, and we aren't even close to providing mental health care to everyone who needs it. Almost 130 million Americans live in areas with less than 1 mental health care provider per 1,000 people. In my home State of Washington, our mental health care workforce is only able to meet 17 percent of our State's needs. Meanwhile, nationwide, less than 1 in 10 people who need treatment for substance use disorder actually get it. And these hardships are not felt equally.

The highest increase in opioid deaths recently has been among Black Americans. Rates of suicide are highest among American Indian and Alaska Native populations, and people with developmental disabilities who are already almost five times more likely to have mental health needs have had their lives upended. Of course, while some communities may face greater behavioral health challenges, this crisis affects all of us.

Even if we aren't personally struggling with mental health or substance use, we all have friends and families who are whether we realize it or not. We all rely on first responders, health care providers, teachers, and other frontline professionals who are facing burnout and trauma. We all have a stake in making sure people can get the help they need.

That is why Democrats passed the American Rescue Plan to provide resources for schools to hire counselors and psychologists, community based behavioral health providers, programs to treat mental health, suicide, burnout, and substance use, and more. But we are not done. Healing the scars of this pandemic won't be quick or easy. This will take years and we must act accordingly. It is time to build on this Committee's bipartisan history of expanding access to mental health services and responding to rising drug overdose deaths like we did in 2016 and 2018.

In my State, I have seen how communities can benefit from some of the critical programs this Committee has worked on, including programs at the Substance Abuse and Mental Health Services Administration. For example, in

Clark County, which saw fentanyl deaths triple in 2020. Lifeline Connections is using a SAMHSA grant to better prepare teachers and school personnel, law enforcement, first responders, and caregivers to respond to mental health crises and refer those in need to appropriate treatment.

Meanwhile, in King County, Federal support has allowed Neighborhood House to provide mental health services for over 150 adults experiencing homelessness. And the Confederated Tribes and Bands of the Yakama Nation are using grant funding from SAMHSA to fight the high rate of suicide in their community by updating their health records and mental health procedures, hiring more therapists, and expanding telehealth services which have been critical to reach people during this pandemic.

If we are going to respond to the behavioral health issues this pandemic has made worse, it is clear we have to build on these efforts. That will take legislative action. So I look forward to hearing from our witnesses about how we can do that and working with Senator Burr and everyone on this Committee on a bipartisan effort to reauthorize, improve, and expand critical Federal programs that address mental health and substance use disorder challenges. I hope that every Member of this Committee and the Senate can work together to bring their priorities forward to us to include.

My goal is to work with Ranking Member Burr to fold these priorities together into a larger package that makes progress on many of the issues that we are going to hear about today, like suicide screening and prevention, youth mental health, the opioids and overdose crisis, and breaking down barriers in access to mental health.

Finally, I want to acknowledge that mental health and substance use disorders do not exist in a vacuum. In addition to this pandemic, there are a lot of issues people are worried about right now, from gun violence to climate change to systemic racism to just making ends meet. As we work to do more to help people struggling with depression, anxiety, and stress, we also need to look for ways to solve the problems that are making things so hard for so many people in the first place.

I hope to continue to work with my colleagues on these root causes as well. I would also like to introduce two letters for the record, one from the American Academy of Pediatrics, the American Academy of Child and Adolescent Psychiatry, and the Children's Hospital Association with recommendations for addressing the National Emergency in Child and Adolescent Mental Health, and the other four members of the American Federation of State, County and Municipal Employees, highlighting the importance of supporting the behavioral health workforce. So ordered.

[The following information was not submitted for the Record:]

The CHAIR. With that, I will turn it over to Senator Murkowski for her opening remarks.

Opening Statement of Senator Murkowski

Senator MURKOWSKI. Madam Chair, thank you for convening the hearing. I appreciate that. I also want to thank Senator Burr for asking me to substitute in as Ranking Member today on this incredibly, incredibly important and certainly timely conversation as we talk about mental health and substance abuse disorders.

Madam Chair, you have outlined well, I think this statistics the challenges that we are seeing. We knew, we have known for years now that mental health and substance abuse disorders have really been at crisis levels in many parts of the country, certainly in my State of Alaska, and we have seen those challenges and those issues only further compounded by this pandemic. Access across the country, access to mental health and substance use care remains severely limited, exacerbating suicide and substance abuse rates.

You have mentioned the statistics in your State, Madam Chair, with regards to mental health providers and facilities. In Alaska, more than 80 percent of our communities do not have sufficient mental health providers while, again, we are seeing this crisis only continue to elevate, and unfortunately it knows no barrier on the spectrum. We are seeing more and more young kids.

I mean, it used to be when we were talking about suicide statistics, we would look at that 25, 45 year age bracket and now the alarm that we are seeing is in 10, 11, 12 year olds who are suffering, and we have an obligation to hear and to respond. Alaska ranks second in the country for suicide deaths. We have seen a sharp increase in drug overdose deaths, just as we have seen across the country this year. Alaska has one of the highest rates of binge drinking. Suicide rates among members of our armed services have doubled. We have seen some very, very disturbing trends of late.

As we have seen across the Nation, our Native people face shockingly disproportionate rates of mental and behavioral health and substance use disorders and suicide. And these are statistics that keep you up at night, not just because they are numbers, but these are real people. These are our constituents. These are people in our neighborhoods, in our communities. They are people who are in pain.

As we will hear from the young woman, Claire Rhyneer, who will be introduced in just a moment, a youth advocate from Anchorage, Alaska, she urges us, she reminds us that these people that are not statistics, but these real people are looking to us, they are watching, the leaders, waiting for us to do something. And I think the message of hope needs to be that we are paying attention, that we are listening, and that we are working together to try to address some of the root causes of what we have seen.

I think just within this Committee, we have seen some strong collaboration on efforts. I have been working with Senator Hassan on the Mainstreaming Addiction Treatment Act, which allows health care providers to prescribe buprenorphine, which can truly, truly save, save lives with the medication assisted treatment.

In addition to lifesaving substance use treatment, we know that we have to invest in wraparound recovery services. I have visited programs in Alaska that focus not just on preventing the overdose deaths, but also really building a community for Alaskans in recovery, because that has to be the follow on. We have worked—we have worked on efforts to reduce fetal alcohol syndrome disorders, to address the mental health needs.

Senator Smith and I are leading both the Mental Health Professional Workforce Shortage Loan Repayment Act to bolster our supply of providers, but also to Telemental Health Improvement Act to ensure that insurance covers these critical services. Senator King and Senator Kelly and I are working on the effective suicide screening and assessment in the Emergency Department Act to provide resources for emergency room personnel to identify, assess, and treat individuals at risk of suicide.

I think unfortunately, we know that is where far too many who are seeking help end up sitting in an emergency room where you don't necessarily have those that are trained to identify and assess. Later this week, I am going to be introducing the Guarding Our Mental Health Act to prevent Coast Guard members who seek help for their mental health from being automatically processed for discharge.

Again, we know we have got to make headway on the stigma issues associated with mental health. And then with Senator Rosen, we are going to be introducing the Youth Mental Health and Suicide Prevention Act to ensure that SAMHSA can provide additional mental health programing to elementary, middle, and high school students. So, Madam Chair, I think we know around the Senate here there is plenty that can divide us.

I would like to think that mental health, substance abuse, these are areas where we really can find true bipartisan consensus and hopefully we can build a package that addresses these issues head on. And I commend the work that you have made along with Ranking Member Burr to do just that.

Again, I am looking forward to being able to introduce the Committee to a bright young Alaskan, Claire Rhyneer. And when it is appropriate, I will do that. But thank you, Madam Chair, and I look forward to the testimony from all witnesses today.

The CHAIR. Thank you. We will now introduce today's witnesses. Senator Burr has joined us, so I will turn it over to him to introduce our first witness, Dr. Prinstein.

Opening Statement of Senator Burr

Senator BURR. Madam Chair, thank you very much for holding this hearing and for the opportunity to introduce Mitch Prinstein to the Committee. Mitch is from Chapel Hill, North Carolina.

Dr. Prinstein is the American Psychological Association Chief Science Officer and responsible for leading the Association's science agenda. Dr. Prinstine also serves as the John Van Seters Distinguished Professor of Psychology and Neuroscience at the University of North Carolina at Chapel Hill.

He began his academic career as an Assistant Professor and later a Director of Clinical Psychology at Yale University Department of Psychology. Dr. Prinstein's research is focused on interpersonal relationships primarily among adolescents, and he has published more than 150 scientific articles and 9 books over the course of his career.

Dr. Prinstein earned his Doctoral and Master's degree from the University of Miami. His bachelor's degree from Emory University. Dr. Prinstein, I thank you for being here today and for all your work on behalf of children and families across the Nation and in our great State of North Carolina. Welcome. Thank you, Madam Chair.

The CHAIR. Thank you, Senator Burr. Next, we have Dr. Michelle Durham. Dr. Durham is the Vice Chair of Education in the Department of Psychiatry and a Clinical Associate Professor of Psychiatry and Pediatrics at Boston University School of Medicine and Boston Medical Center. She is a Board certified physician with a background in pediatrics psychiatry, adult psychiatry, and addiction medicine.

Dr. Durham's public health and clinical roles have always been in marginalized community, and she has been a dedicated advocate for equitable mental health treatment. She is also the Director of Clinical Training for Boston Medical Center's Transforming and Expanding Access to Mental Health in Urban Pediatrics, or the TEAM Up initiative. Dr. Durham, so glad that you could join us today.

I look forward to your testimony. Our next witness is Sarah Goldsby. She is the Director of South Carolina Department of Alcohol and Other Drug Abuse Services. She was confirmed to that position by the South Carolina Senate in February 2018 after serving as Acting Director since August 2016.

Director Goldsby has led South Carolina's response to the opioid crisis and serves as co-chair of the State opioid emergency team, meaning she has been on the frontlines of the crisis we are talking about today. In her role, she has helped expand access to naloxone across South Carolina. She also understands the importance of addressing social determinants of health and making sure people have access to care.

Director Goldsby previously came before this Committee last year to discuss mental health and substance use disorder challenges related to the COVID–19 pandemic. Director Goldsby, welcome back. I appreciate your joining us to share your expertise once again. Our next witness is Jennifer Lockman, Ph.D., is the CEO of the Research Institute at Centerstone in Nashville, Tennessee.

Dr. Lockman oversees all research and program evaluation activities at Centerstone. Her work focuses on developing and testing new interventions to further suicide prevention care. She has been a lead evaluator for multiple Substance Abuse and Mental Health Services Administration grants, focused on suicide prevention in youth and adults, as well as in zero suicide health programs.

Dr. Lockman, thank you for joining us today. I look forward to hearing from you. And finally, I will turn it over to Senator Murkowski once again to introduce our last witness.

Senator MURKOWSKI. Thank you, Madam Chair. I am delighted to be able to introduce to the Committee Claire Rhyneer from Anchorage, Alaska. Claire is an articulate youth advocate. I think she has been able to effectively give voice to so many through storytelling. She has, in this capacity, encouraged others to speak out.

I first came to recognize Claire when her story was printed on the front page of the Anchorage Daily News some months back outlining what she had done as one individual who looked at what was happening around her as a young girl and the lack of availability of services, the questions that she had, and really nowhere to turn but literally the internet.

She had indicated in that article, she says, mental health was just never talked about. It was not talked about in the home. It was not talked about at school. Even in health classes where you would expect to hear it, the discussion was about making sure that you ate the right foods, you got the right sleep, but we don't focus on mental health, and so her advocacy has been one that is truly, truly impressive.

She is a recent graduate of West High School. She is spending her gap year working with the National Alliance on Mental Illness there in Anchorage. She is going to be attending Middlebury College in Vermont this fall.

Claire, thank you not only for being here today and sharing your story, but your advocacy and your voice on behalf of so many. Thank you, Madam Chair.

The CHAIR. Thank you, Senator Murkowski. Ms. Rhyneer, thank you for joining us today to share your story. It is really important that we hear voices like yours about what students are facing, so we appreciate it.

With that, we will begin our witness testimony. Dr. Prinstein, you may begin with your opening statement.

Statement of Mitch Prinstein, Ph.D., ABPP, Chief Science Officer, American Psychological Association, Chapel Hill, NC

Mr. PRINSTEIN. Sorry, can you hear? The CHAIR. Yes, we can.

Mr. PRINSTEIN. Chairwoman Murray, Ranking Member Burr, Senator Murkowski, and Members of the Committee, thank you for the opportunity to testify. I am Dr. Mitch Prinstein, Chief Science Officer of the American Psychological Association.

APA is the largest scientific and professional organization representing psychology in the U.S., with over 130,000 psychological researchers, educators, practitioners, and students. There's been much discussion of a mental health crisis in the U.S.

Today I want to talk briefly about what that crisis looks like. This is an issue that began well before the pandemic, with millions of Americans experiencing emotional and behavioral symptoms that we could have prevented. The U.S. has fared more poorly than most, with the rate of suicide attempts in the United States higher than in any other wealthy Nation on the planet.

There is simply not enough mental health care providers, and there is not enough investment in science to use what we know to prevent mental illness. Today, only one of seven Americans with mental health or substance use disorders is receiving treatment scientifically proven to work. Of course, the COVID–19 pandemic has made this much worse. In 2021 alone, children's hospitals saw a 42 percent increase in self-injury and suicide cases. School principals report that their staff are overwhelmed with children experiencing apathy, hopelessness, anxiety, and thoughts of death.

To say that this is a mental health crisis is not enough. This is an accumulation of decades of neglect, stigma, and unequal treatment of mental health compared to physical health. Now we are at a turning point like we have not seen since World War II, when our country elected to make a serious investment in mental health by building the VA system, investing in mental health workforce, and forming the National Institute of Mental Health. That was over 70 years ago.

The time has come again. Today, we know that bifurcating physical and mental health is based on antiquated notions. It is time to create a mental health system that reflects the 21st century, and we have no time to waste. Here is what you can do immediately to address this national emergency. First, we desperately need a diverse and robust mental health workforce. Today, we have 5,000 psychology trainees who could serve a far greater number of people if Medicare were reimbursed for their work during residency, just as currently occurs for medical residents. This just makes good sense.

Doctoral interns in psychology have an average of over 700 hours of independent direct patient care experience, more than most medical residents, and we can mobilize thousands of mental health care workers quickly. Second, we have the psychological science to deploy preventive interventions through school and community based partnerships.

The Mental Health Services for Students Act and reimbursement for psychologists to guide these partnerships can have multiplier effects, so each member of our current workforce is building resilience with an entire classrooms and schools. Third, we need to expand the integration of primary and behavioral health care because it works, but not with a one size fits all approach. We will need to support all evidence based models and allow primary care providers the flexibility to determine which model best suits their patients' needs.

Fourth, the 2022 Mental Health Parity and Addiction Equity Act Enforcement Report just submitted to Congress indicates that our Federal agencies are struggling. Congress must grant the Department of Labor the authority to assess civil monetary penalties for violations of the law or enforcement will be almost impossible. Now, this will only get us part of the way. We will need long term strategies as well to fix this problem that has been growing for decades. Our country invests $15 billion annually to ensure that we have enough physical health care providers with the appropriate specialties and spread throughout the country, yet we invest less than 1 percent of that amount to build a mental health care workforce.

Congress must authorize, reauthorize and significantly expand the Graduate Psychology Education and Minority Fellowship Programs and enact the Mental Health Professionals Workforce Shortage Loan Repayment Act. It is also critical that we significantly expand our scientific investment in psychological science so we can better understand psychopathology, develop novel treatments, and build resilience before the next stressor occurs.

A $1 billion increase to NIMH and NICHD and NIMHD for youth mental health would still be a very small proportion of the allocation currently offered to study conditions that afflicts far fewer youth than those currently suffering from psychological disorders. Thank you again for the opportunity to speak with you today.

We stand ready to help you with any and all issues dealing with human behavior. We have the expertise to address your Committee's work, and I look forward to answering your questions.

[The prepared statement of Mr. Prinstein follows:]

Prepared Statement of Mitch Prinstein

Chairwoman Murray, Ranking Member Burr, and Members of the Health, Education, Labor, and Pensions Committee, thank you for the opportunity to testify today on the on-going mental health and substance use disorder challenges facing Americans. I am Dr. Mitch Prinstein, Chief Science Officer at the American Psychological Association (APA). APA is the Nation's largest scientific and professional organization representing the discipline and profession of psychology, with more than 133,000 members and affiliates who are clinicians, researchers, educators, consultants, and students. Through the application of psychological science and practice, our association's mission is to have a positive impact on critical societal issues.

The COVID–19 pandemic has placed an enormous strain on individuals, families, and communities. Beyond the very real physical ramifications of the virus, the effects of social isolation, disrupted routines, loss of jobs and income, and grief associated with the death of a loved one have caused significant distress and trauma, which typically have downstream effects on mental health. During the pandemic, about four in 10 adults have reported symptoms of anxiety or depressive disorder, an increase from the one in 10 adults who reported these symptoms from January to June 2019.[1] Data also shows a surge in emergency department visits attributable to a mental health crisis, suicide attempts, and in drug overdoses during the COVID pandemic.[2] Additionally, there have been significant increases in unhealthy behaviors, such as eating disorders, sleep disruptions, alcohol consumption, and illicit drug use.[3,4,5,6] Even these factors, it is likely that the pandemic's mental and physical health impact will be present for generations to come.

To be clear, the need for greater investment in behavioral health care predated COVID–19. According to results from SAMHSA's 2019 National Survey on Drug Use and Health, 26 percent of U.S. adults with any mental illness had unmet mental health needs during the previous year, and over 47 percent of those with serious mental illness report having unmet needs.[7]

---

[1] Panchal, N., et al. The Implications of COVID–19 for Mental Health and Substance Use. Kaiser Family Foundation. (2021). Retrieved from: *https://www.kff.org/coronavirus-covid–19/issue-brief/the-implications-of-covid–19-for-mental-health-and-substance-use/.*

[2] Holland, K. M., Jones, C., Vivolo-Kantor, A. M., et al. (2021). Trends in U.S. Emergency Department Visits for Mental Health, Overdose, and Violence Outcomes Before and During the COVID–19 Pandemic. JAMA Psychiatry, 78(4), 372–379. doi:10.1001/jamapsychiatry.2020.4402.

[3] University of Minnesota Medical School. (2021, April 12). COVID–19 pandemic has been linked with six unhealthy eating behaviors: Study shows a slight increase in eating disorders, one of the deadliest psychiatric health concerns ScienceDaily Retrieved from www.sciencedaily.com/releases/2021/04/210412114740—htm.

[4] Bean, S. R., Khawaja, I. S., Ventimiglia, J. B., & Khan, S. S. (2021, December 1). COVID-somnia: Sleep Disruptions Associated with the COVID–19 Pandemic. Psychiatric Annals 51(12), 566–571. https://doi.org/10.3928/00485713–20211109–01.

[5] Julien, J., Ayer, T., Tapper, E. B., Barbosa, C., Dowd, W. N., & Chhatwal, J. (2021, December 8). Effect of increased alcohol consumption during COVID–19 pandemic on alcohol-associ- ated liver disease: A modeling study. Hepatology. https://doi.org/10.1002/hep.32272.

[6] National Institute on Drug Abuse. (2021, December 20). COVID–19 & Substance Use. National Institutes of Health. https://nida.nih.gov/drug-topics/comorbidity/covid–19-substance use.

[7] Substance Abuse and Mental Health Services Administration. (2020). Key substance use and mental health indicators in the United States: Results from the 2019 National Survey on Drug Use and Health (HHS Publication No. PEP20–07–01–001, NSDUH Series H–55). Center for Behavioral Health Statistics and Quality, Substance Abuse and Mental Health

However, the pandemic has significantly increased the need for services. A recent APA survey of psychologists shows increased demand across all treatment areas, including anxiety, depression, and trauma-and stress-related disorders.[8] Rates of substance use also grew during COVID–19. According to the Centers for Disease Control (CDC), between June 2020 and June 2021, approximately 100,000 people in the U.S. died from an overdose, which is a substantial increase from the previous year.[9]

One of the more alarming trends exacerbated by the pandemic is the impact on youth mental health, including among children who did not previously exhibit symptoms of a behavioral health disorder.[10] The mental health of children is frequently tied to the overall health, safety, and stability of their surroundings. Ongoing national surveys of households with young children have found high levels of childhood hunger, emotional distress among parents, and frequent disruptions in child-care services.[11]

Recent data show that nearly 10 percent of U.S. children lived with someone who was mentally ill or severely depressed.[12] Furthermore, since the start of the pandemic, over 167,000 children have lost a parent or caregiver to the virus.[13] This kind of profound loss can have significant impacts on the

---

Services Ad- ministration. Retrieved from https://www.samhsa.gov/data/sites/default/files/reports/ rpt29393/2019NSDUHFFRPDFWHTML/2019NSDUHFFR090120.htm.

[8] American Psychological Association (2021). Worsening mental health crisis pressures psychologist workforce. 2021 COVID–19 Practitioner Survey. Retrieved from: https://www.apa.org/ pubs/reports/practitioner/covid–19–2021.

[9] National Center for Health Statistics. (2022). Provisional Monthly National and State-Level Drug Overdose Death Counts. Centers for Disease Control and Prevention. Retrieved from: https://www.cdc.gov/nchs/nvss/vsrr/drug-overdose-data.htm.

[10] Osgood, K., Sheldon-Dean, H., & Kimball, H. (2021). 2021 Children's Mental Health Report: The Impact of the COVID–19 Pandemic on Children's Mental Health. Child Mind Institute. Retrieved from: http://wvspa.org/resources/CMHR–2021-FINAL.pdf5555.

[11] Center for Translational Neuroscience. (2021). RAPID-EC Fact Sheet: Still in Uncertain Times; Still Facing Hunger. University of Oregon. Retrieved from: *https://www.uorapidresponse.com/our-research/still-in-uncertain-times-still-facing-hunger; Center for Translational Neuroscience. (2021). RAPID-EC Fact Sheet: Emotional Distress On the Rise for Parents. Again. University of Oregon. Retrieved from: https://www.uorapidresponse.com/emo-tional-distress-on-rise-again'utm—medium=email&utm—source=email—link&utm—content=baby—monitor—11042021&utm—campaign=Q1—2022—Policy+Center—Resources.*

[12] Ullmann, H., Weeks, J. D., Madans, J. H. (2021). Disparities in stressful life events among children aged 5–17 years. National Center for Health Statistics. *https://dx.doi.org/10.15620/cdc:109052.*

[13] Treglia, D., Cutuli, J. J., Arasteh, K., J. Bridgeland, J.M., Edson, G., Phillips, S., & Balakrishna, A. (2021). Hidden Pain: Children Who Lost a Parent or Caregiver to COVID–19 and What the Nation Can Do to Help Them. COVID Collaborative.

mental health of children, leading to anxiety, depression, trauma, and stress-related conditions.

Increases in demand for pediatric inpatient mental health services are also a particularly concerning indicator. Between April and October 2020, the proportion of children between the ages of 5 and 11 and adolescents ages 12 to 17 visiting an emergency room due to a mental health crisis increased by 24 percent and 31 percent, respectively.[14] In recent months, children's hospitals have reported their highest number of children "boarding" in hospital emergency departments awaiting treatment.[15] During the first three-quarters of 2021, children's hospitals reported a 14 percent increase in mental health related emergencies and a 42 percent increase in cases of self-injury and suicide, compared to the same time period in 2019.[16] Faced with such data, in December 2021, the U.S. Surgeon General issued an advisory calling for a unified national response to the mental health challenges young people are facing.[17] Considering the rarity of such advisories, this further underscores the need for action to help stem the long-term impacts of the pandemic on the mental health and well-being of children and adolescents.

Furthermore, the burdens of the pandemic have not been proportionately borne by race and ethnicity. People of color are at a higher risk of infection, hospitalization, and death from the virus as compared to their White counterparts.[18] The pandemic has also shone a light on the historic disparities in access to behavioral health care among populations of color, which has

---

[14] Leeb, R. T., Bitsko, R. H., Radhakrishnan, L., Martinez, P., Njai, R., Holland, K. M. (2020) Mental Health-Related Emergency Department Visits Among Children Aged <18 Years During the COVID–19 Pandemic—United States, January 1-October 17, 2020. Morbidity and Mortality Weekly Report, 69(45), 1675–1680. *http://dx—doi.org/10—15585/mmwr—mm6945a3.*

[15] Children's Hospital Association. (n.d.). Emergency Room Boarding of Kids in Mental Health Crisis. Retrieved from: *https://www.childrenshospitals.org/—media/Files/CHA/Main/Issues—and—Advocacy/Key—Issues/Mentalpercent20Health/2021/Boarding—fact—sheet—121421.pdf.*

[16] Children's Hospital Association. (2021). COVID–19 and Children's Mental Health. Retrieved from: *https://www.childrenshospitals.org/-/media/Files/CHA/Main/Issues—and—Advocacy/Key—Issues/Mental-Health/2021/covid—and—childrens—mental—health—factsheet—091721.pdf'la—en&hash—F201013848F9B9C97FAE1 6A89B01A38547C7C5C7.*

[17] Office of the U.S. Surgeon General. (2021). Protecting Youth Mental Health: The U.S. Surgeon General's Advisory. Retrieved from: *https://www.hhs.gov/sites/default/files/surgeon—general—youth—mental—health—advisory.pdf.*

[18] Centers for Disease Control and Prevention. (2021). Risk for COVID–19 Infection, Hospitalization, and Death By Race/Ethnicity. Retrieved from: *https://www.cdc.gov/coronavirus/2019—ncov/covid—data/investigations—discovery/hospitalization—death—by—race—-eth- nicity.html.*

further harmed their mental wellbeing since the start of this crisis.[19] This includes children and adolescents. Rates of suicide, which have traditionally been high predominantly among White and Native American kids, have risen sharply among Black and African American youth.[20] Black and Hispanic children lost a parent or a caregiver at more than two times the rate of White children, while American Indian, Alaska Native, and Native Hawaiian and Pacific Islander children lost caregivers at nearly four times that rate.[21] Additionally, young people within other marginalized populations, including those who identify as LGBTQ+ and children with developmental and physical disabilities, have been disproportionately impacted.[22]

Even on their own, these data are striking, but taken in aggregate, they could not provide a clearer picture: action is urgently needed. The COVID–19 pandemic continues to be incredibly challenging on an individual and societal level, but it has provided us an opportunity to reevaluate how we deliver mental health services. APA applauds Congress for the COVID-relief funding that has been enacted since March 2020. Congress' swift action was critical to addressing the crisis we were facing and continue to face. However, investments in mental health care cannot just be reactive and made solely on an emergency basis. Consistent, steady, sustainable support is necessary to meet the challenges and growing demand that will continue to arise in the future. We must start the hard work of rebuilding our public health and preparedness and response system now. We cannot afford to wait until the next crisis occurs.

Further, APA supports the recent introduction of the PREVENT Pandemics Act discussion draft, which addresses critical gaps in the way our public health infrastructure responds to pandemics and other public emergencies, particularly as it relates to the roles and responsibilities of the

---

[19] McKnight-Eily, L. R., Okoro, C. A., Strine, T. W., et al. (2021). Racial and Ethnic Disparities in the Prevalence of Stress and Worry, Mental Health Conditions, and Increased Substance Use Among Adults During the COVID–19 Pandemic—United States, April and May 2020. Mor- bidity and Mortality Weekly Report, 70(5), 162–166. *http://dx—.doi—org/10-15585/mmwr— mm7005a3.*

[20] Sheftall, A. H., Vakil, F., Ruch, D. A., Boyd, R. C., Lindsey, M. A., & Bridge, J. A. (2021). Black Youth Suicide: Investigation of Current Trends and Precipitating Circumstances. Journal of the American Academy of Child & Adolescent Psychiatry. *https://doi.org/10.1016/ j.jaac.2021.08.021.*

[21] Treglia, D., Cutuli, J. J., Arasteh, K., J. Bridgeland, J.M., Edson, G., Phillips, S., & Balakrishna, A. (2021). Hidden Pain: Children Who Lost a Parent or Caregiver to COVID–19 and What the Nation Can Do to Help Them. COVID Collaborative.

[22] Morning Consult & the Trevor Project. (2021) Issues Impacting LGBTQ Youth Retrieved from:*https://www.thetrevorproject.org/wp—content/uploads/2021/12/TrevorProject—Public— Final–1.pdf.*

Substance Abuse & Mental Health Services Administration (SAMHSA). However, this is also not enough. APA is hopeful and optimistic that this Committee will also consider comprehensive legislation reflective of the fact that mental health is integral to overall health. As such, APA offers the following recommendations focused on (1) Strengthening the Mental Health Care Workforce; (2) Improving Access to Mental Health Care for Children and Youth; (3) Promoting Integration of Primary Care and Behavioral Health; (4) Continuation of Evidence-Based Mental Health Programs; (5) Ensuring Parity for Behavioral and Physical Health Care; and (6) Investing in Youth Mental Health Research.

Strengthening the Mental Health Care Workforce

A strong mental health workforce is critical to combating the long-term impact of the pandemic and remedying longstanding access gaps. Nationwide, even before COVID–19, the U.S. was facing a serious shortage of mental and behavioral health providers, including psychologists, with every state having documented mental health professionals shortage areas.[23] By 2030, these shortages are projected to worsen significantly,[24,25] with rural communities facing major challenges in recruiting licensed mental and behavioral health care professionals.[26] Despite the need for these services, there are multiple barriers to educating and training psychologists, including the cost of attending graduate school, which most students are increasingly financing by taking on debt. Doctoral psychologists graduate with an average student debt load of between $95,000 and $160,000 from their graduate degrees alone, and close to half of doctoral-level psychologists rely on loans or their own funds

[23] Bureau of Health Workforce (2019) Designated Health Professional Shortage Area Statistics Health Resources and Services Administration; U.S. Department of Health and Human Services Retrieved from *https://data.hrsa.gov/hdw/Tools/MapToolQuick—aspx—mapName— HPSAMH.*

[24] Health Resources and Services Administration. (n.d.). Behavioral Health Workforce Projections, 2016–2030: Clinical, Counseling, and School Psychologists. Retrieved from: *https:// bhw.hrsa.gov/sites/default/files/bureau-health-workforce/data-research/psychologists–2018.pdf.*

[25] Bureau of Labor Statistics. Occupational Outlook Handbook, Psychologists. U.S. Department of Labor. Retrieved from *https://www.bls.gov/ooh/life-physical-and-social-science/psychologists.htm.*

[26] Rural Health Information Hub. (2021). Rural Mental Health. RHIhub. *https:// www.ruralhealthinfo.org/topics/mental-health.*

to pay for graduate school, which takes on average 5–6 years to complete.[27] 27 Data show that psychology graduate students have difficulties affording health care, are concerned about being able to afford completing their training requirements, and have difficulties focusing on their studies as a result of trying to make ends meet.[28] At the same time, student loan-related actions taken by the Federal Government over the last decade have disproportionately impacted graduate students. This includes the imposition of higher interest rates and multiple loan origination fees, as well as the elimination of subsidized Federal loans.[29] These factors further increase the cost of Federal borrowing, particularly when financing graduate education.

Furthermore, as a result of a variety of factors, including lack of generational wealth, students of color, first-generation, and lower socioeconomic status students tend to borrow significantly more, both for their undergraduate and postbaccalaureate degrees.[30] This is true across all fields, but data show that low-income students and students of color working toward doctoral psychology degrees also disproportionately rely on student loans.[31] The prospect of adding further debt often serves as a disincentive to pursuing advanced degrees. Higher student loan debt further impedes workforce diversity, including in mental and behavioral health care fields, where demand for representative, culturally competent providers is high.[32] Finally, research

---

[27] Doran, J., Kraha, A., Marks, L., Ameen, E. & El-Ghoroury, N. (2016). Graduate Debt in Psychology: A Quantitative Analysis. Training and Education in Professional Psychology, 10(1), 3–13.

[28] Lantz, M. M. (2013). Uncovering the graduate student economic landscape: A difficult but necessary dialog. Society of Counseling Psychology Newsletter, 34, 22–23. Retrieved from *http://www.div17.org/wp—content/uploads/SCP17—2013–9.pdf.*

[29] U.S. Department of Education (n.d.) Federal Interest Rates and Fees Federal Student Aid Retrieved from:*https://studentaid.gov/understand-aid/types/loans/interest-rates.*

[30] Miller, B. (2019, December 2) The Continued Student Loan Crisis for Black Borrowers Center for American Progress Retrieved from: *https://www.americanprogress.org/issues/education-postsecondary/reports/2019/12/02/477929/continued-student-loan-crisis-black-borrowers/.*

[31] Wilcox, M. M., Barbaro-Kukade, L., Pietrantonio, K. R., Franks, D. N., & Davis, B. L. (2021). It takes money to make money: Inequity in psychology graduate student borrowing and financial stressors. Training and Education in Professional Psychology, 15(1), 2–17 *https://doi.org/10.1037/tep0000294.*

[32] Sullivan, L., Meschede, T., Shapiro, T., & Escobar, F. (September 2019). Stalling Dreams: How Student Debt is Disrupting Life Chances and Widening the Racial Wealth Gap. Institute on Assets and Social Policy, Heller School for Social Policy and Management at Brandeis University Retrieved from:*https://heller—brandeis—edu/iere/pdfs/racial-wealth-equity/racial-wealth-gap/stallingdreams-how-student-debt-is-disrupting-lifechances.pdf.*

shows that debt also impacts career choice by, for example, reducing the probability that qualified professionals will enter public service careers.[33]

To incentivize qualified providers to pursue careers delivering care to underserved populations, APA encourages the passage of the bipartisan Mental Health Professionals Workforce Shortage Loan Repayment Act (S. 1578), which authorizes a new student loan repayment program for mental health care professionals who commit to working in an area lacking accessible care.

Additionally, to help decrease the reliance on student loans and eradicate some of the barriers obstructing the growth and diversification of this critical workforce, Congress must invest in programs that fund the education and training of future mental health care providers. Unlike physicians, doctoral-level psychologists are not eligible for Medicare-funded residency programs, which provides billions of dollars to support the expansion of the physician workforce through Graduate Medical Education or GME. In addition, although clinical psychology interns go through a training process similar to psychiatry residents, services provided by trainees under the supervision of a licensed psychologist are not reimbursable under Medicare; despite trainees having an average of 500–700 hours of direct patient experience It is policies like these that inhibit the expansion of the mental and behavioral health workforce. Before the COVID–19 pandemic, there was a projected shortage of over 13,000 psychologists by 2030.[34] With the rising mental and behavioral health needs associated with COVID–19, this shortage is expected to grow significantly. Increased funding to the programs below administered by the Health Resources and Services Administration (HRSA) and Substance Abuse and Mental Health Services Administration (SAMHSA) is essential to maintain a steady pipeline of trained psychologists to meet the anticipated mental health needs of the entire nation. APA calls for the expeditious reauthorization of the following programs, which are set to expire at the end of Fiscal Year (FY) 2022:

The Graduate Psychology Education Program (GPE) is the Nation's primary Federal program dedicated solely to the education and training of doctoral-level psychologists. GPE provides grants to accredited psychology

---

[33] Choi, Y. (2014). Debt and college students' life transitions: The effect of educational debt on career choice in America. Journal of Student Financial Aid, 44(1), 3. Retrieved from *https:// ir—library—louisville.edu/cgi/viewcontent—cgi—article—1050&context—jsfa.*

[34] American Psychological Association. (2018). A Summary of Psychologist Workforce Projections: Addressing Supply and Demand from 2015–2030 Retrieved from *https://www.apa.org/ workforce/publications/supply demand/summary.pdf.*

doctoral, internship and postdoctoral training programs to support the interprofessional training of psychology graduate students while also providing mental and behavioral health services to underserved populations in rural and urban communities. APA urges the Committee to reauthorize this important program at $50 million per year, a robust increase commensurate with the scale of mental health and substance use disorder needs and the dangerous shortage in the workforce.

The Minority Fellowship Program (MFP) serves a dual purpose to both increase the number of minority mental health professionals and increase access to mental health services in underserved areas. It provides funding for the training, career development and mentoring of mental and behavioral health professionals to work with ethnic minorities. The program focuses on training students, postdoctoral fellows and residents to be culturally and linguistically competent to adequately address the needs of minorities in underserved areas. It funds trainees in psychology, nursing, social work, psychiatry, addiction counseling, professional counseling and marriage and family therapy.

Decades of psychological research has shown that minority youth report less use of mental health services than non-Hispanic white youth.[35] However, strong barriers for ethnic minorities to access mental health services continue to persist. These include a lack of bilingual providers and lack of culturally competent care. Therefore, the MFP is essential to ensure there are culturally competent behavioral health professionals, as they are a key component to improving health care outcomes for underserved communities. With the shortage of qualified minority psychologists to address the needs of minority populations, the importance of MFP is all the more important.

The Behavioral Health Workforce Education and Training (BHWET) Program supports pre-degree clinical internships and field placements for a broad array of behavioral health professionals, including doctoral-level psychology students, master's-level social workers, school social workers, professional and school counselors, psychiatric mental health nurse practitioners, marriage and family therapists, and occupational therapists. The program is also a key source of support for other mental health training programs and substance use disorder prevention efforts. Preserving this program is key to reaching underserved populations, as well as meeting the

[35] Marrast, L., Himmelstein, D. U., & Woolhandler, S. (2016). Racial and ethnic disparities in mental health care for children and young adults: A national study. International Journal of Health Services, 46(4), 810–824.

needs of patients wherever they are on the spectrum of mental health needs, from mobile crisis services for those with need for immediate intervention to early screening and prevention services for those who may be experiencing minor symptoms of a behavioral health disorder.

The Integrated Substance Use Disorder Training Program (ISTP) expands the number of nurse practitioners, physician assistants, health service psychologists, and/or social workers trained to provide mental health and substance use disorder (SUD), including opioid use disorder (OUD) services in underserved community- based settings that integrate primary care, mental health, and SUD services.

Improving Access to Mental Health Care for Children and Youth

Significant unmet child and adolescent behavioral health needs existed nationwide, even prior to COVID–19.[36,37] Suicide rates among children aged 10 and older have also climbed significantly each year since 2007, making it the second most common cause of death among adolescents before the pandemic.[38] The stakes of untreated mental and behavioral health symptoms for children and adolescents are exceptionally high. Failing to detect and address early indicators of a mental or behavioral health disorder can have profound consequences on the overall trajectory of a child's life, including a greater likelihood of difficulties with learning, addiction to substances, lower employment prospects, and involvement with the criminal justice system of difficulties with learning, addiction to substances, lower employment prospects, and involvement with the criminal justice system.[39] Sacks, V., & Murphey, D. (2018). The prevalence of adverse childhood experiences,

---

[36] Centers for Disease Control and Prevention (2020) Youth Risk Behavior Surveillance Retrieved from:*https://www.cdc.gov/mmwr/volumes/69/su/pdfs/su6901-H.pdf.*

[37] Center for Behavioral Health Statistics and Quality (2018) 2017 National Survey on Drug Use and Health: Methodological summary and definitions. Substance Abuse and Mental Health Services Administration.

[38] Centers for Disease Control and Prevention. (2020). State Suicide Rates Among Adolescents and Young Adults Aged 10–24: United States, 2000–2018. National Vital Statistics Reports. Retrieved from:*https://www.cdc.gov/nchs/data/nvsr/nvsr69/NVSR–69–11–508.pdf.*

[39] Sacks, V., & Murphey, D. (2018) The prevalence of adverse childhood experiences, nationally, by state, and by race/ethnicity. Child Trends. Retrieved from: *https://www.childtrends.org/publications/prevalence-adverse-childhood-experiences-nationallystate-race-ethnicity;*

nationally, by state, and by race/ethnicity. Child Trends. Retrieved from: https://www.childtrends.org/publi-cations/prevalence-adverse-childhood-experiences-nationally state-race-ethnicity;

Even before COVID–19, many young people were already prolific users of social media. Throughout the pandemic, however, for many this became the only means of retaining a sense of connection to their peers and communities. Yet psychological science suggests a darker side to young people's engagement with social media, with results suggesting risks that far exceed the findings revealed in recent months from social media employees themselves. Note that the brain undergoes significant changes at pubertal outset, and emerging research suggests that digital media change neural activation and brain development in long-term and potentially permanent ways. In addition, research demonstrates that youth are highly susceptible to peer influence on social media, they are exposed to more frequent and more severe discrimination online, many teens consume content that actually promotes maladaptive and dangerous behaviors (e.g., cutting, fasting, purging), and like adults, they are prey to mis/disinformation campaigns on social media platforms.[40,41]

To support a multitiered, population health approach, which includes continued clinical care through a more traditional "acute care" model for those experiencing behavioral health disorders, as well as mitigation strategies, such as early detection and intervention, for those at-risk of behavioral health conditions,[42] APA strongly urges the reauthorization of several pediatric mental health programs:

Programs for Children with a Serious Emotional Disturbance provide funds to government entities to deliver comprehensive community-based mental health services to children, youth, and young adults who have a serious emotional disturbance. These programs serve vulnerable, high-risk populations, and have shown to significantly improve the mental, social, and emotional functioning of children and adolescents with severe emotional disturbances through effective evidence-based services and have shown to significantly improve the mental, social, and emotional functioning of children

---

[40] Sherman, L. E., Payton, A. A., Hernandez, L. M., Greenfield, P. M., & Dapretto, M. (2016). The power of the "like" in adolescence. Psychological Science, 27(7), 1027–1035. *http://doi.org/10.1177/0956797616645673.*

[41] S Nesi, J., Telzer, E. H., Prinstein, M. J. (in production). Handbook of Adolescent Digital Media Use and Mental Health. Accepted for Publication, Cambridge University Press.

[42] Evans, A. C., & Bufka, L. F. (2020). The Critical Need for a Population Health Approach: Addressing the Nation's Behavioral Health During the COVID–19 Pandemic and Beyond. Preventing Chronic Disease, 17. *http://dx.doi.org/10.5888/pcd17.200261.*

and adolescents with severe emotional disturbances through effective evidence-based services and have shown to significantly improve the mental, social, and emotional functioning of children and adolescents with severe emotional disturbances through effective evidence-based services.[43]

Pediatric Mental Health Care Access Grants promote behavioral health integration into pediatric primary care by supporting pediatric mental health care telehealth access programs. Data show that psychological factors substantially influence physical health outcomes and efforts to address physical health needs are less likely to be effective without similar attention to behavioral health conditions.[44,45] As such, to maximize the likelihood of a successful intervention, integrating children's physical and behavioral health care is critical. Reauthorizing the Pediatric Mental Health Care Access Grants program would further support the coordination between physicians and behavioral health providers.

Additionally, the Committee should consider the Pursuing Equity in Mental Health Act (S. 1795), which authorizes funding to support research on Black youth suicide, improve the pipeline of culturally competent providers, build outreach programs that reduce stigma, and develop a training program for providers to effectively manage disparities.

Schools also play a critical role in providing health care to many children, particularly as they can be key to both early detection and intervention efforts. In fact, in many communities, they are an essential—and often the only—source of meeting the physical and mental health needs of students and families. While some school districts leverage Medicaid funds to stretch scarce resources and create school-based mental health programs, shortages of school-based behavioral health professionals continue to persist.[46]

Improving the behavioral health and emotional well-being of all students, including by instituting evidence-based comprehensive behavioral health

---

[43] Substance Abuse and Mental Health Services Administration. (2017). The Comprehensive Community Mental Health Services for Children with Serious Emotional Disturbances Program: 2017 Report to Congress. Retrieved from: *https://store.samhsa.gov/sites/default/files/d7/priv/ cmhi–2017rtc.pdf.*

[44] Slavich, G. M., & Cole, S. W. (2013) The emerging field of human social genomics Clinical Psychological Science, 1(3), 331–348. *https://doi.org/10.1177/2167702613478594.*

[45] Australian Institute of Health and Welfare. (2012). Comorbidity of mental disorders and physical conditions 2007. Retrieved from: *https://www.aihw.gov.au/getmedia/05a9c315–7576– 4c3f—aa2a9ccb14964c3e/10953.pdf.*

[46] National Association of School Psychologists. (2017). Shortages in school psychology: Challenges to meeting the growing needs of U.S. students and schools. Retrieved from: *https://www.nasponline.org/resources-and-publications/resources-and-podcasts/school-psychology/shortages-in-school-psychology-resource-guide.*

systems in schools, can help mitigate the impacts of pandemic-related learning loss, pandemic-related learning loss, pandemic-related learning loss, pandemic-related learning loss, pandemic-related learning loss,[47] and reduce the frequency and severity of mental health and substance use disorders.[48] Such a holistic approach provides a full complement of supports and services that establish multitier interventions and promotes positive school environments. They are built on collaborations between students, parents, families, community health partners, school districts, and school professionals, such as administrators, educators, and specialized instructional support personnel, including school psychologists.

Instead of employing resources only when a child experiences a crisis, our behavioral health system must focus resources earlier in life and address the factors that lead to such experiences. Oftentimes, this can be achieved in school-based settings, with the partnership and engagement of parents and families. Schools must receive more support to address these needs by increasing and retaining a highly trained workforce of diverse, culturally competent school-based mental health professionals. APA urges the Committee to pass the following legislation that would increase access to school-based mental health services:

The Mental Health Services for Students Act (S. 1841), which would build partnerships between local educational agencies, tribal schools, and community-based organizations to provide school-based mental health care for students and training for the entire school community to help identify early warning signs of a crisis and prevent its escalation.

The Comprehensive Mental Health in Schools Pilot Program Act (S. 2730), which would provide resources for low-income schools to develop a holistic approach to student well-being by building, implementing, and evaluating comprehensive school-based mental health programs. Integrating evidence-based, culturally competent social and emotional learning programs and trauma-informed approaches to teaching and student well-being help foster positive school climates and develop skills such as motivation and

---

[47] Dorn, E., Hancock, B., Sarakatsannis, J., & Viruleg, E. (2020, December 8). COVID–19 and learning loss-disparities grow and students need help. McKinsey & Company. *https://www.mckinsey.com/industries/public-and-social-sector/our-insights/covid–19-and-learning-loss-disparities-grow-and-students-need-help.*

[48] American Psychological Association. (2020). APA's Guide to Schooling and Distance Learning During COVID–19. Retrieved from: *https://www.apa.org/ed/schools/teaching-learning/recommendations-starting-school-covid–19.pdf.*

engagement, problem-solving, emotional intelligence, resilience, agency, and relationship building.[49]

Such universal programs also help address student behavioral challenges by implementing positive, non-punitive, restorative measures rather than retributive and exclusionary practices.[50]

The Increasing Access to Mental Health in Schools Act (S. 1811) would expand mental health services in low-income schools by increasing the number of school- based mental health professionals, including psychologists. This bill would provide schools with the ability to build long-term capacity to equitably address the mental and behavioral well-being of their students, which can have significantly positive impacts on their academic development and future success.

To further understand the implications of COVID–19 on the education of students, in terms of both their academic achievement and social and emotional development, Congress should invest in increased research and data collection through the Institute of Education Sciences (IES). IES supports research, reports data, and produces evidence-based resources to help improve educational outcomes for all students. Currently, IES is able to fund only one in ten grant applications it receives. Additionally, stronger collaboration and partnerships should be encouraged between the Department of Education, the Department of Health and Human Services, and the Substance Abuse and Mental Health Services Administration with respect to data collection efforts.

Finally, young people of college age face unique challenges when it comes to their mental health. A recent survey of college students finds that a large majority are experiencing emotional distress or anxiety due to the pandemic.[51] Future economic insecurity resulting from the pandemic is among the top concerns of college students,[52] further contributing to stress, anxiety,

---

[49] Coalition for Psychology in Schools and Education. (2015). Top 20 principles from psychology for preK–12 teaching and learning. American Psychological Association. Retrieved from *https://www.apa.org/ed/schools/teaching-learning/top-twenty-principles.pdf.*

[50] Reyes, C., & Gilliam, W. (2021). Addressing challenging behaviors in challenging environments: Findings from Ohio's early childhood mental health consultation system. Development and Psychopathology, 33(2), 634–646. doi:10.1017/S0954579420001790.

[51] TimelyMD (2022). College Students More Concerned About COVID–19 Than Ever, New Survey by TimelyMD Finds. Retrieved from: *https://timely.md/college-students-more-concerned-about-covid–19-than-ever.*

[52] Chegg.org. (2021). Global Student Survey. Retrieved from: https://www.chegg.com/about/wp-content/uploads/2021/02/Chegg.org-global-student-survey–2021.pdf.

and depression.[53,54] Campus counseling centers, which even prior to COVID-19 were the only access point to mental health care for many college students, are seeing significant increases in demand for services, without a corresponding increase in resources, whether through funding, training, or staff.[55] This care is, in part, provided by psychology interns and trainees completing their education, under the supervision of counseling center staff. One of the impacts of the pandemic on college campuses, particularly earlier in the crisis was either the limiting or outright canceling of these internships, which hamstrung the ability of counseling centers to stay operational and continue training future practitioners. APA supports the Higher Education Mental Health Act (S. 3048) that would establish a national commission to study mental health concerns at institutions of higher education, and the reauthorization of the campus suicide prevention programs under the Garrett Lee Smith Memorial Act.

Promoting Integration of Primary Care and Behavioral Health

Psychologists have long been at the forefront of developing evidence-based integrated primary care and behavioral health services. One of the leading models of integrated care is the Primary Care Behavioral Health Model (PCBH), in which primary care providers, behavioral health consultants (BHCs), and care managers work as a team, sharing the same health record systems, administrative support staff, and waiting areas, and collaborate in monitoring and managing patient progress in order to improve the management of behavioral health problems and conditions. In the PCBH model the behavioral health consultant role is often, but not always, filled by a clinical psychologist.

The PCBH model is a truly population-based approach to integrated care, in which the goal is to improve both mental and physical health outcomes for

---

[53] Walsemann, K. M., Gee, G.C., & Gentile, D. (2015). Sick of Our Loans: Student Borrowing and Mental Health of Young Adults in the United States. Social Science and Medicine. 124, 85– 93.

[54] Marshall, G.L., Kahana, E., Gallo, W.T., Stansbury, K. L., & Thielke, S. (2020). The price of mental well-being in later life: the role of financial hardship and debt. Aging & Mental Health, 25(7), 1338–1344. DOI: 10.1080/13607863.2020.1758902.

[55] Center for Collegiate Mental Health. (2021). Part 1 of 5: COVID–19's Impact on College Student Mental Health. Pennsylvania State University. Retrieved from: *https://ccmh.psu.edu/index.php'option=com—dailyplanetblog&view=entry&year=2021&month=02&day=01&id=9:part–1-of–5-covid–19-s-impact-on-college-student-mental-health.*

the clinic's patients—of every age and condition—by managing behavioral health problems and bio-psychosocially influenced health conditions.[56] Generally, the BHC strives to see patients on the same day the primary care provider (PCP) requests help, ideally through a "warm hand-off," and works with the PCP to implement clinical pathways for treatment. An integrated care psychologist's day may include meeting with a parent of a child exhibiting behavioral difficulties or hyperactivity, seeing a new mother experiencing symptoms of depression, helping another patient manage chronic pain or diabetes, and working with another patient who has recently discontinued using his psychotropic medication. Both patients and providers have reported high levels of satisfaction with PCBH model services[57,58] From the patient's perspective, behavioral health services are seamlessly interwoven with medical care, mitigating the stigma often associated with behavioral health services.

The PCBH model is particularly well-suited to use in pediatric care. Interventions and supports to promote children's physical, behavioral, and emotional health can positively influence the long-term trajectory of their health and well-being into adulthood. Almost all children are seen in primary care, and it is estimated that one in four pediatric primary care office visits involve behavioral or mental health problems. Psychologists can be especially helpful in pediatric care because assessing behavioral and emotional issues in children is generally more difficult than in adults, and pediatric education traditionally focuses on children's physical health. In addition to improving treatment in this area, early childhood behavioral health services can help mitigate the effect of adverse social determinants of health. Ideally, integrated pediatric primary care includes a whole-family approach to services that encompasses screening and services for perinatal and maternal depression, domestic violence, and adverse childhood experiences.

Investing in evidence-based integrated primary and behavioral health care across multiple models would help us meet the current crisis, as more than a decade of research has shown that programs implementing the PCBH model,

---

[56] Reiter, J. T., Dobmeyer, A. C., & Hunter, C. L. (2018). The primary care behavioral health (PCBH) model: An overview and operational definition. Journal of Clinical Psychology in Med- ical Settings, 25(2), 109–126.

[57] Petts, R. A., Lewis, R. K., Brooks, K., McGill, S., Lovelady, T., Galvez, M., & Davis, E. (2021). Examining patient and provider experiences with integrated care at a community health clinic. The Journal of Behavioral Health Services & Research, 1–18.

[58] Angantyr, K., Rimner, A., Norden, T., & Norlander, T. (2015). Primary care behavioral health model: Perspectives of outcome, client satisfaction, and gender. Social Behavior and Personality: An International Journal, 43(2), 287–301.

the collaborative care model (CoCM), and blended models of integrated care can increase access to care and achieve the health care triple aim of improving patient outcomes, increasing satisfaction with care, and reducing overall treatment costs. A comprehensive approach to supporting integrated care was just endorsed by the Primary Care Collaborative (PCC), a multi-stakeholder coalition of more than 60 clinician, patient, employer, and health care organizations committed to establishing an equitable, high value health care system based on effective primary care. PCC shared recommendations on integrating primary care and behavioral health in a letter to HHS Secretary Xavier Becerra and CMS Administrator Chiquita Brooks-LaSure, stating:

> "At present, evidence supports multiple integrated behavioral health delivery models in primary care, including the collaborative care model and the primary care behavioral health model. To maximize the number of patients that can benefit from integrated care across diverse practice settings and communities, primary care payment options must be available to support a variety of evidence-based models of integration. Payment policy that supports multiple care integration models has two additional merits. It can support the development of real-world implementation evidence across diverse populations and spur further innovation in behavioral health integration at the practice level and in practice/payer collaboration. For these reasons, PCC supports a multiomponent policy approach to behavioral health integration."[59]

A concerted effort to promote evidence-based integrated primary and behavioral health is needed because unfortunately, implementation of integrated care remains limited. CMS data show that use of the Medicare behavioral health integration billing codes established by CMS in 2017 roughly doubled between 2018 and 2019, with less than a quarter of providers billing using a psychiatrist-based collaborative care model and more than 70 percent of providers using a PCBH or similar model of care. However, it appears that well under 1 percent of Medicare beneficiaries receive care through integrated care model programs between 2018 and 2019, with less than a quarter of providers billing using a psychiatrist-based collaborative care model and more than 70 percent of providers using a PCBH or similar model of care. However, it appears that well under 1 percent of Medicare

---

[59] Primary Care Collaborative. (January 26, 2022). The PCC sends Behavioral Health Integration Recommendation Letter to HHS/CMS (p. 3). Retrieved from: *https://www.pcpcc.org/2022/01/26/pcc-sends-behavioral-health-integration-recommen dation-letter-hhscms.*

beneficiaries receive care through integrated care model programs.[60] Adoption of PCBH and other integrated care models is often challenging for primary care providers, as they face barriers related to physical office space, the need for improved information technology systems, management procedures, clinical staffing and policies, health records and data tracking practices, and provider education and training.

APA supports the provision of Federal financial and technical assistance to aid in the expansion of integrated care, whether provided through partnerships (including state agencies) or through direct aid to primary care providers. Initiatives and incentives to promote integrated care should support implementation of not just PCBH programs, but all evidence-based models of integrated care. Because of differences in providers' patient populations and access to behavioral health providers, there is no "one-size-fits-all" approach to effective integrated primary care. APA urges Congress to continue to give primary care practices the flexibility to choose the model of integrated care that works best for their community and that which will most strongly expand access to integrated primary and behavioral health care, and improve population health.

Continuation of Evidence-Based Mental Health Programs

APA appreciates continued Federal support for the Community Mental Health Services Block Grant, which provides a bedrock of support for community-based mental health screening, evaluation, and treatment programs across all states and communities. The effectiveness of any mental health system depends on its recognition of mental health as existing on a spectrum, and its ability to meet the needs of patients wherever they are on that spectrum and wherever they are in the community. Without access to crisis services, patients often find themselves languishing in emergency rooms or seeking treatment in other inappropriate settings. We strongly support the CAHOOTS Act (S. 764), which incentivizes state Medicaid programs to cover services provided by round-the-clock mobile crisis teams, and Rep. Bustos' Crisis Care Enhancement Act (H.R. 4305), which reserves a higher set-aside amount under the block grant for crisis services. The increased funding for these

---

[60] Centers for Medicare and Medicaid Services. (2021). Medicare Physician & Other Providers—By Provider and Service Dataset. Retrieved from: *https://data.cms.gov/provider-sum- mary-by-type-of-service/Medicare-physician-other-practitioners/Medicare-physician-other-practitioners-by-provider-and-service.*

services provided under these bills will, in addition to improving patient outcomes, increase the efficiency of states' mental health care systems and help enable national initiatives around mental health—such as the 988 National Suicide Prevention Lifeline—to reach their full potential.

Ensuring Parity for Behavioral and Physical Health Care

Enactment of the Mental Health Parity and Addiction Equity Act (MHPAEA) in 2008 promised to end insurance discrimination against individuals with mental health and substance use disorders. Unfortunately, frequent noncompliance with the law and inadequate enforcement has kept us from achieving this promise.

Just last week the U.S. Departments of Labor, Health and Human Services, and Treasury issued their latest joint report to Congress on enforcement of MHPAEA, as required under the law. Importantly, the 2022 MHPAEA enforcement report is the first since Congress established a new enforcement tool under the Consolidated Appropriations Act of 2021 (CAA): the requirement that health plans and issuers perform comparative analyses of their non-quantitative treatment limitations (NQTLs) to demonstrate their compliance with MHPAEA and provide those analyses to the agencies upon request for purposes of determining compliance. Health plans, administrators, and issuers are continuing to apply discriminatory NQTLs (such as preauthorization requirements, admission criteria for provider networks, and reimbursement rates) to mental health and substance use disorder benefits and providers in order to constrain their beneficiaries' use of services.

Most of the responsibility for enforcement has fallen to the Employee Benefits Security Administration (EBSA) within the Department of Labor (DOL), which has jurisdiction over MHPAEA compliance for approximately 2 million health plans covering more than 136 million Americans. Out of this universe, EBSA has issued 156 letters to plans and issuers requesting comparative analyses for their NQTLs. As the report describes, none of the comparative analyses EBSA reviewed contained sufficient information upon initial receipt. EBSA subsequently obtained sufficient information for a review of NQTLs in 30 plans, and in all cases made an initial determination of non-compliance with MHPAEA.

We applaud the agencies' focus on NQTLs and its new enforcement authority, and for prioritizing review of both in-network and out-of-network reimbursement rates for mental health and substance use providers. A 2019

Milliman Research Report compared health plans' in-network reimbursement rates for behavioral health office visits as a percentage of Medicare-allowed amounts with reimbursement rates for medical/surgical office visits, and found that primary care reimbursement rates were nearly 24 percent higher than behavioral health visit rates. Not surprisingly, the same study found that consumers were almost five and a half times as likely to go out-of-network for behavioral health services as for medical/surgical primary care. APA frequently hears from psychologists who have chosen to stop participating in insurance plans because of low reimbursement rates and onerous administrative hassles, and this level of frustration is being exacerbated by the heavy demand for services during the pandemic.

The 2022 MHPAEA Report describes DOL's valiant effort to enforce the law, which we commend, but it is clear stronger tools are needed. We strongly support the agency's request for the authority to assess civil monetary penalties for parity violations—for group health plan, issuers, and administrators—as would be established under legislative language included in the House-passed Build Back Better Act. Congress should enact legislation this year to provide this authority.

In addition, we support the Parity Implementation Assistance Act (S. 1962) to assist states in using the new enforcement authority granted under the Consolidated Appropriations Act to obtain comparative analyses and information from insurers on their implementation of MHPAEA. States have the authority, but often not the resources, to play a role in enforcing MHPAEA.

Finally, we urge the Committee to approve legislation to close the loophole that allows self-funded non-Federal Government-sponsored health plans to opt out of complying with MHPAEA. Sadly, even after all we've experienced with the mental health effects of the pandemic and the acceleration of drug overdose deaths over the past 2 years, these plans covering our public servants are far more likely to claim an exemption from mental health parity requirements than for any other type of coverage requirement. It has been 14 years since Congress passed MHPAEA to end discrimination by diagnosis against those in need of mental health and substance use treatment, and now is certainly the time to do the same for government employees. Congress should also eliminate the ability of self-funded non-Federal Government health plans to opt out of other beneficiary protections, such as benefits described under the Newborns' and Mothers' Health Protection Act of 1996 and the Women's Health and Cancer Rights Act of 1998.

No Surprises Act

APA urges the Committee to investigate the disproportionate impact of the Interim Final Rules issued last year under the No Surprises Act on mental and behavioral health providers. APA and ten of the top mental and behavioral health organizations sent a letter to U.S. Department of Health and Human Services Secretary Xavier Becerra on January 25, 2022, requesting a stay on enforcement of requirements affecting routine mental and behavioral health service.[61] Collectively, we expressed concerns with the impact the IFRs will have on access to mental and behavioral services in communities that have long lacked access to these services. Our practitioners have a long-standing practice of being transparent about fees with their patients as is required under professional ethics codes. We have broad concerns that when CMS develops the rules for Good Faith Estimates (GFEs) for insured patients, insurers will use the information contained in the required Good Faith Estimates (GFEs) as a mechanism or justification to limit treatment beyond the scope of the GFEs. We also urge that those rules do not carry over the flawed Part I dispute resolution provisions identified in the American Medical Association (AMA) and American Hospital Association (AHA) lawsuit. We, and other mental and behavioral organizations, welcome the opportunity to work with the Committee to ensure unnecessary administrative burdens do not take away from the ability of mental and behavioral health providers to provide their patients access to quality treatment.

Investing in Youth Mental Health Research

This is surely the year for Congress to address the growing crisis this Committee has identified by adding significant funds to NIH for an initiative to strengthen youth mental health. APA is calling for a billion-dollar investment in this initiative: this research would pay dividends for decades. Mental health issues, particularly for young people, affect their entire trajectory of life,62 bringing struggles with education, employment, and close

---

[61] American Psychological Association letter to U.S. Department of Health and Human Services Secretary Xavier Becerra. (January 25, 2022). Retrieved from: *https://votervoice.s3.amazonaws.com/groups/apaadvocacy/attachments/Sign-onpercent20letterpercent20No percent20Surprises percent20Act.pdf.*

[62] Veldman, K., Reinjeveld, S. A., Ortiz, J. A., Verhulst, F. C., & Bultman, U. (2015). Mental health trajectories from childhood to young adulthood affect the educational and

relationships. Mental disorders drain our economy through lost productivity and preventable utilization of the healthcare system and add costs within the juvenile justice system, to say nothing of the enormous suffering, the loss, and the personal toll exacted by mental disorders. Through research funded by NIMH, NICHD and NIMHD, we have learned a great deal about how to identify those at risk and engage them in preventive programs. But there is much more to learn and to apply in order to develop interventions, target them appropriately, and treat young people when prevention fails. We need research on primary prevention programs that are ready to be brought to scale, universal socio-emotional skills learning, safe social media interaction, and community-based approaches to support kids' healthy development.

Every year, approximately 1.5 million Americans attempt to end their own lives due to suffering from mental health symptoms. Millions more have significant impairments in their functioning at work and in their relationships as parents and romantic partners. This is largely preventable based on psychological science that could be used to integrate mental health screening, preventions, resilience practices, and evidence-based interventions that we know can significantly reduce mental health symptoms today, and ensure that children are developing with far fewer risks of mental health difficulties in the decades to ensure that children are developing with far fewer risks of mental health difficulties in the decades to ensure that children are developing with far fewer risks of mental health difficulties in the decades to come.[63]

APA is heartened by the focus on mental health in Congress, and eager to work with this Committee and its Members to develop legislation and enact the bills cited above. Your actions now can make all the difference in how many people are treated for their mental health problems and strengthened and fortified against developing problems. Together we can resolve the problems created by an inadequate mental health workforce and improve the capacity of the health care system to serve people who need immediate treatment. Our investment in mental health research now will guide improved prevention and treatment for decades to come. APA is a ready partner and looks forward to working with the Committee to put in place critical changes to our current system of care that will save lives and ensure access to care.

---

employment status of young adults: results from the TRAILS study. J. Epidemiological Community Health, 69(6). 588–593.

[63] Fortgang, R. G., & Nock, M. K. (2021). Ringing the Alarm on Suicide Prevention: A Call to Action. Psychiatry, 84(2), 192–195. *https://doi.org/10.1080/00332747.2021.1907871.*

[Summary Statement of Mitch Prinstein]

During the COVID–19 pandemic, adults' mental and behavioral health needs increased exponentially compared to 2019, and remain unmet for many. For example, over 47 percent of adults with serious mental illness report having unmet needs. Youth mental health is also at an alarming point, with disproportionate impact on youth from communities of color and marginalized communities. Children's hospitals have documented a 42 percent increase in cases of self-injury and suicide, compared to 2019. APA urges Congress to consider the six following issue areas to strengthen existing programs and/ or consider legislation to address these devastating developments.

Strengthening the Mental and Behavioral Workforce

- Pass the Mental Health Professionals Workforce Shortage Loan Repayment Act (S. 1578).
- Reauthorize programs administered by HRSA and SAMHSA, including GPE, MFP, BHWET, ISTP.

Improving Access to Mental Health Care for Children and Youth

Reauthorize:

- Pediatric mental health programs that support children with serious emotional disturbance.
- The Pediatric Mental Health Care Access Grants program.
- Campus suicide prevention programs under the Garrett Lee Smith Memorial Act.

Consider:

- The Pursuing Equity in Mental Health Act (S. 1795).
- The Higher Education Mental Health Act (S. 3048).
- Pass:
- The Mental Health Services for Students Act (S. 1841).

- The Comprehensive Mental Health in Schools Pilot Program Act (S. 2730).
- The Increasing Access to Mental Health in Schools Act (S. 1811).

Promoting Integration of Primary Care and Behavioral Health

- Provide Federal financial and technical assistance to aid in the expansion of integrated primary and behavioral care services provided through use of evidence-based models including the Primary Care Behavioral Health (PCBH) model and Collaborative Care (CoCM) model.

Continuation of Evidence-Based Mental Health Programs:

- Continue support for the Community Mental Health Services Block Grant.
- Consider the CAHOOTS Act (S. 764)
- Consider the Crisis Care Enhancement Act (H.R. 4305).

Ensuring Parity for Behavioral and Physical Health Care

- Enact legislative language included in the House-passed Build Back Better Act to strengthen DOL's enforcement of the Mental Health Parity and Addiction Equity Act (MHPAEA).
- Enact legislation to close the loophole that allows self-funded non-Federal Government-sponsored health plans to opt out of complying with MHPAEA.
- Enact the Parity Implementation Assistance Act (S. 1962)

No Surprises Act

- Investigate the disproportionate impact of the Interim Final Rules issued last year under the No Surprises Act on mental and behavioral health providers.

Investing in Mental Health Research

- Support a Billion-Dollar Investment in IMH, NICHD and NIMHD Funding

The CHAIR. Thank you. Dr, Durham.

Statement of Michelle P. Durham, M.D., MPH, FAPA, DFAACAP, Vice Chair of Education, Department of Psychiatry, Clinical Associate Professor of Psychiatry and Pediatrics, Boston Medical Center, Boston University School of Medicine, Boston, Massachusetts

Dr. DURHAM. Thank you, Chair Mary, Ranking Member Burr, and Senator Murkowski, and distinguished Members of the Senate HELP Committee for holding this hearing and providing me with the opportunity to speak with you today. My name is Dr. Michelle Durham. I am a Pediatric and Adult Psychiatrist at Boston Medical Center and Board Certified in Addiction Medicine. In my over 10 years at BMC and Academic Medical Center in New England's largest safety net hospital, I have never seen our mental health care services stretched so far beyond their capacity as they are now.

Since late December 2021, we have had 30 plus patients in our psychiatric emergency Department, more than four times its capacity, presenting with a much higher level of acuity, some waiting for evaluation, and others boarding a waiting for placement inpatient psychiatric unit. The patients we serve at BMC are predominantly low income, with approximately half of our patients covered by Medicaid or the Children's Health Insurance Program, the highest percentage of any acute care hospital in Massachusetts.

70 percent of our patients identify as Black or Latino, approximately one in three speak a language other than English as their primary language, and over have live at or below the Federal poverty level. BMC has a particular expertise and connecting marginalized communities to health and social services, and yet we still find it happens all too often that our patients with co-occurring mental health and substance use disorders get stuck in a revolving door, falling in and out of mental health and substance use treatment systems, in many cases ending up on the streets either episodically or chronically homeless, only to present repeatedly to our emergency Department.

One of the issues at play is that the necessary supports for these patients are not in place, including affordable low barrier housing and coordinated care integrated with a supportive community. The question is really how do we get people with co-occurring mental health and substance use everything they need to survive and be healthy?

BMC is in the very early stages of implementing a housing first approach in partnership with the city of Boston to get people living on the streets, just steps from our hospital campus, oftentimes living with co-occurring mental health and substance use issues housed first, and then provide wraparound medical services and social supports. Our hope is that this can work to break the vicious cycle for these folks, many of which are BMC patients and eventually can serve as a model for other municipalities replicate.

Our system is also in the process of constructing an 82 bed psychiatric facility in nearby Brockton, Massachusetts, to address the shortage of inpatient psychiatric beds and increase our ability to treat the mental health and substance use needs of our patients from across the region. The facility is expected to provide 56 inpatient psychiatric beds with the capacity to treat patients with co-occurring disorders and 20 26 clinical stabilization service beds.

We estimate that the project will involve a total of $27 million in sunken startup cost, a barrier that the Federal Government could help lower to incentivize capital investments to expand inpatient psychiatric capacity. As a Black, Spanish-speaking psychiatrist waiver to prescribe buprenorphine for opioid use disorder, I am all too aware of the patients our treatment systems are failing to reach.

Preliminary reports from the CDC indicate that the U.S. has eclipsed 100,000 annual drug overdose deaths for the first time ever. While nationally, overdose death rates have increased in every major demographic group in recent years, black men have experienced the largest increases. Even in Massachusetts, where we have seen population wide drug overdose death rates leveled off in recent years, the death rates for black men stand out in stark contrast, having increased astounding 75 percent between 2019 and 2020. Communities of color are suffering disproportionately from COVID–19, and they are dying at disproportionate rates from substance use disorders, bearing the brunt of two compounding public health crises.

At the same time, black men have comparably low rates of mental health and substance use treatment. At BMC, we have launched the Health Equity Accelerator to eliminate the race based health equity gap by utilizing data driven and community based research to inform and change the way we approach care for black people and people of color. While we don't yet have all the answers we seek, we do know that a one size fits all approach doesn't work and that access is strained across the mental health and substance use continuum.

That is why reauthorizing funding to support States and localities responding to mental health and the substance use crisis and flexible ways is crucial. Thank you to the Senate HELP Committee for your commitment to coming together on a bipartisan basis to sustain funding in these critical programs over time. I would like to end by providing a glimpse into the reality of what our patients face every day. In one of my recent shifts in our psychiatric emergency room, a man in his late 20's came in seeking help for his mental health and substance use.

In our short time together, he described his onset of opiate use at 9 years of age. His parents were both using substances. There was minimal supervision in the home. As we see, often the patient had experienced years of substance use, time in the correctional system, death of many family members, and unsuccessful relationships with limited supports.

He has been in and out of treatment over the years as well, but our system as currently designed ultimately exacerbates issues and prevents recovery. In order to make progress, we must work to transform our mental health and substance use care system into one that recognizes relapse as a reality, coordinates care, destigmatizing and decriminalize substance use, and ultimately one that sees the humanity and people with mental health and substance use issues as—that enable—that can enable them to recover and live healthy, fulfilling lives. Thank you for your time and I look forward to the discussion.

[The prepared statement of Dr. Durham follows:]

Prepared Statement of Michelle P. Durham

Thank you Chair Murray, Ranking Member Burr, and distinguished Members of the Senate Committee on Health, Education, Labor, and Pensions (HELP) for holding this hearing and providing me with the opportunity to speak today about mental health and substance use disorders, and the role the Federal Government can play in responding to a growing crisis impacting millions of Americans across all ages.

My name is Dr. Michelle Durham, I am a pediatric and adult psychiatrist at Boston Medical Center (BMC), board certified in adult psychiatry, child psychiatry, and addiction medicine. I am Vice Chair of Education in the Department of Psychiatry at BMC, where I also trained for my residency. I hold a joint appointment at the Boston University School of Medicine as a Clinical Associate Professor of Psychiatry and Pediatrics.

Boston Medical Center is an academic medical center and the largest safety-net hospital in New England. The patients we serve at BMC are predominantly low-income, with approximately half of our patients covered by Medicaid or the Children's Health Insurance Program (CHIP) the highest percentage of any acute care hospital in Massachusetts. 70 percent of our patients identify as Black or Latinx, approximately one in three (32 percent) speak a language other than English as their primary language, and over half live at or below the Federal poverty level. The patients we see at BMC frequently have co-occurring mental health (MH) and substance use disorders (SUD) and oftentimes face numerous health-related social needs linked to poverty, including homelessness and malnutrition. The COVID–19 pandemic, structural racism, and economic crisis has further exacerbated the mental illness, substance use, and trauma experienced by our patients.

In my over 10 years at BMC, I have never seen our mental health care services stretched so far beyond their capacity as they are now. (It's even worse than when I testified on this subject before the Senate Finance Committee in June 2021.) Since late December, we have had 30-plus patients in our psychiatric emergency department more than three to four times its capacity—presenting with a much higher level of acuity, some waiting for evaluation and others boarding awaiting placement in an inpatient psychiatric unit.

- In addition to emergency services, BMC provides a continuum of outpatient and inpatient mental health and addiction services, including:
- The Grayken Center for Addiction at BMC, with 11 clinical programs for substance use disorders, is one of the nation's leading centers for addiction treatment, research, prevention, and education;
- Outpatient Mental Health Clinic, which includes the Addiction Psychiatry Treatment Program (APTP) and the Wellness and Recovery After Psychosis (WRAP) Program;
- Outpatient integrated mental health care within our pediatric and adult primary care clinics and at local community health center partners;

- Mental health urgent care clinic;
- Our Boston Emergency Services Team (BEST) provides community-based evaluations, a mental health crisis stabilization unit, and a jail diversion program;
- BMC Health System is in the process of constructing an 82-bed psychiatric facility in nearby Brockton, MA—including 56 inpatient psychiatric beds with the capacity to treat patients with co-occurring substance use disorder and 26 Clinical Stabilization Services (CSS) beds.

BMC has a particular expertise in connecting marginalized communities to health and social services and yet we still find it happens all too often that our patients with co-occurring mental health and substance use disorders get stuck in a "revolving door," falling in and out of the MH/SUD treatment system, in many cases ending up on the streets, either episodically or chronically homeless, only to present repeatedly to our Emergency Department.

One of the issues at play is that the necessary supports for these patients are not in place:

- Access to affordable, low-barrier housing: For example, where you don't have to maintain sobriety to get a roof over your head. Not enough of these places exist. Though, BMC is in the very early stages of implementing this "housing first" approach, in partnership with the city of Boston, to get people living on the streets just steps from our hospital campus, oftentimes living with co-occurring MH/SUD, housed first, and then provide wrap-around medical services and social supports.
- A good aftercare plan: We think of care transitions as places where patients can fall through the cracks, e.g. leaving detox or an inpatient psychiatric facility to return to the community, but not linking up with outpatient treatment and support. The fact is, more needs to be done on either end to reach patients, understanding that addiction is a relapsing- remitting disease, and recovery is possible.
- A supportive community: When treating co-occurring MH/SUD, the goal is not necessarily to eliminate drug use completely, but how to use substances less so that a person can function in society—i.e. have a job and maintain healthy relationships with family and friends. At

> the same time, overemphasis on medication at the expense of other forms of treatment and support is likely not the answer. The question is really, how do we get people with co-occurring MH/SUD everything they need to survive and be healthy? For so many of our patients, particularly from multicultural/ethnic groups, connection to a supportive community is absolutely essential to recovery. From a care perspective, this can mean integrating community pillars like churches into care plans.

Substance use disorder is in the Diagnostic and Statistical Manual of Mental Disorders (DSM), the mental health field's principal authority for psychiatric diagnoses. It is estimated that about half of people with SUD will develop a MH disorder in their lifetime, and the same is true of people with MH disorders—about 50 percent will develop a SUD in their lifetime.[64] For the patients we treat at BMC, we estimate that the percentage with co-occurring MH/SUD is likely even higher (55–60 percent). The idea that mental health and substance use disorders exist in separate siloes is reflected in how our treatment system is designed—but the distinction is artificial, and is not a reflection of how patients experience MH and SUD, or how as a physician I seek to treat MH and SUD.

As a Black, Spanish speaking psychiatrist, waivered to prescribe buprenorphine for opioid use disorder, I'm all too aware of the patients our treatment systems are failing to reach. Preliminary reports from the U.S. Centers for Disease Control and Prevention (CDC) indicate that the last year for which we have data was the deadliest on record, eclipsing 100,000 drug overdose deaths for the first time ever—a grim milestone.[65] While nationally overdose death rates have increased in every major demographic group in recent years, Black men have experienced the largest increases.[66] Even in Massachusetts, where we've seen population-wide drug overdose death rates level off in recent years, the death rates for Black men stand out in stark

[64] National Institute on Drug Abuse (NIDA) Common Comorbidities with Substance Use Disorders Research Report—Part 1: The Connection Between Substance Use Disorders and Mental Illness, April 13, 2021.*https://nida.nih.gov/publications/research—reports/common—comorbidities—substance—use—disorders/part–1—connection—between—substance—use—disorders-mental-illness.*

[65] U.S. Centers for Disease Control and Prevention, National Center for Health Statistics. Drug Overdose Deaths in the U.S. Top 100,000 Annually. November 17, 2021. *https://www.cdc.gov/nchs/pressroom/nchs—press—releases/2021/20211117.htm.*

[66] Gramlich J. Recent surge in U.S. drug overdose deaths has hit Black men the hardest. Pew Research Center. January 19, 2022. *https://www.pewresearch.org/fact-tank/2022/01/19/recent-surge-in-u-s-drug-overdose-deaths-has-hit-black-men-the-hardest/.*

contrast, having increased an astounding 75 percent between 2019 and 2020 (from 32.6 to 57.1 per 100,000).[67] Communities of color are suffering disproportionately from COVID–19, and they are dying at disproportionate rates from SUD, bearing the brunt of two compounding public health crises. The COVID–19 pandemic has exacerbated all the inequities those of us practicing in mental health and SUD care have known for decades—workforce shortages, lack of coordinated care, lack of parity, and low reimbursement.

At the same time, Black men have comparably low rates of MH/SUD treatment. Racism and discrimination in all facets of life for these communities have not only made accessing care difficult, but once in treatment, unfair and inequitable systems and practices cause folks to quickly disengage from the treatment they so rightly deserve and need in order to recover.

At BMC, we have launched the Health Equity Accelerator to eliminate the racebased health equity gap by utilizing data-driven and community-based research to inform and change the way we approach care for Black people and people of color.[68] We are going directly to people in the community for answers and centering their experience seeking MH/SUD treatment to inform our interventions and program- ming moving forward.

While we don't yet have the answers we seek, we do know that a one-size-fits-all approach doesn't work and that access is strained across the MH/SUD continuum. That is why reauthorizing funding to support states and localities responding to MH and SUD crises in flexible ways is crucial including through State Opioid Response Grants, Substance Abuse Prevention and Treatment Block Grants, and Community Mental Health Services Block Grants. Thank you to the Senate HELP Committee for your commitment to coming together on a bipartisan basis to sustain funding in these critical programs over time.

I would like to end with providing a glimpse into the reality of what our patients face every day. In one of my recent shifts in our psychiatric emergency room, a man in his late 20's came in seeking help for his mental health and substance use disorder. In our short time together, he described his onset of opioid use at 9 years of age—his parents were both using substances

---

[67] Massachusetts Department of Public Health. Opioid-Related Overdose Deaths, All Intents, MA Residents—Demographic Data Highlights. November 2021. *https://www.mass.gov/doc/opioid-related-overdose-deaths-demographics-november–2021/ download.*

[68] Dayal McCluskey P. Boston Medical Center launches new plan to address racial disparities in health care. Boston Globe. November 16, 2021. *https://www.bostonglobe.com/ 2021/11/16/ metro/boston-medical-center-launches-new-plan-addressing-racial-disparities-health-care/.*

and there was minimal supervision in the home. As we see often, the patient had experienced years of substance use, time in the carceral system, death of many family members, and unsuccessful relationships with limited to no supports. He has been in and out of treatment over the years as well, but a system that does not allow relapse, a system that does not coordinate care, a system that stigmatizes substance use, a system that criminalizes substance use ultimately exacerbates issues and prevents people from being able to recover and live healthy, fulfilling lives.

Because whether we're talking about mental health or substance use disorders, or co-occurring MH/SUD, I think the question we're seeking to answer is how do we as a society continue to see the humanity in people with mental illness and/or who are using substances, and shape our policies and programs intended to treat and support people with MH/SUD accordingly.

Thank you for your time. I look forward to the discussion.

[Summary Statement of Michelle P. Durham]

In my over 10 years at Boston Medical Center (BMC), an academic medical center and the region's largest safety-net hospital, I have never seen our mental health care services stretched so far beyond their capacity as they are now. Since late December 2021, we have had 30-plus patients in our Psychiatric Emergency Department—more than three to four times its capacity—presenting with a much higher level of acuity, some waiting for evaluation and others boarding awaiting placement in an inpatient psychiatric unit.

BMC has a particular expertise in connecting marginalized communities to health and social services and yet we still find it happens all too often that our patients with co-occurring mental health (MH) and substance use disorders (SUD) get stuck in a "revolving door," falling in and out of the MH/SUD treatment system, in many cases ending up on the streets, either episodically or chronically homeless, only to present repeatedly to our Emergency Department.

One of the issues at play is that the necessary supports for these patients are not in place, including affordable, low-barrier housing and coordinated care integrated with a supportive community. The question is really, how do we get people with co-occurring MH/SUD everything they need to survive and be healthy?

As a Black, Spanish speaking psychiatrist, waivered to prescribe buprenorphine for opioid use disorder, I'm all too aware of the patients our treatment systems are failing to reach. Preliminary reports from the CDC indicate that the U.S. has eclipsed 100,000 annual drug overdose deaths for the first time ever. While nationally overdose death rates have increased in every major demographic group in recent years, Black men have experienced the largest increases. Even in Massachusetts, where we've seen population-wide drug overdose death rates level off in recent years, the death rates for Black men stand out in stark contrast, having increased an astounding 75 percent between 2019 and 2020. Communities of color are suffering disproportionately from COVID–19, and they are dying at disproportionate rates from SUD, bearing the brunt of two compounding public health crises. At the same time, Black men have comparably low rates of MH/SUD treatment.

At BMC, we have launched the Health Equity Accelerator to eliminate the race-based health equity gap by utilizing data-driven and community-based research to inform and change the way we approach care for Black people and people of color. While we don't yet have the answers we seek, we do know that a one-size-fits-all approach doesn't work and that access is strained across the MH/SUD continuum. That is why reauthorizing funding to support states and localities responding to MH and SUD crises in flexible ways is crucial. Thank you to the Senate HELP Committee for your commitment to coming together on a bipartisan basis to sustain funding in these critical programs over time.

In order to make progress, we must work to transform our MH/SUD care system into one that recognizes relapse as a reality, coordinates care, destigmatizes and decriminalizes substance use, and ultimately, one that sees the humanity in people with MH/SUD and enables them to recover and live healthy, fulfilling lives.

The CHAIR. Thank you very much. Director Goldsby.

Statement of Sara Goldsby, MSW, MPH, Director, South Carolina Department of Alcohol and Other Drug Abuse Services, Columbia, SC

Ms. GOLDSBY. Good morning, Chair Murray, Ranking Member Burr, Senator Murkowski, and Members of the Committee. My name is Sara Goldsby and I serve as Director of South Carolina's Department of Alcohol and Other Drug Abuse Services. I also serve as President of the National Association of State Alcohol and Drug Abuse Directors, or NASADAD, and it is a privilege to join you today.

I would like to begin by thanking you for your work to pass the Comprehensive Addiction and Recovery Act, or CARA, and the 21st Century Cures Act and the Support Act. In addition, thank you for providing historic Federal investments and programs housed within the Substance Abuse and Mental Health Services Administration, including the Substance Abuse Prevention and Treatment or SAPT Block Grant.

As you mentioned earlier, our country continues to experience the devastating impact of substance use disorders, and the number of overdose deaths is simply staggering. In my home State of South Carolina, overdose deaths have increased by 60 percent over the last 5 years, and more of those deaths occurred in the last 2 years, with the increased use during COVID–19, and the incredibly potent illicit fentanyl supply we have been inundated with.

Overall, almost one-third of individuals admitted to treatment in our country's publicly funded addiction system, excuse me, cited heroin or prescription opioids as their primary substance abuse. Yet we also know substance use disorders impact different States, counties, and communities in different ways. In South Carolina, for example, we are seeing a rise in admissions to treatment for alcohol use disorder, where 42 percent of people admitted to treatment reported alcohol as their primary problem.

There is no doubt that the COVID–19 pandemic contributed to increases in problems related to substance use disorders, yet we have all worked to adjust. States and providers have developed innovative approaches to prevention, treatment, and recovery programing. Federal agencies and Congress have worked to provide important flexibilities through program guidance and communication.

In addition, Congress and the Administration worked to provide critical funding for prevention, treatment, and recovery, along with lifesaving overdose reversal medication. As I observe the work moving forward in the field, I continue to be amazed and inspired by the incredible commitment, courage, and resolve that I see on a daily basis. I am particularly grateful for our frontline providers.

Even though they are exhausted, they are stretched thin, they continue to serve, they continue to help, and they continue to save lives, and they continue to help find a road for recovery for everyone they serve. And I offer a number of recommendations as we continue our work together. First, we ask that

Federal policy ensures a strong SAMHSA as the lead Federal agency on substance use disorders service delivery.

We believe SAMHSA should be the default agency for all Federal substance use disorder programing, and we applaud Dr. Miriam Delphin-Rittmon, Assistant Secretary for Mental Health and Substance Use as a leader of SAMHSA. Second, please work to ensure that Federal policy initiatives and Federal funding for substance use disorders flows through State alcohol and drug agencies, given our work to ensure quality and evidence based services, and to ensure effective planning, implementation, oversight, and accountability.

Third, we hope for continued support of the SAPT Block grant. The flexibility afforded in the Block grant allows States to target resources where they are needed more based on data and the conditions on the ground. Our country faces a giant workforce problem. We are struggling to find people to do the job. And while we appreciate HRSA, we need an all hands on deck approach.

We can—we hope this Committee will give SAMHSA and its programs full statutory authority to immediately help with our workforce challenges. We appreciate this Committee's work to help reduce suicide and improve our Nation's response to people experiencing crisis. Since this time, SAMHSA has been actively working with stakeholders to prepare for the July 2022 launch of 988. And as we move forward, we ask that Congress and others specifically elevate and specifically reference substance use disorders as a core focus of work related to crisis response.

We believe this approach is needed given the many distinct and unique considerations that accompany service delivery for people with substance use disorders and substance driven crisis. Finally, we hope Congress continues to work with stakeholders and the Administration to maintain certain flexibilities that were granted in connection with the public health emergency.

I am happy to review other recommendations with the Committee as time permits. In the meantime, thank you for the opportunity to testify today, and I look forward to questions you may have.

[The prepared statement of Ms. Goldsby follows:]

Prepared Statement of Sara Goldsby

Chair Murray, Ranking Member Burr, and Members of the Committee, my name is Sara Goldsby, and I am the Director of the South Carolina Department of Alcohol and Other Drug Abuse Services (DAODAS). I also serve as the President of the National Association of State Alcohol and Drug Abuse Directors (NASADAD). NASADAD represents State agency directors across the country that manage their respective State alcohol and drug prevention, treatment, and recovery systems.

It is an honor to testify before you today regarding the ways in which the Federal Government, states, communities, and families have been working together to address substance use disorders. I appreciate the opportunity to share perspectives.

We continue to see the devastating impact of substance use disorders across the country. The number of overdose deaths is staggering. In 2020, 93,331 individuals died from drug overdoses in the United States, the highest number ever recorded in a 12-month period and a 30 percent increase from 2019. Approximately 75 percent of overdose deaths involved synthetic opioids and illegally manufactured fentanyl (Centers for Disease Control and Prevention (CDC), 2021). In my home State of South Carolina, overdose deaths have increased by 60 percent over the past 5 years.

Overall, almost one-third (30.3 percent) of individuals admitted to treatment in our country's publicly funded addiction system cited heroin or prescription opioids as their primary substance of use (TEDS/SAMHSA, 2019). We also know substance use disorders impact different States, counties, and communities in many different ways. In South Carolina, for example, we are seeing a rise in admissions to treatment for alcohol use disorder. In particular, approximately 42 percent of treatment admissions reported a primary substance of alcohol or alcohol with a secondary drug (TEDS/SAMHSA, 2019).

There is no doubt that the COVID–19 pandemic contributed to increases in problems related to substance use disorders. For example, the National Institute on Drug Abuse (NIDA) cited research that found increases in the number of positive urine drug tests ordered by health care providers and legal systems (NIDA, 2022). The reports analyzing the drug screen results indicated an increase in fentanyl, cocaine, heroin, and methamphetamine compared to previous years (NIDA, 2022).

While the pandemic presented challenges to service delivery, we all worked together to adjust. States and providers developed innovative approaches to prevention, treatment, and recovery programming. Federal agencies and Congress worked to provide States and providers important flexibilities through program guidance and communication. In addition, Congress and the Administration worked to provide critical funding for prevention, treatment, and recovery along with life-saving overdose reversal medication. I had the privilege of testifying before this Committee in April 21 to share some of this work.

There is no doubt that the pandemic continues to present challenges. We have a great deal of work ahead of us.

Please know that the support from this Committee, the House, the Senate, and the Administration has been vital. Thank you.

As I observe the work moving forward in the field, I continue to be amazed and inspired by the incredible commitment, courage, and resolve I see on a daily basis. I am particularly grateful for our frontline providers. Even though they are exhausted and stretched thin, they continue to serve; they continue to help; they continue to save lives; and they continue to improve lives. We should all find a moment to thank and recognize our providers any chance we get.

I will review a number of recommendations for the Committee's consideration at the end of my remarks. All of these observations are critical. At the same time, it is my hope that extra energy is directed at addressing the many challenges related to our nation's substance use disorder workforce.

Critical Role of the State Alcohol and Drug Agency: I would like to step back and describe the role of each State's alcohol and drug agency. These agencies oversee and implement the publicly funded prevention, treatment, and recovery service system.

Planning: All State alcohol and drug agencies develop a comprehensive plan for service delivery and capture data describing the services provided. Our agency does this in a number of ways. Each year, we require a strategic plan to address alcohol and other drug issues from each county alcohol and drug authority. These plans are required to follow the strategic prevention (or planning) framework and must consider the most updated data available for a needs assessment.

As we understand each county's unique needs, capacity, and strategies to address substance use issues, we then create a State plan for service delivery supported by Federal and State funds available through our office. Additionally, we support the State Epidemiological Outcomes Workgroup (SEOW), composed of statisticians, epidemiologists, and data holders across State agencies. The SEOW's annual reports on prevalence and burden of substance use in our State inform priorities for planning and are shared with stakeholders statewide. Finally, we co-lead the State's Opioid Emergency Response Team that develops and manages the emergency plan to address the opioid epidemic across sectors in the State.

Working to support providers to ensure quality and delivery of evidence-based practices: An important focus of State alcohol and drug agency directors across the country is the promotion of effective, high-quality services. In South Carolina, we expect our providers to implement evidence-based screening tools and to use American So- ciety of Addiction Medicine (ASAM) placement criteria to ensure patients are placed in the appropriate level of care. All of our contracted treatment providers are required to maintain either accreditation by the Commission on Accreditation of Rehabilitation Facilities (CARF) or the Joint Commission on Accreditation of Healthcare Organizations (JCAHO).

We also conduct real-time compliance checks year-round with ongoing reviews of the clinical charts of all our contracted treatment providers. This is to ensure compliance with best practices and Medicaid standards. We require our providers to use evidence-based services across the continuum—including prevention services and support community programs that use the strategic prevention framework process.

We ensure our contractors' use of evidence-based data from trusted sources and informed practices that we approve. We support our providers year-round with training and technical assistance as requested and as we deem appropriate.

Coordinating with other State agencies on programs and services across prevention, treatment and recovery: State alcohol and drug agencies work collaboratively across State governments to ensure that addiction issues are addressed with a coordinated, cross-agency approach. For example, the State alcohol and drug agencies work with State departments of mental health, criminal justice, child welfare, education, and more. Because alcohol and drug issues cross every sector and impact citizens statewide, we partner closely with the other public health and social service agencies in South Carolina. We engage in daily communication with the S.C. Department of Health and Environmental Control (SCDHEC) for situational updates, data sharing, and on a number of joint projects, including HIV education and early intervention services, as well as overdose prevention programming for law enforcement officers and firefighters.

We also employ liaison staff that bridge our agency with others. Our Certified Peer Support Specialists are employed by DAODAS but are stationed at the S.C. Department of Corrections (SCDC) as they conduct peer trainings for inmates and coordinate inmates' access to treatment and services upon their re-entry to the community. The liaison who works between our agency and the S.C. Department of Social Services (SCDSS) helps develop policy and programming for children and families in the social services system who are affected by alcohol and other drugs. This bridge has helped align best practices and good policy across two large public systems.

Our liaison at the S.C. Department of Mental Health (SCDMH) is responsible for coordinating training for co-occurring mental and substance use disorders across the State's community mental health centers and our county alcohol and drug authorities. This work is helping our State achieve a "no wrong door" approach to serving citizens experiencing both mental health and substance use issues. Furthermore, we have a formal partnership for projects to address veterans with our State Department of Veterans' Affairs (SCDVA). Additionally, we have a contract with the S.C. Department of Probation, Parole, and Pardon Services (SCDPPPS) to train their officers on substance use disorders and evidence-based screening. Finally, I am in contact most days with the Major over Narcotics at the S.C. Law Enforcement Division as we share information on trends, trafficking, and State policy.

Communicating with, and acquiring input from, providers and local communities and stakeholders: State alcohol and drug agencies play a critical role in supporting the substance use disorder provider community. Our staff are in regular and routine contact with staff at provider organizations. Leadership at DAODAS meets monthly with all of the directors of the county alcohol and drug authorities during their monthly association meeting. The managers of DAODAS' Divisions of Treatment & Recovery Services and Prevention & Intervention Services meet quarterly with the local Treatment Directors and Prevention Coordinators, respectively, for training and global communication, but they also connect one-on-one for assistance and support as needed.

Our State Opioid Treatment Authority (SOTA) meets quarterly with the directors of the State's opioid treatment programs (OTPs) to discuss services and policy related to methadone services. Additionally, these directors and their program coordinators are routinely in touch with the SOTA for one-on-one assistance as needed.

Our Finance & Operations team meets quarterly with the treatment providers' finance managers, and they make time twice a year for one-on-one calls to answer questions regarding bookkeeping, reimbursement, and other financial operations issues.

Our Recovery Services coordinator is in close contact with the leaders of the recovery community organizations (RCOs) around the State, offering support and technical assistance as they establish programs and grow. Before the COVID–19 pandemic, our staff often traveled to provider sites for visits and in-person program reviews.

In South Carolina, we consider our agency and our providers to be a system with mission-driven connectivity that cannot be broken.

State alcohol and drug agencies appreciate action taken by Congress to address substance use disorders in general, and the opioid crisis: NASADAD is appreciative of this Committee, along with Congress and the Administration in general, for the work done to address substance use disorders in general, and the opioid crisis in particular. In addition, we appreciate passage of the Comprehensive Addiction and Recovery Act (CARA), 21st Century Cures Act, and the SUPPORT Act.

We highlight a few of the many programs below:

Substance Abuse Prevention and Treatment (SAPT) Block Grant (21st Century Cures, Section 8002): The SAPT Block Grant is NASADAD's No. 1 programmatic priority. This program is the cornerstone of States' substance use disorder prevention, treatment, and recovery systems. The SAPT Block Grant serves approximately 2 million people annually.

Federal statute requires State alcohol and drug agencies to allocate at least 20 percent of SAPT Block Grant funds toward primary substance use prevention. This "prevention set-aside" is a core component of each State's prevention system. In particular, SAPT Block Grant funds make up more than 60 percent of primary prevention funds managed by State alcohol and drug agencies. In 14 States, the prevention set-aside represents 75 percent or more of the State agency's substance use prevention budget. In six States, the prevention set-aside represents 100 percent of the State's primary prevention funding.

We sincerely appreciate recent action by Congress to allocate historic investments in the SAPT Block Grant. These investments were made in the fiscal year 2021 omnibus appropriations bill (P.L. 116–260) and subsequently in the American Rescue Plan (P.L. 117–2). Prior to these significant investments, the SAPT Block Grant remained essentially level-funded for a number of years. In particular, from 2011 to 2021, SAPT Block Grant funding did not keep up with health care inflation, resulting in a 24 percent decrease in purchasing power.

Account for the State Response to the Opioid Crisis (21st Century Cures, Section 1003): We sincerely appreciate the creation of an account for the State opioid response to the opioid crisis (Section 1003). This $1 billion fund for fiscal year 2017 and fiscal year 2018 helped State alcohol and drug agencies to significantly enhance treatment, prevention, and recovery services along with overdose reversal activities. This funding, initially known as the State Targeted Response to the Opioid Crisis Grants (STR), now known as the State Opioid Response Grants (SOR), provided a substantial level of support for innovative and lifesaving programs in States across the country. The Substance-Use Prevention that Promotes Opioid Recovery and Treatment (SUPPORT) for Patients and Communities Act re-affirmed the importance of grants to States to address the opioid crisis through Section 7181.

Priority substance abuse treatment needs of regional and national significance within SAMHSA's Center for Substance Abuse Treatment (CSAT) (21st Century Cures, Section 7004): CSAT works closely with State alcohol and drug agencies to help expand access to treatment for and recovery from substance use disorders. CSAT focuses on work to improve the quality of substance use treatment services through its Addiction Technology Transfer Center (ATTC). NASADAD recognizes Dr. Ingvild Olsen, Acting Director of CSAT, for her leadership of the Center. Further, we wish to recognize the Division of State and Community Assistance (DSCA) for their support of NASADAD's members in working to implement State-based awards including the Substance Abuse Prevention and Treatment (SAPT) Block Grant. In addition, the Division of Pharmacologic Therapies (DPT) is a key component of SAMHSA that works with State Opioid Treatment Authorities (SOTAs) and State agency directors to ensure effective programming related to medications for substance use disorders, including those moving forward within our nation's opioid treatment programs (OTPs).

Priority substance abuse prevention needs of regional and national significance within SAMHSA's Center for Substance Abuse Prevention (CSAP) (21st Century Cures, Section 7005): As noted by SAMHSA, CSAP provides national leadership in the development of programs, policies, and services to prevent the onset of illegal drug use, prescription drug misuse, and underage alcohol use and tobacco use. CSAP also works to help promote evidence-based practices through structures like the Prevention Technology Transfer Centers (PTTC). We applaud Dr. Jeff Coady, Acting Director of CSAP, for his direction. In addition, we recognize CSAP's Division of Primary Prevention (DPP) for their work with States.

A NASADAD priority program within CSAP is the Strategic Prevention Framework—Partnerships for Success (SPF-PFS) initiative. This program allows State alcohol and drug agencies to utilize cross-agency collaboration to address prevention priorities through a data-driven process. State alcohol and drug agencies partner with anti-drug coalitions to implement this important work at the local level. At the national level, NASADAD partners the

Community Anti-Drug Coalitions of America (CADCA) to help foster these relationships and promote best practices in prevention.

Evidence-based prescription opioid and heroin treatment and interventions demonstration grants (CARA, Section 301): The evidence-based opioid and heroin treatment and interventions demonstration grant was authorized in CARA to help State alcohol and drug agencies increase access to Food and Drug Administration-approved medications for opioid use disorders in order to ensure clinically appropriate care. The authorization requires SAMHSA to fund only those applications that specifically support recovery services as a critical component of the program involved.

Improving Treatment for Pregnant and Postpartum Women (CARA, Section 501 and SUPPORT Act, Section 7062): CARA reauthorized the Residential Treatment for Pregnant and Postpartum Women program to help support comprehensive, family centered treatment services where women and their children can receive the help they need together in a residential setting. CARA also created a pilot program to afford State alcohol and drug agencies flexibility in providing new and innovative family centered substance use disorder services in non-residential settings. The SUPPORT Act reauthorized both programs from 2019—2023 and increased the funding level from an authorization of $16.9 million to $29.9 million.

Community Coalition Enhancement Grants (CARA, Section 103): This section authorized the Office of National Drug Control Policy (ONDCP), that coordinates with Centers for Disease Control and Prevention (CDC), to make grants to community anti-drug coalitions to implement community-wide strategies to address their local opioid and methamphetamine problem. States work with community anti-drug coalitions daily to engage in key primary prevention efforts at the local level.

Building Communities of Recovery (CARA, Section 302): The BCOR initiative authorized SAMHSA to award grants to recovery community organizations (RCOs) to develop, expand and enhance recovery services. RCOs across the country are doing an excellent job of helping persons in recovery regain positive and productive relationships with their families, employers, and communities. NASADAD is a strong partner of Faces and Voices of Recovery (FAVOR) and its Association of Recovery Community Organizations (ARCO) as efforts are made to expand access to recovery support services in the publicly funded system.

Medicare Coverage of Certain Services Furnished by Opioid Treatment Programs (Section 2005, SUPPORT Act): This section amended the Social Security Act to expand Medicare coverage to include treatment services provided by SAMHSA-certified opioid treatment programs (OTPs). The covered services include medication assisted treatment (MAT), counseling, drug testing, and individual and group therapy.

Plans of Safe Care (SUPPORT Act, Section 406): This provision amended the Child Abuse Prevention and Treatment Act (CAPTA) to make grants to help State child welfare agencies, State alcohol and drug agencies and others facilitate collaboration in developing, updating and implementing plans of safe care. Plans of safe care are tools that inventory and direct services and supports to ensure the safety and well-being of an infant impacted by substance use disorders, withdrawal, or fetal alcohol spectrum disorders, including services for the infant and their family/ caregiver. The grant funds may also be used to support developing agency-to-agency memoranda of understanding (MOU), training, developing and updating technology to improve data collection, and more.

Recommendations for Consideration

Promote and ensure a strong SAMHSA that serves as the lead Federal agency across the Federal Government on substance use disorder service delivery: We support maintaining investments in SAMHSA as the lead agency within HHS focused on substance use disorders. The nation benefits from a strong SAMHSA given the agency's longstanding leadership in the field. A strong SAMHSA includes a vibrant role for each of its centers—the Center for Substance Abuse Treatment (CSAT), Center for Substance Abuse Prevention (CSAP), Center for Mental Health Services (CMHS), and Center for Behavioral Health Statistics and Quality (CBHSQ).

NASADAD expresses our support for Dr. Miriam E. Delphin-Rittmon, Assistant Secretary for Mental Health and Substance Use and leader of SAMHSA, as she guides the agency and works across HHS to promote a unified Federal approach to substance use disorders. We strongly believe SAMHSA should be the default home of substance use disorder discretionary grants and programming related to prevention, treatment, and recovery. This requires financial resources but also the human resources needed to provide this leadership.

Ensure that Federal policy and resources related to substance use disorders are routed through the State alcohol and drug agency: State alcohol and drug agencies play a critical role in overseeing and implementing a coordinated prevention, treatment, and recovery service-delivery system. These agencies develop annual statewide plans to ensure an efficient and comprehensive system across the continuum. Further, State alcohol and drug agencies promote effective systems through oversight and accountability. Finally, NASADAD members promote and ensure quality through standards of care, technical assistance to providers, and other tools. As a result, NASADAD prefers Federal funding, programs, and policies designed to address substance use prevention, treatment, and recovery flow through the State alcohol and drug agency. This approach allows Federal initiatives to enhance and improve State systems and promotes an effective and efficient approach to service delivery. Federal policies and programs that do not flow through or at least coordinate with the State agency run the risk of creating parallel or even duplicative publicly funded systems and approaches.

Continued investment in the Substance Abuse Prevention and Treatment (SAPT) Block Grant while maintaining maximum flexibility: NASADAD's top programmatic discretionary grant program priority is the Substance Abuse Prevention and Treatment (SAPT) Block Grant. We sincerely appreciate the work of this Committee on this important program. In addition, we appreciate recent historic financial investments made by Congress in the SAPT Block Grant. In the context of reauthorization, NASADAD prefers to maintain as much flexibility as possible in the use of SAPT Block Grant funds consistent with the nature of, and benefits related to, the block grant mechanism. The flexibility afforded in the SAPT Block Grant allows States the opportunity to target resources based on the conditions on the ground as opposed to pre-ordained spending requirements.

Promote sustained and predictable funds through three-to 5-year discretionary grants: In addition to adequate resources, State alcohol and drug agencies note that sustained and predictable resources are absolutely critical. They allow States to partner with sub-State entities, providers, and others to plan activities in a systematic manner. One-and 2-year programs, with only a short-term commitment, can create an environment of uncertainty related to the future of a critical initiative that provides lifesaving services. It can be difficult, if not impossible, to successfully plan and operate programs with an eye on continuity of services if providers are not confident that resources will be available to serve their patients. NASADAD strongly supports the National Governors Association's (NGA) call to extend the duration of Federal grants beyond the typical one-or 2-year funding cycle to either a three-or 5-year cycle.

Ensure new Federal initiatives and funding complement and enhance the current system: NASADAD appreciates the many Federal legislative efforts to address substance use disorders that were found in the Comprehensive Addiction and Recovery Act (CARA), 21st Century Cures Act, and the SUPPORT Act. In the process, the Association has been partnering with Congress, the Administration, and non-governmental organizations to implement many of these initiatives. This includes work related to program management and implementation, data collection/ reporting, and engagement in the many day-to-day activities that ensure programs are managed effectively and efficiently. As a result, we recommend policies that complement or enhance the work that has already been done in order to leverage our collective response in an efficient and effective manner.

Continue to work to address the opioid crisis but also elevate efforts to address all substance use disorders, including those linked to alcohol and other substances: The opioid crisis is one of the worst public health tragedies in our nation's history. The sheer volume of death linked to this epidemic is difficult to grasp. We also know this country faces distinct challenges related to all substances whether it is prescription drug misuse, heroin, alcohol, marijuana, methamphetamine, cocaine or others. According to SAMHSA's National Survey on Drug Use and Health (NSDUH), alcohol remains a distinct problem in the country, with 28.3 million Americans battling an alcohol use disorder. As we look at those receiving publicly funded treatment, 31 percent of all admissions to treatment had a primary alcohol use disorder; 30 percent had a primary heroin or other opiate problem; and 11 percent had primary marijuana use disorder. State directors in certain States are also observing increases in problems related to methamphetamine and cocaine. As a result, NASADAD promotes policies and grant programs that are flexible yet also address the specific needs associated with the current opioid crisis. The flexibility included in the SAPT Block Grant also affords States the opportunity to target resources to address all substances.

Provide SAMHSA the authority and resources to help address the nation's substance use disorder workforce crisis: State alcohol and drug agency directors across the country are observing distinct workforce challenges. Quite simply, my colleagues note difficulties finding enough people to support prevention, treatment, and recovery programming. We understand the issue is complex. We also know there are many steps that need to be taken to buildup our workforce to meet the variety of needs related to substance use disorders. These steps include initiatives around recruitment, access to all levels of education, training, retention, salaries, and continuing education. There are strategies that can help loan repayment; scholarships; and early outreach in schools promoting a career that helps address substance use prevention, treatment and recovery. We recommend action to give SAMHSA the full statutory authority to help address our challenges related to the substance use disorder workforce. This includes action clarifying that SAPT Block Grant funds may be used to help States address workforce needs. Further, we support a specific proposal in CARA 3.0—Section 211—that would authorize a grant in SAMHSA's CSAP to State alcohol and drug agencies in order to bolster our nation's substance use prevention workforce needs as we are not aware of any Federal programs that currently address this.

Ensure that initiatives designed to implement 988 and crisis services improvement to specifically include programs and strategies to address substance use disorders: In 2020, the National Suicide Hotline Designation Act of 2020 was signed into law. The Act incorporated 988 as the new National Suicide Prevention Line (NSPL) and Veterans Crisis Line (VCL). We wish to express our appreciation for working to draft and approve this important piece of legislation to help reduce the number of suicides and improve our response to people experiencing a crisis. Since this time, SAMHSA has been actively working with stakeholders to prepare for the July 2022 launch of 988. This work includes the release of funds designed to help strengthen and expand existing Lifeline operations and telephone infrastructure along with funds to buildup staffing across States' local crisis call centers.

SAMHSA is partnering with States, providers, people with lived experience, and others to hold convenings in an effort to prepare for 988. These efforts include the complex task of strengthening our nation's service-delivery system for crisis services. We understand the launch of 988 is the beginning of a long journey that promises to help improve our approach to helping people experiencing a crisis. As we move forward, we ask that Congress and others elevate and specifically reference substance use disorders as a core focus of work related to crisis response. We believe this approach is needed given the many distinct and unique considerations that accompany service delivery for people with substance use disorders.

Maintain Recent Flexibilities to Ensure Access to Substance Use Disorder Services: The regulatory changes seeking to ensure continued substance use disorder service delivery during the COVID–19 pandemic should be maintained at least 1 year after the Federal Government determines the United States is no longer operating under a public health emergency. At this point, these policies should be further evaluated. These actions include the flexibilities regarding take-home doses of methadone for certain patients; the ability to initiate buprenorphine treatment for opioid use disorders without a face-to-face appointment; reasonable flexibilities related to HIPAA rules in order to allow service providers to utilize a variety of communication tools for service delivery; and others.

State alcohol and drug agencies play a critical role in the prevention, treatment, and recovery of substance use disorders and I look forward to working with the Committee on ways the Federal Government, States, communities, and families can work together to address this very important issue.

Thank you again for the opportunity to testify today and share my perspective. I look forward to any questions you may have.

[Summary Statement of Sara Goldsby]

Continued challenges with overdose deaths: Our country continues to see the devastating impact of substance use disorders across the country. The number of overdose deaths is staggering. In 2020, 93,331 individuals died from drug overdoses in the United States, the highest number ever recorded in a 12-month period and a 30 percent increase from 2019. Approximately 75 percent of overdose deaths involved synthetic opioids and illegally manufactured fentanyl (Centers for Disease Control and Prevention (CDC), 2021). In my home State of South Carolina, overdose deaths have increased by 60 percent over the past 5 years.

Challenges with many substances: Overall, almost one-third (30.3 percent) of individuals admitted to treatment in our country's publicly funded addiction system cited heroin or prescription opioids as their primary substance of use (TEDS/ SAMHSA, 2019). We also know substance use disorders impact different States, counties, and communities in many different ways. In South Carolina, for example, we are seeing a rise in admissions to treatment for alcohol use disorder. In particular, approximately 42 percent of treatment admissions reported a primary substance of alcohol or alcohol with a secondary drug (TEDS/SAMHSA, 2019).

Working through the pandemic: There is no doubt that the COVID–19 pandemic contributed to increases in problems related to substance use disorders. While the pandemic presented challenges to service delivery, we all worked together to adjust. States and providers developed innovative approaches to prevention, treatment, and recovery programming. Federal agencies and Congress worked to provide States and providers important flexibilities through program guidance and communication. In addition,

Congress and the Administration worked to provide critical funding for prevention, treatment, and recovery along with life-saving overdose reversal medication. I had the privilege of testifying before this Committee in April 21 to share some of this work.

Extra support and attention to help workforce challenges: I offer a number of recommendations below as we continue this work. All of these observations are critical. At the same time, it is my hope that extra energy is directed at addressing the many challenges related to our nation's substance use disorder workforce.

Recommendations:

- Ensure that Federal policy and resources related to substance use disorders are routed through the State alcohol and drug agency
- Promote and ensure a strong SAMHSA that serves as the lead Federal agency across the Federal Government on substance use disorder service delivery
- Provide SAMHSA the authority and resources to help address the nation's substance use disorder workforce crisis
- Ensure that initiatives designed to implement 988 and crisis services improvement to specifically include programs and strategies to address substance use disorders
- Promote sustained and predictable funds through three-to 5-year discretionary grants
- Continue to work to address the opioid crisis but also elevate efforts to address all substance use disorders, including those linked to alcohol and other substances
- Maintain Recent Flexibilities to Ensure Access to Substance Use Disorder Services

The CHAIR. Thank you. Dr. Lockman.

Statement of Jennifer D. Lockman, Ph.D., CEO, Centerstone Research Institute, Nashville, TN

Ms. LOCKMAN. Thank you.

The CHAIR. You want to make sure your mic is on?

Ms. LOCKMAN. Can you hear me now?

The CHAIR. No. We have a staff person—or Senator Burr?

Ms. LOCKMAN. Is that okay?

The CHAIR. There you go. Yes——

Ms. LOCKMAN. Okay, thank you for the help. I would like to thank Chair Murray and Ranking Member Burr and this Committee for your dedication to seeking solutions to the growing mental health and substance use crisis our country is facing today.

I would also like to thank Senator Braun for his leadership for the State of Indiana, which is one of the States we are proud to serve in. I am honored to be here as the voice of my colleagues at Centerstone, and most importantly on behalf of the people we serve. Centerstone is the Nation's largest nonprofit mental health company. Centerstone provides community based behavioral health care, substance abuse treatment, and intellectual and developmental disability services.

At Centerstone Research Institute, a Centerstone company, we conduct research to prevent and cure mental illness and addiction. We also work to translate data into meaningful clinical tools and practices, thereby reducing the research to practice gap. We applaud this hearing today because unfortunately deaths due to suicide, overdose, and drug and alcohol related disease are all too prevalent. As of 2020, suicide was the 12th leading cause of death in the United States for adults and the third leading cause of death for youth.

Between 40 percent and 50 percent of Americans have been exposed to suicide during their lifetime. This means that at least half of us sitting in this room today are likely to have been personally affected by the loss of someone that we loved to suicide. For this reason, Congress, in partnership with the Substance Abuse and Mental Health Services Administration, created the Garrett Lee Smith National Strategy for Suicide Prevention, Zero Suicide, and COVID–19 Emergency Response suicide prevention grants.

Centerstone Health Care System is honored to share our experience and the outcomes from some of our SAMHSA grants we have received. For our Zero Suicide SAMHSA grant, we are now working to spread evidence based practices known to decrease suicide throughout our entire health system and using data to make them even better. For example, we have updated our suicide prevention pathway to ensure everyone in our health care system gets evidence based suicide screening, risk management, and treatment.

We have moved toward a new screening system that first asks more about upstream risk factors for suicide, such as thwarted belongingness, perceived burdensomeness, and acquired capability for suicide, and then also asked about suicide directly through the PHQ–9 and C-SSRS. We anticipate the screening process helps us identify and treat drivers of suicide risk earlier and with better outcomes. We have also piloted a suicide prevention specialty care clinic, the first known and community mental health centers in the United States.

We expect all of our Centerstone clinicians to be able to identify and treat suicide risk. However, it is difficult and costly to keep all of our clinicians up to date on suicide specific treatments as fast as the science changes. In medicine, we have seen that people often get better outcomes at cost when at high risk by seeing medical specialists like cardiologists and oncologists.

Thus, through our grant, we are creating a referral system so that persons at the highest risk for suicide can also be seen by a specialist, someone who is trained in multiple suicide specific treatments, the very best that science has to offer. Our grants have also provided a crisis follow-up program for youth and adults during care transitions from inpatient facilities, a high risk period for suicide attempts and re-attempts.

Our data suggest this Federal program helps individuals reestablish connectedness, decrease their sense of burdensomeness, reduce suicidal ideation, and successfully linked to outpatient care 70 to 90 percent of the time. These services would be unbillable and impossible without the Federal SAMHSA grants.

Knowing this program works to save lives is especially timely given the July 2022 launch of 988 as a three digit dialing code for the National Suicide Prevention Lifeline. As we look toward launching 988, we must also continue to evaluate strategies to ensure services are funded and available nationally. This is why we also support the Behavioral Health Crisis Services Expansion Act as a crucial component to financing a crisis care continuum.

Another grant program that has been a lifeline is a Certified Community Behavioral Health Clinic, Medicaid demonstration, and CCBHC SAMHSA grant program. CCBHCs allow consistent care for those with mental health or substance use conditions and a place to go in times of crisis. This model is helping to address some of the dire workforce challenges our field has faced even prior to the pandemic.

We recommend continued investment in the CCBHC program. Centerstone is also pleased to be one of the only few comprehensive opioid recovery center grant recipients in the Nation. We recommend continued investment in this promising program. Of all the things you might take away from my testimony today, please be sure to hear this, Federal funding works. Federal funding saves lives. Federal funding helps prevent suicide and substance related deaths, uses program evaluation to help make evidence based programs even better, and helps individuals recover and contribute in their communities.

In the words of one of our clients, "there is no way to define a future if you are not there for it, and everyone is really focused on making sure that you stay there for it. Stay alive, stay safe. It has been really helpful for me to develop my own path. It has made a lot of difference."

It has been one of the great joys of my life to watch people go from a place of deep despair to go on to rediscover their talents, their strengths, and go on to build a life that they really want to live. Thank you, and I look forward to your questions.

[The prepared statement of Ms. Lockman follows:]

Prepared Statement of Jennifer Lockman

I would like to thank Chair Murray and Ranking Member Burr and this Committee for your dedication to seeking solutions to the growing mental health and substance use crisis our country is facing today. I'd also like to thank Senator Braun for his leadership for the State of Indiana, which is one of the states we are proud to serve in. I'm honored to be here as the voice of my colleagues at Centerstone and most importantly on behalf of the people we serve.

Centerstone is the nation's largest nonprofit mental health company. Centerstone provides community-based behavioral health care, substance-abuse treatment, and intellectual and developmental disabilities services in Florida, Illinois, Indiana, and Tennessee. At Centerstone's Research Institute (CRI), a Centerstone company, we conduct research to prevent and cure mental illness and addiction. We also work to translate data into meaningful clinical tools and practices, thereby reducing the research-to-practice gap.

We applaud this hearing today because unfortunately, deaths due to suicide, overdose, and drug and alcohol related disease are all too prevalent. As of 2020, suicide was the 12th leading cause of death in the United States for adults, and the 3d leading cause of death for youth. For every suicide death, there are approximately 1.1 million suicide attempts, or about one every 27.5 seconds (Drapeau & McIntosh, 2021). Between 40 percent to 50 percent of Americans have been exposed to suicide during their lifetime (Cerel et al., 2014; Feigelman et al., 2017). This means that at least half of us sitting in this room today are likely to have been personally affected by the loss of someone we loved to suicide. Although suicide deaths decreased approximately 3.4 percent between 2019 and 2020, perhaps due to a "pulling together effect" we have seen before during national crises, the deeply painful impact of suicide deaths on American individuals, families, and communities remains high (Drapeau & McIntosh, 2021; Joiner et al., 2006).

For this reason, Congress in partnership with the Substance Abuse and Mental Health Services Administration (SAMHSA) created the Garrett Lee Smith, National Strategies for Suicide Prevention, Zero Suicide, and Covid–19 Emergency Response suicide prevention grants. Centerstone's healthcare system is honored to share our experience and the outcomes from some of the SAMHSA grants that we have received.

Through our Zero Suicide SAMHSA grant, we are now working to spread evidence-based practices known to decrease suicide throughout our entire health system, and using data to make them even better. For example, we have updated our Suicide Prevention Pathway to ensure everyone in our healthcare system gets evidence-based suicide screening, risk management, and treatment. We have moved toward a new screening system that first asks about more "upstream" risk factors for suicide (such as thwarted belongingness, perceived burdensomeness, and acquired capability for suicide; Joiner et al., 2005), and then asks about suicide directly (PHQ–9; C-SSRS). We anticipate this screening process helps us identify and treat drivers of suicide risk earlier, with better outcomes (Louzon et al., 2016: Richards et al., 2019).

We have also piloted a suicide prevention specialty care clinic, the first known in Community Mental Health Centers in the United States. We expect all of our Centerstone clinicians to be able to identify and treat suicide risk; however, it is difficult and costly to keep all of our clinicians up to date on suicide-specific treatments as fast as the science changes. In medicine, we have seen that people often get better outcomes at cost, when at high risk, by seeing medical specialists (e.g., cardiologists, oncologists). Thus, through our grant, we are creating a referral system so that persons at the highest risk for suicide can be seen by providers who are trained in multiple suicide-specific treatments—the best that science has to offer.

Our grants have also provided a Crisis follow-up program to youth and adults during care transitions from inpatient facilities, a high-risk period for suicide attempts and re-attempts (Chung et al., 2017). Our data suggest this program helps individuals re-establish connectedness, decrease their sense of burdensomeness, reduce suicidal ideation, and successfully link to outpatient care (70–90 percent of the time). These services would be unbillable, and impossible, without the Federal SAMHSA grants. Knowing this program works to save lives is especially timely given the July 2022 launch of "988" as the three-digit dialing code for the National Suicide Prevention Lifeline (NSPL). As we look toward launching 988 we must also continue to evaluate strategies to ensure these data-supported services are funded and available nationally. This is why we also support the Behavioral Health Services Crisis Expansion Act (S. 1902) as a crucial component to financing a crisis care continuum.

Another grant program that has been a lifeline is the Certified Community Behavioral Health Clinic (CCBHCs) Medicaid demonstration and CCBHC SAMHSA grant program. CCBHCs allow consistent care for those with mental health or substance use conditions and a place to go in times of crisis. This model is helping to address some of the dire workforce challenges our field has faced even prior to the pandemic. We recommend continued investment in the CCBHC program. Centerstone is also pleased to be one of only a few Comprehensive Opioid Recovery Center grant recipients in the Nation. We administer this grant in Indiana, where we were able to train over 467 professionals in evidence-based practices and open a recovery house for women. We recommend continued investment in this promising program.

Out of all the things you might take away from my testimony today please be sure to hear this: Federal funding works. Federal funding helps prevent suicide and substance-related deaths, uses program evaluation to help make programs better, and helps individuals recover and contribute in their communities. Thus, it's critically important that future Federal grants to require evidence-based programs and data-driven program improvements. It has been one of the great joys of my life to watch our SAMHSA grant programs help individuals who previously did not want to live, rebuild a life based on their values, talents, and strengths, often overcoming psychosocial barriers and past trauma to do so. In the words of one of our clients: "There's no way to define a future if you are not there for it. And everyone is really focused on making sure that you stay there for it, stay alive, stay safe. It's been really helpful for me to develop my own path, and feel supported, but feel directed in ways that need to be. It's made a lot of difference."

Thank you, and I look forward to your questions.

I would like to thank Chair Murray and Ranking Member Burr and this Committee for your dedication to seeking solutions to the growing mental health and substance use crisis our country is facing today. I'd also like to thank Senator Braun for his leadership for the State of Indiana, which is one of the states we are proud to serve in. I'm honored to be here as the voice of my colleagues at Centerstone and most importantly on behalf of the people we serve.

At Centerstone's Research Institute (CRI), we conduct research to prevent and cure mental illness and addiction. We also work to translate research into meaningful clinical practices and implement research-based strategies in real-world settings, thereby reducing the research-to-practice gap. CRI's workforce is interdisciplinary and comprised of Physicians, Psychologists, Dissemination and Implementation Scientists, Counselor Educators, Program Evaluators, Social Workers, Public Health Advisors, Biostatisticians, Clinical Transformation Specialists, Design Thinking Experts, and others. Centerstone's Research Institute is a company of Centerstone, the nation's largest nonprofit mental health company who provides community-based behavioral health care, substance-abuse treatment and intellectual and developmental disabilities services in Florida, Illinois, Indiana, and Tennessee.

We applaud this hearing today because unfortunately, our rates of deaths of despair are rising. Deaths of despair are deaths by suicide, overdose, and disease due to excessive drug or alcohol use. Over the last 10 years, deaths of despair have increased nearly twofold to over 185,000 deaths in 2020 (CDC, 2022). Deaths of despair have increased so drastically that they have substantially impacted our life expectancy in the United States in 2015, marking the first decrease in life expectancy in decades; all of this occurring BEFORE the pandemic.

Today, mental health and addiction services are needed now more than ever as the COVID–19 pandemic has increased the prevalence and incidence of behavioral health disorders in adults and children/adolescents. Nationwide, 2020 was the deadliest year on record for fatal overdoses.[69] Within the pediatric population—children's emergency room visits related to mental health spiked dramatically—up 24 percent for kids 5 to 11 years old and 31 percent for teenagers 12 to 17 years old.[70] Even before the pandemic, 75 percent of U.S. counties experienced severe shortages of mental health providers.[71] As demand for behavioral health services continues to rise, and workforce challenges increase, providers around the Nation are struggling to meet the demand.

---

[69] https://www.politico.com/news/2021/07/14/covid-pandemic-drug-overdoses–499613.

[70] https://www.cdc.gov/mmwr/volumes/69/wr/mm6945a3.htm.

[71] Macher, D., Seidman, J., Gooding, M., & Diamond, C. (2020, May 11). COVID–19 is Stressing a Fractured Mental Healthcare System in the US. https://avalere.com/insights/covid–19- is-stressing-a-fractured-mental-healthcare-system-in-the-us.

As one of the nation's leading not-for-profit providers of behavioral health—we are acutely aware that mental health and substance use disorder challenges are a growing concern within our communities. We see it with our teachers, healthcare workers, our firefighters and police, our returning military service personnel, and our own families. To this end, in addition to our oral testimony, we offer several policy recommendations to address the nation's growing behavioral health needs that we believe are realistic, bipartisan, and aligned with the best science of care.

1. Advancing the Best Science of Care Relative to Suicide Prevention and Intervention; Particularly as the Nation Prepares to Launch 9- 8-8 in July of '22

In 2020, nearly 46,000 people died by suicide a slight decrease from the year before. However, this doesn't tell us the whole story. Deaths of despair have been rising dramatically in the US over the past decade. Deaths of despair is defined as all deaths by suicide, overdose, and disease due to excessive drug or alcohol use; it is a term often used because of their shared underlying factors and the difficulty to parse apart one death from the other (that is, suicides are often misclassified as overdoses). Over the last 10 years, deaths of despair have increased nearly twofold to over 185,000 deaths in 2020 (CDC, 2022). Deaths of despair have increased so drastically that they have substantially impacted our life expectancy in the United States in 2015, marking the first decrease in life expectancy in decades; all of this occurring BEFORE the pandemic (see table 1 and table 2).

In response to these alarming trends, Congress in partnership with the Substance Abuse and Mental Health Services Administration (SAMHSA) created the Zero Suicide Initiative and other grant programs aimed at suicide prevention. Indeed, research suggests that up to 90 percent of individuals at risk for suicide interact with healthcare systems within the year before there death, such that healthcare systems are an ideal place for suicide prevention and treatment (Ahmedani et al., 2019). Centerstone's healthcare system is honored to share our experience and the outcomes from some of the SAMHSA grants that we have received. I hope to illustrate that through national funding efforts, evidence-based practices, and data-driven program innovation, suicide deaths can be prevented.

Through our Zero Suicide SAMHSA grant, we are now using existing evidence- based practices known to decrease suicide throughout our health system, and using data to make them even better. For example, through our grant, we have updated our Zero Suicide Pathway to ensure everyone in our healthcare system gets evidence-based suicide screening, risk management, and treatment. Specific to suicide screening, we have realized through Centerstone data surveillance that the Columbia Suicide Severity Rating Scale (C-SSRS; Posner et al., 2011) works well at identifying many people who are suicidal and need care—but does not identify a group of individuals who may be most likely to die by suicide. For this reason, we have moved toward a new screening system that first asks about more "upstream" risk factors for suicide (such as thwarted belongingness, perceived burdensomeness, and acquired capability for suicide; Joiner et al., 2005), and then asks about suicide directly (PHQ–9; C-SSRS). In this way, we are building on the existing evidence to cast a "wider net," to potentially prevent and treat drivers of suicide risk earlier in the course of illness, and identify a unique cohort of individuals who may be at the highest risk for suicide who may not disclose if asked directly (Louzon et al., 2016: Richards et al., 2019).We were able to find this out due to data monitoring strategies enacted with Zero Suicide funding. As a result, we are able to apply lessons learned from this data by going upstream, testing new research ideas and asking different questions that target the DRIVERS of suicidal thinking (i.e., disconnection, burdensomeness) but not suicidal thinking directly.

Through our Zero Suicide SAMHSA grant, we have also piloted a suicide prevention specialty care clinic, the first known in Community Mental Health Centers in the United States. Whereas we expect all of our Centerstone clinicians to be able to identify suicide risk, manage risk at the appropriate level of care, and know at least one frontline evidence-based treatment for suicide, we realize it is difficult and costly to train all of our providers in multiple suicide-specific treatments and keep them up to date as fast as the science changes. In medicine, we have seen that people often get better outcomes at cost, when at high risk, by seeing a medical specialists (e.g., cardiologists, oncologists). It is possible, then, that the same may be true for suicide risk. Through our grant, we are creating a referral system to where persons at the highest risk can be seen by providers in our specialty clinic for their care. Our providers in this clinic have been well-trained in over six, modern, evidence-based, suicide-specific treatments and are well-equipped to manage high risk conditions and co-occurring diagnoses. Thus far we've had really great feedback and outcomes—both from the clinicians we've trained as well as the clients we're serving. As one of our clinicians stated recently: "My perspective on suicide prevention has changed significantly since I started being part of this clinic . . . I believe being part of this [specialty] clinic has helped me gain confidence in treating clients, reduced the fear in treating suicidal ideation/behavior, and start to have in-depth . . . conversations with clients about how to manage their crisis and explore steps toward a life worth living."

Table 1

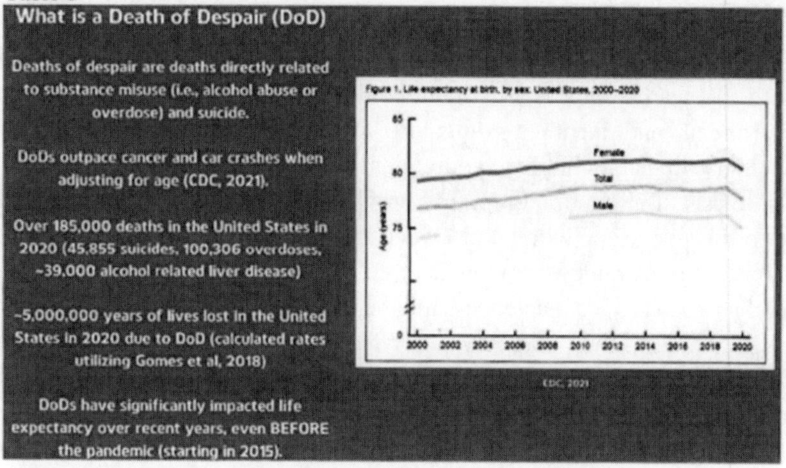

Table 2

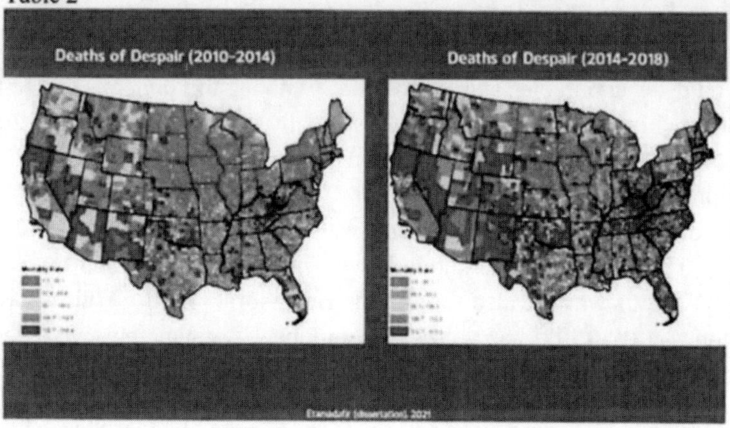

An additional area where we've applied our Zero Suicide funding is what is referred to as *"implementation science."* We know that a lot of treatments that are studied in the lab or university—as great as they are—once you put them in a real- world environment often times do not work in the way they were designed. This is because there are systems level barriers to where it may be harder to use those therapies or treatments in the ways that were studied. Implementation science helps us to truly understand how these approaches are implemented and how we can navigate workflow challenges and other community-level barriers to change our treatments so that they can be modified to truly work in real world practice settings.

We have also participated in several SAMHSA grants, such as the Garrett Lee Smith and National Strategy for Suicide Prevention Grants (GLS; NSSP) that have allowed us to provide suicide crisis follow-up services to adults and youth. Research suggests that individuals discharged from emergency departments and inpatient units are at high risk for suicide and often experience difficulty linking to outpatient care services (Chung et al., 2017). Our Crisis Follow-up Program provides phone calls to clients and a supportive phone app within the 4 weeks post-discharge. Our program uses an evidence-based framework (Joiner et al., 2005) to help adults and youth re-establish a sense of connectedness to others, re-discover and apply their talents and life values—such that they don't feel that they are a burden to others, monitor their suicide risk using a phone app, and successfully link to outpatient care. Data outcomes from our program suggest statically significant and clinically meaningful outcomes, including reductions in suicidal ideation, increases in self-efficacy to prevent suicide, and that between 70 percent to 90 percent successfully link to outpatient care (compared to the national average of 40 percent). It's critically important to note that, because adults and youth in this program are experiencing care transitions, these services provided to them would be unbillable, and impossible, without the Federal SAMHSA grants. Knowing this program works is especially timely given the July 2022 launch of "988" as the three-digit dialing code for the National Suicide Prevention Lifeline (NSPL).

As we look toward launching 988 we must also continue to evaluate strategies to ensure these data-supported services are funded and available nationally, this is why we also support the Behavioral Health Services Crisis Expansion Act (S. 1902) as a crucial component to financing a crisis care continuum. With appropriate funding and resources—we know we can prevent deaths and save lives. That's why this grant is so important. Additionally, we encourage Congress's consideration of longer term, more sustainable financing mechanisms.

As we look toward launching 988, we must continue to evaluate strategies to ensure these data-supported services are funded and available nationally. To that end, we recommend:

Passage of the Behavioral Health Services Crisis Expansion Act (S. 1902) as a crucial component to financing the crisis care continuum; and That the final Conference Report for the fiscal year 2022 Labor-HHS Appropriations bill include: 10 percent set-aside for mental health crisis systems in the Mental Health Block Grant (MHBG) program; $100 million to establish the Mental Health Crisis Response Partnership Pilot Program to help communities create mobile crisis response teams that divert the response for mental health crises from law enforcement to behavioral health teams; and $375 million to provide grants to Certified Community Behavioral Health Clinics (CCBHCs) to provide treatment for those with mental health illness.

Ultimately, we believe that our nation's ability to respond to behavioral health crises in the same way we respond to other medical emergencies—with prompt, effective, and culturally competent care—is essential to our collective well-being. With the new three-digit crisis number becoming universally available in July 2022, it is essential to act quickly to fund and implement important components of the overall 988 system.

Addressing the behavioral health workforce shortage, while increasing care integration/access

There are other community behavioral health and substance use disorder grants that have also made a meaningful impact on the people we serve. For example, a program that has been a lifeline is the Certified Community Behavioral Health Clinic (CCBHCs) Medicaid demonstration and CCBHC SAMHSA grant program. Our CCBHC program also allowed us, when the COVID–19 Pandemic hit, to examine if our clients were getting good outcomes via tele-health and phone compared to face-to-face treatment. Our evidence indicated they were, which has increased our continued application of telehealth throughout our operations to ensure patient access and outcomes.

On the whole, Certified Community Behavioral Health Clinics (CCBHCs) can play a transformative role in addressing historically dire workforce shortages, creating a more seamless/integrated care delivery system, and bolstering the nation's 988 preparedness; all while ensuring providers meet quality metrics. Specifically, these entities are designed to provide a comprehensive range of mental health and substance use disorder services to vulnerable individuals in a single location. CCBHCs are responsible for providing nine types of services, implementing evidence-based practices, coordinating care, and integrating with physical healthcare services.

To date, there are two types of this model—the grantees, which are in the pilot phase, and CCBHC Medicaid demonstrationsites which have permanently expanded the model and adopted a new payment methodologies, more akin to the FQHCs, to support on-going services.

Nationally, the CCBHC model has generated the following outcomes.

*Indiana Outcomes (*Pilot/Grantee Phase)*

The CCBHC model in Indiana has helped ensure positive outcomes among Centerstone clients, including:

73 percent of adult clients reported little/no depressed feelings 93 percent reduction of clients hospitalized for mental health reasons in previous 30 days 100 percent reduction of clients who utilized an emergency room for behavioral health issues in previous 30 days 64 percent increase in adult clients reporting their symptoms were not bothering them.

*Illinois Outcomes (*Pilot/Grantee Phase)*

The CCBHC model in Illinois has helped ensure positive outcomes among Centerstone clients, including:

50 percent decrease in homelessness 60 percent reduction of clients who utilized an emergency room for behavioral health 50 percent decrease in nights spent in jail

New York

New York officials reported that CCBHCs had a 54 percent decrease in the number of individuals using inpatient behavioral health services, which translated to a 27 percent decrease in associated monthly costs.

Texas

The CCBHC model in Texas is projected to save $10 billion by 2030; In 2 years, there were no wait lists at any CCBHC clinic; and

40 percent of clients treated for co-occurring SUD and SMI needs, compared to 25 percent of other clinics

Missouri

Overall access to mental health and addiction treatment services increased 23 percent in 3 years, with veteran services increasing 19 percent; and

Missouri found a 76 percent reduction emergency room visits and hospitalizations where CCBHCs were embedded in those facilities. In those same CCBHC areas, Missouri law enforcement saw a 55 percent decrease in interactions with people with behavioral health conditions.

Additionally, data from providers across the Nation has found that the CCBHC model significantly addresses workforce challenges.[72]

Specifically, the payment methodology associated with CCBHCs allows providers to reimburse for services they may not have a direct reimbursement for—i.e., assistance with addressing social determinants of health, robust care coordination, crisis services, and covering positions (i.e., peer support specialists) that may not be recognized by all payer types, etc. Many of these non-billable services and provider types are critical in providing coordinated care that results in increased patient outcomes as well as a financial model that supports the existing workforce.

It's estimated that as of January 2021 CCBHCs added 9,000 new positions nationwide; and On average, this resulted in 41 new jobs per clinic.

Given the growing need for improved access, bolstered workforce, and assurances that consumers received evidenced based treatments; *we support the passage of The Excellence in Mental Health and Addiction Treatment Act of 2021—S. 2069* led by Senators Stabenow (D-MI) and Blunt (R-MO) which would allow every State the option of joining the innovative Certified Community Behavioral Health Clinic (CCBHC) Medicaid demonstration and authorize grant (pilot) investments in the model for current and prospective CCBHCs.

II. Expanding Access to Telehealth Services for Behavioral Health Care

While we applaud inclusion of the telemental health services provision in the December 2020 end of year COVID relief package (Consolidated Appropriations Act of 2021, Section 123), we believe putting service restrictions on telehealth access for mental health services through in-person requirements undercuts the very tenets around the flexibility and access afforded by telehealth and other virtual care modalities. For example, under this new rule a beneficiary who—during the PHE was seeing a provider several hours from their home via telehealth—will have to now see their provider in-person, at least one time per year, to maintain continuity of care after the pandemic. This will most certainly delay or fully eliminate access to care for some consumers. Furthermore, the new requirement for an

[72] https://www.thenationalcouncil.org/wp-content/uploads/2021/05/052421—CCBHC—Impact Report—2021—Final.pdf—daf—375ateTbd56 (p. 7).

in-person visit applies only to mental health treatment, whereas Medicare beneficiaries seeking treatment for substance use disorder (SUD) via telehealth are not subject to this requirement. Given the elevated occurrence of SUD with mental health comorbidities, and recent reports indicating that 2020 was the deadliest year for overdoses,[73] this requirement ultimately creates new barriers which could result in significant delays in access to lifesaving care. Last, this requirement will further encumber already overworked providers to arbitrarily delineate between their patients on "who gets what type of service" based on diagnosis, rather than clinical presentation and best practice. This approach is counter to the gold standard of providing.

With regard to program integrity—telehealth, by design, is a transparent and accountable means of care delivery. Technology platforms that provide telehealth are currently capable of capturing a range of data points from telehealth and telephonic encounters that can offer transparency to the delivery of virtual care and protect against fraudulent actors. Unlike in-person care, telehealth encounters conducted over platforms such as Electronic Health Records (EHRs) or other tech-enabled landscapes that automatically capture the time call took place, duration, patient information, and other details that can be used to strengthen compliance efforts. As long as the provider is utilizing a technology platform that records relevant data, it does this for every connection—making the engagements recordable, auditable, and actionable.

In order to address this telemental health access gap, we recommend passage of The Telemental Health Care Access Act—S. 2061 led by Senators. Smith (D-MN), Cassidy (R-LA), Cardin (D-MD), and Thune (R-SD). The Telemental Health Care Access Act would provide continuity in behavioral health care access by removing the statutory requirement that Medicare beneficiaries be seen in person within 6 months of being treated for a mental health service via telehealth.

In summary, Federal funding works. Through these grants, our clients are establishing safer, better lives they are wanting to live, and we couldn't provide this treatment without these grants. We need to continue to ensure that SAMHSA grants require the implementation of evidenced-based services, so we can test these models and iterate based on lessons learned. Additionally, we need to look toward nation-wide, sustainable means of funding for areas where the data has indicated need and benefit to consumers.

---

[73] https://www.politico.com/news/2021/07/14/covid-pandemic-drug-overdoses–499613 the "rig ht care at the right time" to improve patient and population health outcomes.

Broadening insurance and telehealth coverage for the full continuum of behavioral health services—and, in particular, crisis care—as well as advancing CCBHCs can play a transformative role in meaningfully addressing our nation's growing behavioral health crisis.

Thank you for your continued focus on this important matter, if there are any additional questions and/or data we might be able to provide—please do not hesitate to reach out by contacting either myself or Lauren Conaboy, VP of National Policy, Centerstone at *lauren.conaboy@centerstone.org.*

[Summary Statement of Jennifer Lockman]

As of 2020, suicide was the 12th leading cause of death in the United States for adults, and the 3d leading cause of death for youth. For every suicide death, there are approximately 1.1 million suicide attempts, or about one every 27.5 seconds (Drapeau & McIntosh, 2021).

For this reason, Congress in partnership with the Substance Abuse and Mental Health Services Administration (SAMHSA) created the Garrett Lee Smith, National Strategies for Suicide Prevention, Zero Suicide, and Covid–19 Emergency Response suicide prevention grants.

Through our Zero Suicide SAMHSA grant, we have updated our Suicide Prevention Pathway to ensure everyone in our healthcare system gets evidence-based suicide screening, risk management, and treatment. We have moved toward a new screening system that first asks about more "upstream" risk factors for suicide (such as thwarted belongingness, perceived burdensomeness, and acquired capability for suicide; Joiner et al., 2005), and then asks about suicide directly (PHQ–9; C-SSRS).

We have also piloted a suicide prevention specialty care clinic, the first known in Community Mental Health Centers in the United States. Through our grant, we are creating a referral system so that persons at the highest risk for suicide can be seen by providers who are trained in multiple suicide-specific treatments—the best that science has to offer.

Our grants have also provided a Crisis follow-up program to youth and adults during care transitions from inpatient facilities, a high-risk period for suicide attempts and re-attempts (Chung et al., 2017). Our data suggest this program helps individuals re-establish connectedness, decrease their sense of burdensomeness, reduce suicidal ideation, and successfully link to outpatient care (70–90 percent of the time).

These services would be unbillable, and impossible, without the Federal SAMHSA grants. Knowing this program works to save lives is especially timely given the July 2022 launch of "988" as the three-digit dialing code for the National Suicide Prevention Lifeline (NSPL).

Another grant program that has been a lifeline is the Certified Community Behavioral Health Clinic (CCBHCs) Medicaid demonstration and CCBHC SAMHSA grant program, which allow consistent care for those with mental health or substance use conditions and a place to go in times of crisis.

Centerstone is pleased to be one of only a few Comprehensive Opioid Recovery Center grant recipients in the Nation. We administer this grant in Indiana, where we were able to train over 467 professionals in evidence-based practices and open a recovery house for women.

All the things you might take away from my testimony today please be sure to hear this: Federal funding works. Federal funding helps prevent suicide and substance-related deaths, uses program evaluation to help make programs better, and helps individuals recover and contribute in their communities. We need to continue to ensure that SAMHSA grants require the implementation of evidenced-based services, so we can test these models and iterate based on lessons learned. Additionally, we need to look toward nationide, sustainable means of funding for areas where the data has indicated need and benefit to consumers.

The CHAIR. Thank you very much. Ms. Rhyneer, we will turn to you.

Statement of Claire Rhyneer, Mental Health Youth Advocate, Anchorage, AK

Ms. RHYNEER. Chair Murray, Ranking Member Burr, Senator Murkowski, and Members of the Committee, thank you for having me here to testify today. My name is Claire Rhyneer, and I am from Eagle River, Alaska. In high school, I was a storyteller and facilitator for mental health advocacy through storytelling.

This organization is a youth led, youth founded group of Anchorage students working to decrease stigma and increase access to mental health resources. Last year, I worked as a program and outreach coordinator for NAMI Anchorage, the Alaska affiliate for the National Alliance on Mental Illness.

I am here today to advocate for youth who have or currently are experiencing mental health conditions. I am advocating for myself, for my peers, for Alaskan youth, but also for youth across the Nation to give them a voice. To be completely clear, the people who most need the services are least able to be here advocating. I am representing the tip of the iceberg.

A few years ago, I experienced a difficult and dark period of depression. But more than being difficult and dark, my experience was governed by confusion. I was self-harming and all I felt was uncertainty. I asked myself, do I need help? How should I know? I turned to Google, taking dozens of are you depressed quizzes. However, Google is not a doctor and is in no position to diagnose a middle school girl or anyone. It left me more confused. Each night, I wondered what was wrong, and in hindsight, it is terrifying to know that I was physically harming myself and still unsure if I needed support. What I uncovered online and on social media was horrifying.

The photos, videos, and stories were disturbing, but it was even more disturbing to discover that I was attracted to it and found myself going back to it. No one bullied me or neglected me. From an external perspective, my life was perfect. But mental health was never discussed at school, at home, or even in my health classes beyond the, take care of yourself, get sleep, eat well, and exercise spiel.

I kept telling myself everything was okay, Why should I feel sad? Why should I feel lost? I am so fortunate. How could I possibly feel this way? Ultimately, I didn't seek help because I didn't know if anything was wrong. And I am more than an anecdote. When I tell a roomful of people that I was confused or that I turned to Google for help, I see a course of nods.

I need more than one hand to count the number of close friends who have experienced suicidal ideation. And barriers to care do not discriminate. They infiltrate every home, regardless of ethnicity, class, or geography. Compared to most, I am privileged. Finding a community of peers let me know that I was not alone. I was once again able to be focused on school, sports, my family and friends. I learned how to maintain my wellness. And I am proud to be able to say, I know where you are coming from, and this pain can be temporary and to know that it is true.

The people who did not find these supports, unlike me, are not here. Many of them will never be able to tell us their story. So we have an obligation to these youth to make a difference. We need to support school counselors, station social workers in schools, fund wellness programs at universities, and introduce mental health curriculum into health classes where they belong.

We must reflect on the way we separate academic success from mental well-being. We need to make care more affordable, and insurers incorporated into primary care and that it is covered by insurance. We need culturally competent health care workers and diversity among providers. We need to reduce stigma, promote early intervention, normalize mental health conversations early, and educate our youth, teachers, and parents.

Those of us who know suicide and mental illness are preventable are watching the leaders of this country and waiting for you to do something. And the ones who think suicide and suffering is inevitable, they need you. Vulnerability is contagious and powerful.

I am here in the hopes that my story might inspire change, both for all of us to work toward healthier communities, but also to inspire other young people who may be listening. If you are suffering, I urge you to speak up. Thank you.

[The prepared statement of Ms. Rhyneer follows:]

Prepared Statement of Claire Rhyneer

Chair Murray, Ranking Member Burr, Senator Murkowski, and Members of the Committee: Thank you for having me here today to speak from the perspective of a young person who understands the importance of mental health awareness.

My name is Claire Rhyneer, and I am from Eagle River, Alaska. In high school I was a storyteller and facilitator for MHATS (Mental Health Advocacy through Storytelling). MHATS is a youth-led, youth-founded group of Anchorage students working to decrease stigma and increase access to mental health resources through true, personal, short stories of mental health struggle and triumph. Last year, following my work with MHATS, I worked as Program and Outreach Coordinator for NAMI Anchorage, the Alaskan affiliate for the National Alliance on Mental Illness.

I'm here today to advocate for youth who have, or currently are experiencing mental health conditions. I'm advocating for myself, for my peers, for Alaskan youth, but also for youth across the Nation to give them a voice.

To be completely clear, the people who most need the services are least able to be here advocating. I am representing the tip of the iceberg.

A few years ago, I experienced a difficult and dark period of depression. But more than being "difficult" and "dark" my experience was governed by confusion. I was self-harming and all I felt was uncertainty. I asked myself: Do I need help? How should I know? I turned to Google, taking dozens of "Are You Depressed?" quizzes.

However, Google is not a doctor and is in no position to diagnose a middle school girl—or anyone. It left me more confused. Each night I wondered not only what was wrong, but if something was wrong at all. In hindsight, it is terrifying to know that I was physically harming myself and still unsure if I needed support. No one bullied me or neglected me. From an external perspective, my life was perfect. I was getting good grades, my parents loved and cared for me, and I had friends I could talk to. But mental health was never discussed at school, at home, or even in my health classes, besides the "take care of yourself, get sleep, eat well, and exercise" spiel.

In the absence of relevant information, I turned to online communities. What I uncovered on social media was horrifying. I could find images, drawings, stories, even videos of intense self harm. It was disturbing to find, but it was even more disturbing to discover that I was attracted to it and found myself going back to it.

I still cannot look back at the journal entries from those years, but I know I wrote down "I don't know what is happening to me" over and over and over again. I kept telling myself everything was okay. *Why should I feel sad? Why should I feel lost? I'm so fortunate, how could I possibly feel this way? Maybe I'm making this all up in my head,* I thought.

Ultimately, I didn't seek help because I didn't know if anything was wrong. I didn't believe myself. It's like having a broken leg and telling yourself that you're just imagining the pain, it will go away on its own, and there's no bother in telling anyone because it's probably not a real problem. I told myself my self harm was just for attention.

I am more than an anecdote. When I tell a roomful of people that I was confused, or that I turned to Google for help, I see a chorus of nods. I can count on more than one hand the number of close friends who have experienced suicidal ideation. Starting in middle school, there were nights when I wasn't sure if I would see my friend the next day at school.

In suicide prevention, we emphasize that there is no one reason that someone dies by suicide. There are always a multitude of factors. Not only do college and university therapy offices have months-long waitlists, but private practitioners are cost-prohibitive and aren't covered by insurance. High school counselors are scarce and ill-equipped. Many youth never even reach the point of asking for help. They are like me. They doubt and diminish their experience. They don't believe anything is wrong. They're scared to reach out. They're worried about what their community will say. They think their family will crack jokes or not take them seriously. They expect their parents to blame themselves. They're afraid they'll be seen as "weak," "crazy," "attention-seeking," "wacko," "broken," or a "lost cause."

These barriers to care do not discriminate. They cross every border and infiltrate every home, regardless of race, class, or geography.

However, living in Alaska poses unique challenges. First, Alaska's dark winters make SAD (Seasonal Affective Disorder) more prevalent. In areas near the equator, only 1 percent of the population experiences SAD. In Alaska, that number is closer to 10 percent. Second, the generational trauma our Alaska Native populations suffer from colonization contribute to higher rates of substance use and mental health conditions. Third, the prevalence of guns in Alaska generate higher suicide rates. Alaska Native men between the ages of 15–24 have the highest rate of suicide among any demographic in the country. Fourth, providers are few and far between, especially in rural areas and small villages. Youth who need services must fly 2 hours away from their home, leaving behind their family and support systems. While telehealth has become more accessible, good weather, power, wifi, and service are not guaranteed. Fifth, the services Alaska does have are limited. They are overwhelmed, underfunded, and exhausted. While I worked at NAMI, I had to tell people they would be on a waitlist for 9–12 months before they'd receive care from a case worker. It would be 3 months before the patient would even be contacted to confirm they were accepted as a patient. It would be another 6 months after that before they could talk to a case worker and begin care. And last, transportation is especially onerous in Alaska, even in its central hub, Anchorage. People who signed up for NAMI recovery programs canceled after they realized it wasn't virtual. They couldn't afford transportation for the few miles between their home and our centrally located office building.

The Covid–19 pandemic exacerbated and introduced new issues. During typical high school classes, a teacher is one of the first lines of defense. They can catch changes in a student's behavior, performance, and attitude. But during zoom classes, I stared at a screen of gray squares. Questions from the teacher were met with silence. Teachers found fewer opportunities to ask, "Hey, are you okay?" "How are things going at home?" "You seem a little off, is there anything you want to talk about?" Furthermore, during the first year of online school, student support programs disappeared. Suicide prevention trainings and presentations were put on hold. General clubs moved online and lost attendance. Sport games and races barred spectators and family members. Students in unsafe families couldn't find the security they typically found at school.

Compared to most, I am privileged. In my Junior year, I was introduced to YANA (You Are Not Alone) Club, suicide prevention trainings, and MHATS. It was my own friends at MHATS who taught curriculum related to mental health and helped me tell my story. It's because of these resources and education that I opened up to my parents last year. I am now able to be focused on school, on sports, on my family and friends, and maintain my wellness. I am proud that I am now able to point my friends in the right direction when they express similar feelings. I am proud to be able to say "I know where you're coming from," or "I know how that feels." I am proud to be able to say "this pain can be temporary" and to know that it is true.

But this is only true because of the education and support I received. We need to support school counselors, station social workers in schools, fund wellness programs at universities, and introduce mental health curriculum into health classes where they belong. We must reflect on the way we separate academic success from mental well-being. We need to make care more affordable, ensure it's incorporated into primary care, and that it's covered by insurance. We need culturally competent health care workers and diversity among providers. We need to reduce stigma, promote early intervention, normalize mental health conversations early, and educate our youth, teachers, and parents.

We cannot be satisfied with allowing our children and youth to be educated by mental health through social media and searching online. We cannot be complicit in allowing my friends and classmates and your kids and neighbors to suffer in silence. We cannot knowingly let our students experience the confusion, doubt, and harm that I felt.

I am here because I am a privileged voice. The people who are failed by this system aren't here. They can't be. They are busy going to school, they are caring for their families, they are working multiple jobs. They are searching "Am I depressed?" on Google and are self harming in their bedroom. Their friends are filling in as therapists, sacrificing their own well-being to listen and support.

Those of us who know suicide and mental illness are preventable are watching the leaders of this country and waiting for you to do something. And the ones who think suicide and suffering is inevitable? They need you.

Thank you for inviting me to testify. I would not have been here without my peers at MHATS, the people at NAMI, my parents, and the friends and family who have been generous enough to share their stories with me and the rest of the world. Vulnerability is contagious and powerful. I'm here in the hopes that my story might inspire change—both for all of us to work toward a healthier community, but also to inspire other young people. If you are suffering, I urge you to speak up. Thank you.

[Summary Statement of Claire Rhyneer]

In high school, I was a storyteller and facilitator for MHATS (Mental Health Advocacy through Storytelling). MHATS is a youth-led, youth founded group of Anchorage students working to decrease stigma and increase access to mental health resources through true, personal, short stories of mental health struggle and triumph.

Last year, following my work with MHATS, I worked as Program and Outreach Coordinator for the Alaskan affiliate of the National Alliance on Mental Illness (NAMI) in Anchorage.

I am here today to advocate for youth who have or currently are experiencing mental health conditions. I am advocating for myself, for my peers, for Alaskan youth, but also for youth across the Nation to give them a voice.

Mental health was never discussed at school, at home, or even in my health classes, besides the "take care of yourself, get sleep, eat well, and exercise".

I didn't seek help when I was experiencing mental health issues, because I didn't know if anything was wrong. I did not believe myself. I told myself my self harm was just for attention.

The Covid–19 pandemic exacerbated and introduced new issues. During online school, teachers found fewer opportunities to ask, "Hey, are you okay?" "How are things going at home?" "You seem a little off, is there anything you want to talk about?"

At school, I was introduced to YANA (You Are Not Alone) Club, suicide prevention trainings, and MHATS. It is because of these resources and education that I opened up to my parents last year.

I am now able to focus on school, on sports, on my family and friends. I learned how to maintain my wellness.

We need to support school counselors, trained social workers in schools, fund wellness programs at universities, and introduce mental health curriculum into health classes where they belong. We must reflect on the way we separate academic excellence, success and mental well-being. We need to make care more affordable, ensure it's incorporated into primary care, and that it is covered by insurance.

We need culturally competent health care workers and diversity among providers. We need to reduce stigma, promote early intervention, normalize mental health conversations early, and educate our youth, teachers, and parents.

The CHAIR. Thank you very much. I want to thank all of our witnesses, but Ms. Rhyneer, thank you so much for your very compelling personal story, your courage, and you are making a difference. We all appreciate it. With that, we are going to begin a round of 5 minute questions. I again ask my colleagues to keep track of the clock and stay within those 5 minutes.

I will begin with Dr. Prinstein. And as we all know, the last 2 years have been incredibly difficult in so many ways, but especially on children and youth. They have faced huge disruptions in their own lives. They have lost loved ones, including their parents. They have missed out on valuable time with their friends and teachers.

It has become so dire that some of our leading experts have declared a "national emergency" when it comes to child and adolescent mental health. You know, as a mother, myself, a grandmother, and as a former preschool teacher, I am really worried about our kids right now. And we just heard very compelling story from one of them. I know parents from my home State of Washington all the way to here to the Capitol are really concerned about this.

I think it is really important to address the effects of trauma, substance use, grief, and other stressors on our kids. And I wanted to ask you today to talk with us about the best practices for identifying trauma and other stressors among our children.

Mr. PRINSTEIN. Thank you. We have a number of assessment tools that we can use to screen kids and to understand what their experiences may be or even before they experience a crisis. We need the support to be able to launch those tools and also to do research to examine how we can use technology to really make the most use of the kinds of passive screening or opportunities to intervene and offer mental health tips, anything that we can do.

In particular, this is really important when we think about underserved and underrepresented youth. It is absolutely critical that we are discussing mental health in schools that we are building into our curriculum social emotional competence.

We have the tools to build kids' resilience. We just need the opportunity to be able to teach what we know to all of those teachers and counselors and administrators so we can help them to identify kids before they reach a moment of trauma.

The CHAIR. Thank you. Dr. Durham, Dr. Goldsby, I want to talk about inequality within our health care system. It has really led to disparities in our health care access and outcomes and resources, and behavioral health is obviously no exception. When trying to get care, people of color often face systemic barriers and are less likely to complete treatment or even get appropriate services. Individuals with disabilities are five times more likely to have mental health needs, often can't find providers to get the care they need.

Meanwhile, in our rural communities, we face significant provider shortages, and members of the LGBT community are more likely to experience mental health and substance use disorders. So as this Committee now considers legislation to improve mental health and substance use disorder outcomes, we have to do everything we can to address those disparities.

Dr. Durham, I wanted to start with you. Your work is at a safety net hospital, and you see parents experiencing—patients experiencing mental health and substance use crisis. What barriers to care do your patients experience and how do they impact behavioral health outcomes and access?

Dr. DURHAM. Thank you, Senator Murray, for that question. You described a lot of things in your opening statement that are inequitable in substance use and mental health treatment in general. I think largely what many of us, as witnesses have said during our testimony so far, is that there is a huge inequity in just the workforce issue. Having mental health providers that maybe don't want to work with people with substance use issues, having folks with— that focus on substance use issues that don't want to work with the mental health aspect of the patient.

I think that adds a complexity when people want to go for care that they have to go to many different providers to get the treatment that they need. We need to stop siloing in health care in general and in the mental health care. This distinction that our physical health is separated from our mental health.

We see often that people get lost because they go from one provider to another trying to get the treatment they need and deserve, and they can't find one provider to do all of those things. The second thing I would say is that just in general, getting access to care is very hard for our patients. There are a lot of barriers when we start thinking about what substance use treatment programs only want to give medication versus thinking about other psychotherapeutic interventions.

How people get into treatment is very difficult sometimes. Unfortunately, providers will say, well, you need to go to the emergency room intoxicated to get a detox bed. If not, they are not going to accept you.

This is the reality of how patients get treatment in the system because of bed availability, because of the way reimbursement happens, because of the way insurers operate. And last but not least, I do want to think about how do we think about substance use in general, the inequity in that.

I think it is probably the only disorder that we consider a crime. You can get stopped, you can get pulled over for simply using or possessing this, and we don't treat it like other mental health or physical health issues. I do believe it is a brain illness. It is chronic. It is relapsing and remitting. And it deserves the full treatment like anybody with diabetes, hypertension, or any other condition.

The CHAIR. Thank you. And I am out of time with Goldsby. I am going to come back to you, if I can, later on to ask you that question. And I will turn it over to Senator Murkowski.

Senator MURKOWSKI. Thank you, Madam Chair. Claire, thank you. Thank you for your testimony. Very, very compelling and thank you for your voice, your leadership in this very important area.

I recall a visit that I made out to rural Alaska some years ago. It was a town hall meeting with Native leaders and young people from neighboring village had come to the town hall and asked to be recognized, and they raised the issue of suicide. None of the adults in the room wanted to talk about it.

The young people, one young man said suicide is becoming normal within our village as far as the youth were concerned, which was shocking and troubling. But it was almost as if there was a generational disconnect. The kids wanted to speak about it, needed to speak about it, and the elders in the room were afraid. They were afraid, I believe, that if they spoke about it, it might be encouraged.

You have been involved in suicide prevention trainings in school, peer to peer. Share with me a little bit, if you will, and the Committee, not only the importance of increasing access to these trainings and the recommendations for how we can reach out to kids, because again, it is younger—it seems younger and younger children are feeling these sense of depression and despair and crisis and suicidal ideation.

It is important how we speak to one another so that it is heard. Can you address how we can provide for more in the curriculum that is actually meaningful to kids? How can we provide for counselors who understand how to speak the language? Because I fear that there is a disconnect there.

Ms. RHYNEER. Absolutely. Thank you. Yes, suicide is a huge issue in Alaska and actually one thing Alaska does the CUBS Behavior Survey, and they show that the percentage of students attempting suicide has grown significantly in the past few years. So in 2019, 25 percent of all students in the school district seriously considered suicide and 20 percent of them attempted—20 percent of them attempted it, and so that is one-fifth of my classmates. But like, how many parents do you think knew about it? Do you think one-fifth of parents really knew that their student had seriously attempted suicide?

One thing that prevents students from talking about it is honestly the stigma that parents have. So they never even reach the point of asking me out or asking for help because they doubt and diminish their experience. They don't believe anything is wrong. They are scared. They think their family will crack jokes or not take them seriously, or they expect their parents to blame themselves.

They are afraid they will be seen as weak or crazy or attention seeking wacko, broken, a lost cause, any of those things. So reducing stigma in general, one of those things that we can do. Like in Alaska, what we are trying to do is pass a bill that would help bring mental health education into K–12 schools. So by talking about mental health in schools, specifically in health classes, we begin conversations early and allow space for people to share.

Health classes currently cover topics like nutrition and physical health, exercise, dental health, all these sorts of things, cancer prevention, and so mental health deserves to be a topic in one of those classes. It is just as important. And guidelines for this kind of curriculum would be developed with local and statewide and national agencies to make sure we are safe and age appropriate.

Of course, we wouldn't be teaching the same thing to high schoolers as elementary school kids, but it would help see symptoms and recognize them, and then what to do about them and reach out for help. So that is one really important thing.

Also, in terms of suicide prevention, just like clubs like you are not alone club, that those suicide prevention trainings in schools and goes around to classes and talks about it. That is a really important thing, too. So all of those things working together.

Senator MURKOWSKI. Thank you, Claire. Madam Chair, I am almost out of time, but I think every one of the witnesses in one way or another has talked about the need for workforce, and whether it is school counselors, those that can work with kids in programs, or whether it is all the way to the other end with a full psychiatric care that is available.

My hope is, is that we build out a package of focus on mental health. We really key in on the workforce issues because I think we recognize that in all our States, we are sorely, sorely lacking.

The CHAIR. Thank you very much. I look forward to working with you on that. Senator Casey.

Senator CASEY. Chair Murray, thank you for the hearing. And I want to thank you and Senator Murkowski and Ranking Member Burr, and of course our witnesses. I want to start with Director Goldsby with a question regarding plans of safe care.

This is an issue I have worked on for years to support both infants and families affected by substance use disorder. We know that infants and their parents need what I think most would refer to as non-punitive services, as well as treatment and support as parents navigate both recovery and parenting a young child. But despite longstanding Federal law, plans of safe care remain very much underutilized.

I appreciate the work of this Committee in the CAPTA legislation and authorization over time to address some of the issues that have contributed to these plans of safe care being underutilized.

Too many families are slipping through the cracks, and so in particular, I appreciate the effort to establish a reporting mechanism when an infant needs a plan of safe care that is separate from the child welfare system.

But Director Goldsby, I would ask you, what steps can we take in Congress, especially here in the Senate, to help States and communities adopt public health driven approaches to substance use in both pregnancy and as well as to reach more families in need of support?

Ms. GOLDSBY. Senator Casey, I am glad you asked. You know, I think thanks to the work of this Committee and CAPTA work that we have underway. We are currently engaged in some in-depth technical assistance with my agency and our South Carolina social services agency as we work hand in hand to develop a plan to address your exact concern.

Our Plan of Safe Care Workgroup is focusing on moving intervention services upstream, a more public health approach to support all pregnant individuals who might or may or may not have a substance use issue. But the screening earlier, having that universal screening brief intervention and referral to treatment for everyone earlier in pregnancy and often in pregnancy really minimizes additional prenatal substance exposure.

We have decided to call our plan of safe care a family wellness support plan because our aim will really be to initiate that prenatal plan sooner and as soon as the mother is identified, either with toxicology or the screening, so that we are offering a non-punitive, supportive set of services across our systems to include mental health and substance use treatment and all the wraparound services.

For some who have severe substance use diagnosis, this plan might include a referral to one of our family care centers, which is our residential treatment centers for women and children that are supported by the Substance Abuse Prevention and Treatment Block Grant, so that mothers can really stay engaged in services and supported through the delivery of their child. And that way, health care providers know that they are engaged, know that they are in treatment.

This is all going to lead to more likely results of family remaining unified at the time of delivery so that the mother and the children can continue on in that residential treatment or be discharged home to community based services.

But a lot of education has to be done among our health care community for them to understand that, like we mentioned, substance use disorders is not a moral failing, but is a health care issue, a disease State, and that people with mental health and substance use issues really shouldn't be further stigmatized but assisted.

I will just note that all of this work is supported by our Pregnant and Parenting Women program through SAMHSA, our expert work supported by SAMHSA discretionary grants and, of course, our Block grant.

Senator CASEY. Director, thank you for your work, and I appreciate your answer. I wanted to turn to Dr. Prinstein. On page 16 in your testimony, you note that implementation of integrated care, where primary care and behavioral health care providers work as a team, remains unfortunately limited.

While there are a lot of models that integrate physical and mental health care, many physicians still don't have the ability to seamlessly connect patients to a mental health provider.

You mentioned some of the barriers, whether it is physical space or IT issues or clinical staffing. What should we do in terms of our focus to help more primary care providers move toward integrated care, and how can telehealth support the shift?

Mr. PRINSTEIN. Thank you. Integrated care is, in fact, an excellent way to go. As we just heard before, it is very hard for people to find a health care provider and a mental health care provider. And due to stigma, sometimes even pursuing that in person is difficult.

But walking into your physician's office is not attached to stigma. Three things to remember with integrated care. One, it is a lot more than just sticking to mental health care provider into the office of a physician.

This is really about the time and the funding that is required for cross training so that way physicians and mental health care providers can speak different language—each other's language, share records, share billing processes. These are usually not the traditional 1 hour sessions with the mental health care provider, so new billing processes are needed.

Two, substantial infrastructure costs are required to successfully integrate the integrated behavioral care, to implement that. So it is important to incentivize physicians to do so. And finally, a one size fits all approach is just not going to work with integrated behavioral care.

We have evidence that all approaches can be very effective, and primary care providers needs to be the folks to decide how best to set it up in a way that meets their needs, their patients, and their community.

Senator CASEY. Thank you, Doctor. Thank you, Chair Murray.

The CHAIR. Thank you.

Senator Collins.

Senator COLLINS. Thank you, Madam Chair. Dr. Prinstein, I want to discuss with you the impact that the prolonged COVID pandemic has had on our children's mental health. I was struck by two recent columns and the New York Times, written by David Leonhard, in which he makes the point very well. He writes, "the pandemic's disruptions have led to loss learning, social isolation, and widespread mental health problems for children.

Many American children are in crisis"—and here is the important point—"as the results of pandemic restrictions rather than the virus itself." We know, as Senator Murray has mentioned, that three medical groups representing pediatrics, child psychiatrists, and children's hospitals have recently declared a national emergency in child and adolescent mental health.

The New York Times columnist has concluded that remote schooling has failed and that there is little evidence that shutting schools leads to fewer COVID cases among children.

Given that the pandemic has persisted for 2 years, which is a good portion of many children's lives, what should we be doing as policymakers to balance pandemic response policies with the serious concerns that many parents have expressed to me about their children's—the impact on their children's mental health, the social isolation, the remote learning, the restricted activities that they are seeing directly are harming their children's social and mental development?

Mr. PRINSTEIN. Thank you for raising that, Senator Collins. APA joined with HIA and AAP in declaring that national emergency, and we agree. The science is telling us that kids are experiencing mental health difficulties for a whole host of reasons. One is, of course, the major stressor that has occurred in their lives. They are watching relatives that are passing away or being so ill that they need to go to the hospital. They have tremendous disruption of their roles and routines.

They see polarization in leaders with disagreements between parents and schoolteachers on what it is that they are supposed to do. And they are having a very difficult time also with social isolation, but not necessarily because of the isolation per se, but because of the time that kids are spending on social media instead, which we now know has incredibly dangerous effects not only on kids development but on the development of kids' brains during that time.

This is a very big issue and very concerning. It also is an opportunity. This is a time when we have people talking about mental health like they have never talked about before, and people are recognizing the need for us to be addressing mental health before it reaches the acute crisis, excuse me, of people needing to go and get outpatient or inpatient treatment.

This is an opportunity for us to really build into the fabric of how we educate, how we talk within our communities, the importance of mental health and resilience programs. Our entire mental health system right now is built for adults. It is built also for people who are already at the point in a crisis and need treatment. That is not what the science suggests. What we could be doing now and what this presents us with an opportunity to do is to pay attention to all of those folks who are at risk or who have not even shown any psychological symptoms yet and build the resilience necessary to ensure that they will never need outpatient or inpatient treatment.

That is what we are seeing with kids right now. There is a wide openness to talking about these issues, and kids, just as Ms. Rhyneer was talking about so eloquently, want us to step up and teach them information about mental health so they can learn the skills before they reach a crisis point.

Senator COLLINS. Thank you. Dr. Goldsby, my time is almost expired, but an estimated 636 people in Maine died from drug overdoses last year. That is a terrible and alarming record high.

But what it obscures is the actual number of overdoses which was in the neighborhood of 8,000 overdoses in the State of Maine, where thanks to the heroic efforts of first responders, medical professionals, and sometimes bystanders, they were saved.

How can we ensure that non-fatal overdose patients are not just a statistic, but receive the care that they need to prevent a subsequent and potentially fatal overdose?

Ms. GOLDSBY. Senator Collins, we talk about overdose reversal in South Carolina as an intervention. And it is in that moment when somebody has faced a life threatening situation that they may be best reached by someone who offers them hope, hope to live, hope to a path to recovery, and I think those intervention services are key as we do more outreach, as we have our first responders saving lives, taking advantage of this critical crisis moment to engage people in services that will lead them on a path to long term recovery.

That can look at a number of ways with a number of different programs, but I think it is taking advantage of that moment, that lifesaving moment that we really engage in treatment services.

Senator COLLINS. Thank you.

The CHAIR. Thank you.

Senator Baldwin.

Senator BALDWIN. Thank you, Madam Chair. In 2019, I introduced the bipartisan National Suicide Hotline Designation Act, which was signed into law in 2020. Converting from the existing 10 digit number to 9–8–8 will make it easier for Americans to get the help they need, and I am proud of the investments included in the American Rescue Plan to support this transition.

Dr. Lockman, as you know, the 988 dialing code will be available nationally for calls, texts, or chat beginning in July 2022. What else should we be doing in Congress right now to make sure that the lifeline is equipped to facilitate real access to care? And how can we make sure that the lifeline reaches those in greatest need, including our LGBTQ youth?

Ms. LOCKMAN. Thank you so much for that question and thank you for your support. As you know, the advent of 988 opens up a whole new opportunity for people to have ready access to mental health care providers and paraprofessionals in ways that they haven't before. There is a couple of things that I think of in terms of what we can do to make sure that we are prepared for this transition.

The first one is to make sure that everyone has access on the crisis hotline to the very best in training. We know that the science advances so fast and there needs to be continued training and retraining to make sure we are using the very best practices to take care of people. For example, we rarely use language such as committed suicide anymore because it denotes that it is a crime. Instead, we say, died by suicide, and that is important for someone to know.

We also talk about things such as it is important to not die, not just for the sake of not dying, but for the sake of having time to transition to recovering the life that you really want to live. So one thing is making sure that there is continued investment and support and making sure that every single person, whether you are the person that they call or that they text, is ready and equipped to provide evidence based practices, interventions, and the language around suicide, safer care.

The other thing that I think about in terms of making sure that everyone is equipped to reach a care provider who cares about them, including our LGBTQ community, is making sure that we are using inclusive language and the messaging around 988 and making sure that everyone knows that they have a safe place to go when they are talking about suicide.

We have seen in our own SAMHSA grant programs, including serving this community, that talking about connectedness, talking about mental health wellness, talking about meaningful living, and as others have testified, moving the language more upstream to where everyone has a place to grow and become their very best self, this language is likely as important as talking about reducing suicide.

Thank you for your attention to this very important transition. The third thing I will say is that we need to make sure that we are building out the entire crisis continuum. 988, as we know, is the starting place.

But there also are plans to go into making sure that our mobile crisis services are well-equipped and well-trained, and also making sure that we are standing up other crisis infrastructure. For example, and there is over 600 CSUs, or Crisis Stabilization Units, operating in the United States right now. That provides a really important and critical part of the crisis continuum to make sure that there is diversion from emergency Departments.

The emergency Departments are wonderful in terms of being able to, when people are well-trained, to address and prevent suicide. But CSUs have a different model. They have a living room model to where you are coming in and treated from a standpoint of recovery from the beginning, and also treated with peer support, with a focus on growing and wellness and recovering from suicide or substance abuse or other host of other concerns.

I thank you for your support and making sure that we are building out the entire continuum to make sure that someone reaches someone well-trained who can respond to their immediate need, but also can put them on the path to long term growth, wellness, and well-being.

Senator BALDWIN. Thank you. Dr. Prinstein, it sounds like you would like to also reply. Please do.

Mr. PRINSTEIN. Thank you. I have spent the last 22 years doing research on suicidal youth, those who are at most risk, and thank you so much for the work you have done to establish 988. It is incredibly important that when folks call, of course, they are getting treatment that is likely to work.

We now only have science to support one approach to treatment, and the vast majority of folks are not trained in that approach. It is very, very important that we increase the training of providers. In addition, it is important that we have culturally competent providers, so folks are able to call and understand the embeddedness of suicidal thoughts within their communities.

When I have done that research, we found that suicidal participants would call 10, 12 outpatient providers and not be able to find anyone who would take their case. We need more people trained in suicide.

We need more people trained to deal with the scientifically evidence-based approaches to suicide, in particular. Happy to help in any way that we can.

The CHAIR. Thank you. Senator Cassidy.

Senator CASSIDY. Thank you all. Dr. Durham, great to see you.

Dr. DURHAM. Great to see you as well.

Senator CASSIDY. For my colleagues, Dr. Durham is a former student, and despite my training, heard has done very well.

[Laughter.]

Senator CASSIDY. And is the only one in the room who recognizes that I am wearing a Mardi Gras tie and trained in New Orleans. Everybody else thinks I can't match colors. Dr. Durham, you mentioned you opened a 56 bed facility. Now, I understand that Massachusetts has a waiver from the IMD exclusions.

IMD, which says that you can only have 16 beds in your facility. And the issue here is both cost, but the perception of going back to the bad old days when we just put people in a big warehouse of the mentally ill and not let them out.

But you mentioned as a positive that you are going beyond the 16 beds to 56 beds. Can you speak to the importance of that waiver or that ability to go above 16? Because I assume these are Medicaid patients?

Dr. DURHAM. Yes, many of them will be—thank you, Senator Cassidy. Again, good to see you as well. Many of them are Medicaid, Medicare, and we do see a very small number of privately insured folks at BMC. But the—BMC is a large safety net hospital for the city of Boston and beyond Boston, and we have never had our own inpatient psychiatric unit.

That has caused increased boarding in our own psychiatric emergency room, in our emergency room period, for decades. So a big investment of the hospital is like where do we send our patients who are on Medicaid or Medicare, because many of the facilities in and around Boston are also full in at capacity? And so it was an investment for our patients essential.

Senator CASSIDY. So just to be sure, unlike the kind of stereotype and the criticism that if you go beyond 16 beds you are just warehousing, here, you find that you are able to provide needed services that otherwise would not be available, correct?

Dr. DURHAM. I am not familiar with what you are talking about exactly, but what I can say is that we do need a continuum of care for mental health.

Senator CASSIDY. Sounds good.

Dr. DURHAM. So we need investment in community, in intermediate resources, and in inpatient level of care, so across the continuum.

Senator CASSIDY. And over 16 beds allows you to get an economy of scale as well as to provide more services. I will add that editorial because that is something for we policymakers to consider just to say that.

Dr. Lockman, in your full testimony, you mentioned the telemental health bill that we are trying to push out, and can you kind of comment upon the ability of allowing telemental health to address the person power shortage of providers that was previously referred to?

Ms. LOCKMAN. Absolutely. So when the pandemic hit at Centerstone, we had never used telling mental health widely, and we couldn't actually find research to understand the degree to which it would be effective, particularly in our population. Our population has a lot of community based needs, a lot of psychosocial barriers, and there was a great need to be able to reach them quickly.

We have done our own research in terms—and actually in part through the SAMHSA grant, so we are so thankful for that Federal funding. And we have seen that providing services via phone or telehealth has about the same outcomes as being seen face to face.

This has allowed us incredible mobility during the time of the pandemic. It has allowed our providers to see more patients, and it has also allowed more people to come and have better access to care that really transverses a lot of psychosocial barriers.

Senator CASSIDY. I am running out of time. To cut to the chase, you would highly recommend that Congress pass my bill.

[Laughter.]

Ms. LOCKMAN. We highly support telehealth services and phone based services for mental health services.

Senator CASSIDY. Sounds great. Dr. Prinstein, you highlight the importance of programs such as the programs for children with a serious emotional disturbance, which Senator Murphy and I were able to get passed as part of a bigger piece of legislation. And the Community Mental Health Block Grant targeting funds that children with serious emotional disturbances.

Now we have heard from States that because it is perceived in the regs that the child has to have a diagnosis of serious emotional disturbance before they would qualify to benefit from these funds, that we should make it clear that the funds could be used for preventive services to prevent a child from developing SED, if you will. Any comment on that?

Mr. PRINSTEIN. Yes. First of all, thumbs up on the toll the Mental Health Improvement Act. Excellent. Science supports that that is working.

Second, yes, there is a huge backlog right now for folks who are waiting to get an individualized education plan from a school psychologist, sometimes waiting years until they can get that diagnosis so they can access those funds.

I agree that having the ability to access funds for preventive services would be fantastic.

Senator CASSIDY. Okay, I am almost up. Now, Mr. Rhyneer, thank you so much for what you do. As someone whose family has being affected by suicide by a young person—I am sorry to be emotional.

Thank you. I yield back.

The CHAIR. Thank you. Senator Murphy.

Senator MURPHY. Thank you to this tremendous panel. Thank you, Madam Chair, for convening this hearing. Thank you, Senator Cassidy, for your heroic work, standing up for people with mental illness and learning disabilities. And if I can just for a moment lift up a piece of legislation that Senator Cassidy and I worked on and this Committee supported, we passed legislation through this Committee making real the mental health parity legislation that Congress passed decades ago.

The reality was we told plans to cover mental health just like you cover health the rest of the body, but it didn't work out that way. Plans ended up putting up all sorts of barriers and bureaucracy and red tape in front of getting reimbursement for mental health that they didn't for an orthopedic procedure or an operation on your heart or lungs.

One of the things we did a few years ago is require the Department of Labor and Department of Health and Human Services to do an audit of a select group of insurance plans. And we just got the report. It is both defeating and encouraging. It basically came to the conclusion that not a single insurance plan that they reviewed was in full compliance with parity.

But through these audits, they actually got the plans to change their practices and parameters such that now tens of thousands of mental health consumers are now actually getting what they paid for when they paid their insurance premiums. You know, an example is one insurance plan was covering nutritional therapy for diabetes, but was not covering it for anorexia, bulimia, or binge eating.

Another example was a plan was requiring prior authorization for all outpatient procedures for mental health and substance abuse but was not requiring it for a broad range of orthopedic procedures.

We are finally getting this right, and I wanted to maybe pose this question to you, Dr. Durham, to talk a little bit about your experience in dealing with insurance companies and families who are trying to get reimbursement, and the differences that you see in a big medical system in the way that barriers are put up when it comes to mental health and substance abuse that just don't exist when you are going to get the follow-up treatment on an operation on your knee.

I think we are making progress here thanks to this Committee, but I think we still have a long way to go.

Dr. DURHAM. Thank you, Senator Murphy, for your question. I agree completely that none of this is new to us that are on the front lines that are serving patients day in and day out. That—I have not read the report fully, but I understand that all in all that insurers are not allowing us to treat people with the best evidence and at all times, whether that is medication, whether that is therapy, whether that is trying to get them into another facility for more intense care.

What happens in our emergency room, for an example, is that we do have to get what we call a prior off, prior to sending someone to an inpatient psychiatric facility. You would never do that with someone who comes in with a heart attack to the emergency room. They immediately go and get the help they need on the medical floor and no questions asked.

We spend hours, sometimes, our social work colleagues, ourselves, our case managers in the emergency room just trying to get someone placed, and at times to the level of where someone like me as a physician has to do a doc to doc to essentially say our case, why do we want this patient to go into an inpatient psychiatric unit?

There are times where we are denied, and we have to figure out another level of care. In the outpatient world as well. I am a child psychiatrist and I see kids in the clinic, and I have been on the phone with an insurer as well when a medication adjustment needs to be made for hours.

My time in the clinical setting, where I should be seeing patients, is spent on the phone trying to essentially get a kid that was always on a medicine, but the formulary changed, and I wanted them to continue that medicine.

We need a lot of help in this area. We need to have parity for physical and mental health and not have to be at the beck and call, if you will, of these prior off.

Senator MURPHY. Very well said. And this is an issue I know that there will be bipartisan agreement on because we are just ask- ing for compliance to the existing law. We don't have to pass a new requirement to insurers. We just have to give the tools to the Departments to make sure that the insurers comply.

I am going to submit a question for the record to the panel with respect to how we get more professionals who are in contact with kids, a little bit of extra learning on mental health first aid and mental health diagnosis.

We spend billions of dollars on training for teachers, for pediatricians, and we could do better by giving a little bit additional help on identifying some of the root causes. And last, let me just say thank you to you, Ms. Rhyneer.

Thank you for speaking truth to power on this issue and for standing up for kids. I am a parent to a teenager and a pre-teen, and so I see the rabbit hole that kids can go down when they are experiencing those first signs of crisis given out online some pretty toxic information and influences are, and I think you have opened our eyes to that with your testimony today. Thank you, Madam Chair.

The CHAIR. Thank you. Senator Braun.

Senator BRAUN. Thank you, Madam Chair. In March 2021, American Rescue Plan was signed into law, $4 billion to address the opioid epidemic. But with that the lack of anything substantive in terms of trying to crack down on the source. Fentanyl is mostly made in China, trafficked through Mexico. Listen to these statistics. I want the public to hear it mostly.

100,000 Americans have died in the last year due to overdoses. Many of them, if not most of them, from fentanyl. This is the part that is most shocking.

In the age group 18 to 45, we have lost more young people from overdoses than COVID, car accidents, and suicides.

It is another example of where spending money was not a solution without real teeth, real substantive directives at the source of it. We visited the Southern border a little less than a year ago and we were going from record low illegal crossings to about 70,000 to 75,000. That is now leveled out at about 170,000.

I mean, appalling. I have got two questions, both for Ms. Goldsby. When it comes to not only the impact on losing lives, but along with workforce to boot, I think we have lost close to 2 million prime age workers due to the fact that they are contending with opioid issues, how much of this issue is directly related to the policies we have on our Southern border where illegal crossings are up, fentanyl comes along with it. How much is that contributed to this tragic loss of life?

Ms. GOLDSBY. Senator Braun, thank you for your question. You know, a couple of things, my expertise rests with prevention, treatment, and recovery service delivery, but from 2018 to 2019 in South Carolina, we were really making headway and saw the number of overdoses leveling off due to all of our efforts and all of the Federal funding with State targeted and State opioid response funds.

Since then, and in the last 2 years, our overdoses have sky-rocketed, and we are estimating about 63 percent of our overdose fatalities in 2020 were a direct result of the extremely potent illicit fentanyl and the drug supply.

I think in the last 2 years, we have pivoted to doing everything we can to keeping people alive and implementing evidence based harm reduction and intervention services. We have got naloxone everywhere that we can get it. The lifesaving antidote. With the flexibilities and the funding support from SAMHSA, we have been able to distribute fentanyl test strips to those individuals who may not know what substances they are ingesting as the illicit fentanyl has gotten into the methamphetamine supply and the cocaine supply.

The evidence suggests that people are better able to prevent an unintended overdose death if they use these fentanyl test strips, they are using less of the drug. And every interaction to get these supplies to people on the streets where they are is an opportunity to engage them in treatment services and get them on the path to recovery.

That is where our efforts are focusing so heavily now, and I will say we are not feeling defeated, but it has been a major setback in the last couple of years with how dramatically things have shifted.

Senator BRAUN. Well, thank you. I think without directly saying so by deduction, you can relate what is happening on the Southern border to what you are grappling with. Senator Markey and I have got two pieces of legislation about increasing provider and patient education.

One is the Label Opioids Act and the other the Safe Prescribing of Controlled Substances Act. Through your work in addressing the opioid epidemic, can you speak to the importance of provider inpatient education and how these bills might impact that? Ms. Goldsby.

Ms. GOLDSBY. Senator Braun, thank you. Sorry. I think the patient and provider education is key and we have a long way to go, especially with our provider education in all of our health care workforce.

I think that has been a theme today that we have talked about folks not understanding addiction and mental health issues as disorders, addiction issues as chronic diseases, and the evidence based services, interventions, and treatment models that address these disorders successfully. And so we have come a long way.

We have invested a lot in our response and in engaging the workforce as such. But I know that we have a long way to go, especially as we contemplate access and what that means for people who are approaching health care providers who don't or don't know how or don't address addiction appropriately.

Senator BRAUN. Thank you. I would like you and the other members of the panel to take a look at these two bills. It would be a small step in at least trying to get more information out there and to weigh in on maybe endorsing both of these pieces of legislation. Thank you.

The CHAIR. Thank you. Senator Kaine.

Senator KAINE. Thank you, Chair. What an excellent panel of witnesses and my colleagues have asked very, very good questions. I want to first put a challenge on the table that I may be asking my colleagues to help us resolve. Two officers who were here defending the Capitol on January 6 died by suicide in the days right after that attack. Howard Lieberman good was a Capitol Police officer, Jeffrey Smith was a Metro Police officer.

Two other Metro Police officers died by suicide a number of months later. I don't mention them because their families have not reached out and asked for help, and I don't want to presume their intentions. But the families of Officers Smith and Lieberman have reached out for help.

Law enforcement officers, Federal, and State local are generally accorded a death benefit should they die in the line of duty. But law enforcement officers death benefits usually State that a death by suicide cannot be a death in the line of duty. That is a significant injustice that is directly tied to antiquated notions of suicide.

It is often hard to determine whether a death is in the line of duty. If the law enforcement officer dies of cancer, usually the administrators of these plans have to go back and determine, well, was the officer exposed to a toxic substance in the line of duty, or is it related to something else? But to declare categorically that no death by suicide can ever be a line of duty death is a fundamental injustice, and both the Smith and Lieberman good families are now taking that up with the respective benefit plans under which they served.

In the military, military suicides are not excluded as line of duty deaths. In fact, an overwhelming percentage of death by suicide of active duty military, they get investigated and the overwhelming percentage of these cases, they are determined to be a line of duty deaths. So this is a really important mental health issue for law enforcement. There is an unjust and antiquated view of suicide affecting these line of duty death determinations.

There are two who served at this Capitol and died by suicide in the days right after the January 6 attack, and they have ongoing proceedings going before the relevant authorities. And so it may be slightly premature, but we may need to address this as a matter of law in the same way that we have allowed active duty military to have a suicide determined to be in the line of duty, law enforcement officers should not be shut off from them.

I want to ask each of you about a passion of mine that has been shared by Members of the Committee and that is the mental health of our healers, keeping our healers healthy. Mental—medical professionals prior to the pandemic had very dramatically escalating rates of suicide compared to the general population, and many medical professionals feel some significant stigma about seeking mental health counseling because of worrying about its effect on credentialing at hospitals or licensing at the State level or what colleagues might think.

Committee colleagues have joined together with me in a bipartisan way to pass the Lorna Breen Act, which I introduced with others on this Committee, named to commemorate a very talented emergency room physician in New York, a Virginia native who died by suicide at the beginning of the real wave of pandemic in April 2020.

But what can we do in the profession to help our healers feel more able to get the help they need?

Mr. PRINSTEIN. Sure. Thank you, Senator Kaine, for bringing that up and thank you for your work in this area. It is, in fact, very important. We are definitely seeing burnout. The mental health care providers are frontline workers too, of course. And we are seeing major burnout and concern among mental health care providers.

In partnership with the CDC, the American Psychological Association has been providing some services for health care providers who are not only experiencing burnout and need psychological first aid training, but also are quite angry and are feeling really challenged by the amount of harassment that they are getting, the amount of victimization that they are being subjected to for treating folks due to COVID, for offering vaccines.

A remarkable amount of frustration that they are experiencing for their patients that they can't get the opportunity to treat because they are overrun with folks who are experiencing COVID and are unvaccinated. There are a variety of things that can be done. As you ask providing concrete support, modeling self-care, psychological first aid training, as I mentioned.

Excuse me, but I wanted to thank you for both of your points really raising this issue of stigma that is still pervading the way that we think about mental health issues versus physical health issues.

I hope that this Committee can be very, very clear that that is sometimes also even reflected in the amount of funding that we provide to develop a workforce in mental health versus physical health care, and that just has to stop. Thank you.

Senator KAINE. My time has expired. Thank you, Chair Murray.

The CHAIR. Thank you. Senator Marshall.

Senator MARSHALL. Thank you, Madam Chair. I want to lock in on prior authorization for a second. And my first question is for Dr. Durham. Prior authorization is the No. 1 administrative burden facing physicians today across all specialties. Prior authorization, the No. 1 administrative burden facing all physicians across all specialties.

As a physician myself, I knew of the frustration of having to do this. Talk to a person who may be a non-specialist who wasn't from my area, so I couldn't imagine trying to do a prior off with you on a patient in the E.R., your years of experience, and as an obstetrician, I am trying to tell you who doesn't have—needed inpatient management.

Couldn't imagine doing that. But this burnout is leading to early retirement. It ties up nurses. It is frustrating to nurses as well. It makes us all less productive. I guess my question—and you spoke about this earlier, prior authorization.

My question is, do you ever feel that prior authorization is used to ration care or to delay the care of the patient needs?

Dr. DURHAM. Thank you so much for your question, and as a fellow physician that you understand sort of what we are going through. I do think it delays care. Absolutely, especially in the emergency room context.

We have literally two to 3 hours sometimes just to get someone a bed because we are waiting for the insurance to respond, to give the okay that yes, what you have presented to us meets the criteria for us to get a patient, an inpatient psychiatric bed.

Without a doubt, it delays care. And when we are thinking about an emergency room, we have a lot of patients we need to see. I talked briefly in my testimony about we have been beyond capacity in our emergency rooms, and I think that that is not unique to BMC, but across the Nation during this crisis that people are going in for emergency services.

Awaiting beds, awaiting placement just clogs the system, if you will.

Senator MARSHALL. Thank you. My next question for Dr. Prinstein. We are going to stay on the same subject prior authorization. If there was a streamlined solution, would it be helpful to your specialty—streamlined meaning I would suppose that 10 diagnosis account for 80 or 90 percent of the issues that need to be prior off.

We have Senate Bill 3018. It is bipartisan, bicameral as well. We have 17 sponsors, including 8 Democrats, 9 Republicans, 450 national and State organizations are sponsoring this legislation, which would streamline the prior authorization. Would it be helpful for members in your specialty?

Mr. PRINSTEIN. Yes, I think it would, and thank you. Psychiatry represents, of course, a small percentage, just 10 percent of the mental health workforce. The rest of us are psychologists, social workers, counselors, marriage and family therapists, and thinking of solutions that include all mental health providers is appreciated.

Senator MARSHALL. Thank you. You bet. My next question for Ms. Goldsby. You work in the Department of Alcohol and Drug Abuse Services. Does prior authorization ever impact your patients, especially does it delay care or ration care?

Ms. GOLDSBY. Senator Marshall, we do sometimes see prior authorizations delaying care, particularly for some patients who have insurance benefits when they are needing to be placed on medications.

Senator MARSHALL. And a streamlined approach to those patients would be beneficial to your staff?

Ms. GOLDSBY. Yes, absolutely. No barriers to treatment, yes.

Senator MARSHALL. Okay, Dr. Lockman, kind of same issue,

prior authorization in your world. I know you are doing research, more research based. Do you ever sit there and think about some of that where your research leads you to that, will patients have access to it? Are you worried about an insurance company deciding as opposed to evidence based medicine deciding what that patient should be receiving?

Ms. LOCKMAN. Absolutely. I concur. You know, every single hour that we spend navigating pre-authorization to get a patient the evidence based treatment that he or she needs is an hour that could be spent on something else.

You are delivering the care that changes people's lives. It can be spent on also doing the training that you have mentioned is critical. So I think any way that we can cut down on the processes would be helpful so that we can just get people the treatment that they need.

Senator MARSHALL. Okay, thank you so much. I will go to Ms. Rhyneer. Ms. Rhyneer, I am not going to ask you about prior authorization, so that is a good thing. I guess my question for you is, have you experienced some of the mandates, whether it is a mask mandate or vaccine mandate closing down school, how has that impacted the mental health of your students?

Ms. LOCKMAN. I think there has been some silver linings, and of course, I think COVID has exacerbated and introduced new issues. So during typical high school classes, a teacher is one of the first lines of defense. They can catch, you know, changes in a student's behavior, performance, or attitude. But during Zoom classes, I stared at a screen of gray squares. And so the teachers found fewer opportunities to ask, like, hey, are you Okay? How are things going at home? You seem a little off, is there anything you want to talk to or talk about? So that is kind of one bad thing.

But a silver lining, on the other hand, is like, I think the conversation around mental health has become a little bit more comfortable. And so teachers have been like, if you need a self-care, take the day off, go take a walk, do your own thing. You know, let's take the Zoom class off for today, and that was something that was totally okay to do. So I think there is good and bad.

I think I am willing to stay at home for the safety of our community. I also know that for some families, that makes it really hard. And for some families, it is not safe for the student to stay at home.

School is kind of like the safety net or this security blanket to be away from that. And that makes it tough. I don't know if there is a way to say that it was all bad or all good.

Senator MARSHALL. Thank you so much. I yield back.

The CHAIR. Thank you.

Senator Hassan.

Senator HASSAN. Thank you, Madam Chair, and I thank you and the Ranking Member for organizing and approving today's hearing. And to all of the witnesses, thank you so much for being here and for the work that you do. I want to start with a question to you, Dr. Prinstein. Young patients are being forced to wait in emergency rooms for up to a month, hoping an inpatient psychiatric bed will open up. And sometimes in my State, it is more than that.

They have written to me recounting their experiences waiting in hospitals. They describe truly horrific experiences, such as being kept in isolation and going weeks without showers, let alone mental health care.

The situation is so severe that New Hampshire used Federal funds to purchase a local hospital to take these children out of the emergency room. But we know there is more work that still needs to be done.

Even with the purchase of this hospital and now additional beds, there are still long waits in our emergency rooms. What concrete steps can Congress take to effectively reduce youth wait times for urgent mental health care?

Mr. PRINSTEIN. Thank you so much for the question, Senator. I appreciate it. It is the case that once someone, especially a child, is experiencing imminent risk charges themselves and others, they do need to be in a hospital. They do need the constant surveillance. And we might think that adding more hospital beds is the answer. It certainly is an opportunity to make sure we have enough emergency services.

But the problem truly has to be addressed by offering more outpatient providers that can make sure that kids never get to that level of crisis. We have the treatments, we have the science to show that it works. We just need more people to administer those treatments and keep kids from getting to that emergency stage.

750 times more funding to make sure we have enough physicians in this country than what we are providing for our entire mental health care workforce. If we had that, if we treated the likelihood that one out of every five young women will experience a major depressive episode before the age of 25, as we heard Ms. Rhyneer say, in Alaska, one out of every four young people are going to experience severe suicidality, think what we would do if that was a physical health disorder?

We would be training people what to expect. We would be training parents and teachers to spot the warning signs. We would be making sure that everyone had access to treatment the minute that they started showing any symptoms of a physical health illness whatsoever.

But it is happening for depression. And the reason why we are seeing all of this overrun in the hospitals is because we haven't provided the workforce to make sure that we can provide outpatient treatment before we reach that crisis stage.

Senator HASSAN. Well, thank you. And let me follow-up on the points you are making with Ms. Rhyneer and Dr. Durham. It is important that we acknowledge the stigma around mental health in schools. Ms. Rhyneer, you were just talking a little bit about things opening up a little bit and people talk more about it.

I received a letter from a student from Candy in New Hampshire sharing her experience with what she considers is a real lack of awareness in her school. She wrote in part, schools and workplaces are not taking mental health seriously. We do not learn about mental health in school, nor the workplace.

I have seen firsthand the way that these disorders can affect people. It is not seriously talked about, not taken seriously enough. It is powerful to hear students like this young woman talk openly about mental health, and we need to do more to support them. Points you all have been making.

Dr. Durham and Ms. Rhyneer, how can we work with students to end the stigma around mental health? And I will start with Dr. Durham, and then we will go to Ms. Rhyneer.

Dr. DURHAM. Thank you for that question. You know, when I think about the patients I see at BMC in particular, I talked about under-resourced communities, mostly low-income Black and Latinx folks that come and see us.

There is a huge stigma and ethnic minority communities, and we need to start, like many of people have said here in schools at home, but also partnering with other community organizations, the church, other systems of care that people go to other than health care systems, that we can start opening that dialog and thinking more openly, sort of like Claire has done today, telling our stories.

We have a lot of initiatives even within Boston Medical Center, of reaching out and partnering with our local churches. We have people in our Department that are doing some of that work to start breaking down barriers and stigma so people can come in for treatment.

Senator HASSAN. Well, thank you. Ms. Rhyneer.

Ms. RHYNEER. Yes, I totally agree. I was going to say the same thing, we can support community and local organizations. Some of the ones that I was in was, I was introduced to Aiyana club, suicide prevention trainings, but also MHATS, Mental Health Advocacy Through Storytelling, and that encouraged me to tell my story.

The program is youth led. It is youth founded. A group of incorporated school students working to decrease stigma and increase access to mental health resources through true personal short stories of mental health struggle and triumph. And we run a program, a 12 week program, twice a year, aiming to teach and guide conversations on mental health and storytelling, and then help participants develop their own stories on mental health.

Then all of our participants share the story they have developed at a final live storytelling event, kind of in the style of a moc radio hour or anything else like that. So helping organizations in promoting them and encouraging them and funding them and things like that is really, really important.

It was my own friends at this organization who taught curriculum and helped me tell my story, and it is because of those resources and that education that I opened up to my parents last year and the reason why I am here today.

Senator HASSAN. Well, thank you. And I realize I am out of time. I will follow-up, Ms. Goldsby, with the question to you about telehealth and medication assisted treatment. Thanks so much, Madam Chair.

The CHAIR. Thank you. Senator Smith.

Senator SMITH. Thank you so much, Madam Chair. And I would like to start by asking unanimous consent to submit, for the record, a letter from AFSCME Council 5 and AFSCME Council 65 in Minnesota on the need for sustainable solutions and long term investments in the mental health care workforce.

The CHAIR. So ordered.

[The following information can be found on page 75 in Additional Material:]

Senator SMITH. Chair Murray and Senator Murkowski, I am so grateful for you holding this hearing and bringing together these experts and colleagues to dig into mental health and substance use disorder challenges. I mean, this is an epidemic, as we have heard today, that is traumatizing our country.

Dr. Prinstein said it so well in his opening remarks, that this emergency is related to COVID, but it is the result of decades of systemic neglect and lack of attention and bifurcating mental and physical health to the detriment of our whole health.

I can tell you, of course, I hear about this from Minnesotans every single day, educators and parents and students especially who are grappling with significant mental health conditions. And I want to share that this is personal for me for two reasons.

The first is that my mentor, Paul Wellstone, who once held the seat that I have today, led on this issue with Senator, New Mexico Senator Pete Domenici. And through their leadership, Congress passed legislation to get parity for mental and physical health reimbursements in the insurance system.

Now, as we have heard today, we are still climbing up that mountain to get compliance for mental health parity, and we won't stop until we do. But I want to just note their leadership, which was instrumental. And the second reason that this issue is personal to me is that I experienced depression when I was a young person, starting in college and then again when I was a young mom.

I know a little bit about what it feels like to feel like there is something fundamentally wrong with you and there is nothing that can be done about it. There is no solution. And you know, I share my story because I want to—I am thinking about people who are currently suffering from mental health challenges and feel like they are all alone and nobody knows—nobody knows, and that they can't talk about it because of the stigma.

Ms. Rhyneer, I want to particularly thank you for your testimony and for sharing your story. Senator Murkowski knows that I actually also went to East Anchorage High School, so we have a little bit of Anchorage in common as well. But let me go, I am going to stay with you, Ms. Rhyneer. I want to just talk a little bit about mental health care in schools.

Last month, the University of Minnesota released some data, which said that 71 percent of principals in Minnesota are saying that more mental health resources for students would be the most important support that they could get. And I visited schools, and I have seen how this works and what a difference it can make.

Ms. Rhyneer, could you talk to us about why in-school services are important, why they work for students, and kind of how you see they might get it the stigma challenges and other challenges that students have accessing the mental health care that they need.

Ms. RHYNEER. Sure, yes. So school is a great place, just because it is a place where all students are going to be, and you can do a lot of different things in school. You can have the community, you can have the teaching, you can have peers, you can have a door to all working together and your parents too.

Also, we have counselors and—or we want to have counselors and therapists in schools. But alsohaving the curriculum around is really important. You know, I have talked to numerous students who say they didn't realize how bad of the situation they were until years later. Like they never recognized their own systems. They never reached out for help.

Having curriculum in schools is great to have people recognize their own symptoms and be like, oh, I think something is going on. I need to reach out to somebody. That person that they need to reach out to is, ONC 130, this room down the hall that they can walk down there and say, hey, I really need some help.

That counselor can call the parent and be like, hey, I talked to your kid. Maybe you should talk to them. So it is a really great place to have all those services in one place.

Senator SMITH. It is such a great way of describing what difference it makes. And also, I would say how we can—you are really integrating physical and mental health because maybe you go in to see the school nurse about a stomachache and then the school nurse ask some questions and understands that what you really need there is some underlying issues you need to address around anxiety or depression, and it happens all in one place in the kind of integrated care that we have heard the experts and physicians on the panel talk about.

Madam Chair, as you know—I am sure you know that I have several bills that I have been working on that would expand access to mental health care services in schools, and I am going to be very interested in pursuing these bills and this legislation as we go forward for exactly the reasons that I am Claire just described. Thank you so much.

The CHAIR. Thank you. Senator Rosen.

Senator ROSEN. Thank you, Madam Chair. And thank you, Senator Murkowski, for holding this really important hearing today, and of course, for the witnesses, for being here. I want to build on what Senator Smith was talking about because it is important that we equip schools with the comprehensive mental health and suicide prevention resources we know are so critical because not just under Smith, but we have heard from everyone this morning schools, our students, we are just facing such a growing mental health crisis.

In the American Academy of Pediatrics, they recently declared a national State of emergency in children's mental health. And in Nevada's Clark County School District, we tragically lost 20 students, 20 students to suicide since the onset of the pandemic in 2020. Those families will never be the same. And so we must do more to keep our students safe, to promote their mental health and their well-being.

Which is why, as Senator Murkowski noted earlier, I am working with her on bipartisan legislation to help provide additional resources to support K-through–12 mental health. And currently the Substance Abuse Mental Health

Services Administration, or SAMHSA for short, does not, does not have the authority to provide funding assistance directly to school districts to promote comprehensive health and suicide prevention services.

Dr. Prinstein, given the current mental health crisis in our schools, would legislation authorizing SAMHSA to directly provide targeted and timely resources to K through 12 schools help prevent the mental health challenges before they occur, and of course, address suicide attempts and prevent a suicide from taking place?

Mr. PRINSTEIN. Yes, Senator Rosen. Thank you so much. Hurray, this is a great step and very, very important. The opportunity to make sure that schools themselves can use their local expertise and their knowledge of what their community needs is a fantastic idea. I will say, please do keep in mind that school staff are currently overwhelmed and usually turning to psychology and as well as other mental health care providers to teach them about the skills that are needed. Psychologists often do this just out of the goodness of their own heart. There is no reimbursement mechanism.

This starts to become hopefully a far more widespread practice of schools instituting preventive programs throughout entire communities, please do think about ways that psychologists and other mental healthcare providers can be as helpful and dedicate as much time as possible to help teach the school staff what is needed, to use our evidence based assessments to screen for risk, and to use our evidence based interventions to reach and help as many people as possible.

We have many prevention programs ready to deploy, and this is a very exciting opportunity that you are speaking of. Thank you. Senator ROSEN. Well, you set me up perfectly for my next question, because all 17 counties in Nevada are designated as health professional shortage areas. And so that is why I am really proud of the work being done by University of Nevada Reno, the Master's level students, they are providing mental health counseling services to K through 12 students in nearby Churchill County and hopefully doing some of that other training when they are in the schools that you speak of.

This partnership allows our UNR interns to gain real world experience in a supervised setting while also increasing the access and just the knowledge base for everyone in those schools, particularly right now in Churchill K-through–12 students.

Again, back to Prinstein, this is a model. We are using it in Nevada. How might this model or others that you see, not just in Nevada—how can we lead the way in helping to promote these kinds of partnerships that will address the burnout and critical shortages and get those benefits to the students and teachers as well counselors?

Mr. PRINSTEIN. I think it would be terrific if we had the workforce to be able to do that in all States. Imagine that there were school psychologists enough to deploy and consults with every school out there, not just one per school districts or one per county, sometimes with kids waiting for years before they are able to get an evaluation, meanwhile their parents watch them failing grades and experiencing difficulties, just waiting for that school psychologist to join in.

There are sometimes only one mental health care provider for an entire county or for a 100 mile radius, which makes it very hard to consult with all the school districts that ask us to really play a role in just the way that you are describing.

I think that this approach, coupled with a substantial increase in the workforce, could really be a wonderful model for us to try and change the way that we are thinking about mental health from a prevention approach as well as an intervention approach.

Senator ROSEN. Well, thank you. I appreciate that, and I look forward to working with all of you and my colleagues to promote workforce training in the mental health space. We really need it in so many areas. Thank you, Madam Chair.

The CHAIR. Thank you. And we do have two votes called so that as all the Senators who have questions. Senator Murkowski, do you have any closing remarks?

Senator MURKOWSKI. Just very quickly, Madam Chair. And again, I agree this has been an excellent, excellent panel. You know, when we think about the issue of the issues of mental health and substance use disorders, so much of the response has to be when the individual is ready for it, it needs to be the intervention at that moment, and I was struck—I keep going back to reading Claire's testimony.

Claire, you indicate, you said, while I worked at NAMI, the National Association of Mental Illness, I had to tell people they would be on a waitlist for 9 to 12 months before they would receive care from a caseworker, 3 months before the patient would be even contacted to confirm they could be accepted, another 6 months before they could talk to a caseworker and begin care.

When we talk about the workforce issues, we cannot have a situation, an emergency, a crisis, and have an individual be told it will be 3 months before we know whether you can even receive care. So a lot of focus on the mental health issues.

I will tell you, Dr. Prinstein, when you when you indicated that the United States is No. 1 in the world for suicide rates, we think that money can solve a lot of things, but apparently, we are not directing the resources to these very critical areas of mental health like we need to.

Apparently, we haven't dedicated the resources for the workforce. Apparently, we haven't connected with the younger people and really all across the spectrum, we haven't addressed some of the racial issues that you have pointed out here. So we obviously have a great, great, great deal to do here.

I think that today's witnesses have provided us great insight, but it is a reminder that we have so much to do. So thank you to all of our witnesses and look forward to working on these problems.

The CHAIR. Senator Murkowski, thank you, and thank you for helping us put this together. Thank you to all of our witnesses. Senator Murkowski, you talked about workforce. That clearly is an issue. A number of other issues were addressed. But I think you actually identified one at the very beginning, which we don't talk about enough, and that is, how do we talk about suicide?

I think there is, as you stated, among young people a willingness, a desire, understanding that this cannot be a taboo topic that in fact, we need to have an understanding of it. We need to have a discussion of it.

But it is so hard for so many people to talk about it, as she said, because they fear that they are going to encourage somebody to do it. We all have a lot of learning to do, and we have a lot of learning within our schools and across our communities to deal with this issue.

I look forward to working with you, Senator Murkowski, on that and all of our colleagues. That will end our hearing today. Again, I want to thank Senator Murkowski for joining me today. For all of our colleagues, for a very insightful discussion.

I really want to thank all of our witnesses, Dr. Prinstein, Dr. Durham, Director Goldsby, Dr. Lockman, and Ms. Rhyneer for sharing your time and experience with us.

For any Senators who wish to ask additional questions, questions, for the record will be due in 10 business days, February 15th at 5 p.m.

This Committee will next meet February 8th for a hearing on employment opportunities and challenges for people with disabilities. Committee stands adjourned.

Additional Material

COUNCIL 5, AFSCME,
COUNCIL 65, AFSCME,
January 31, 2022.

The Honorable TINA SMITH
U.S. Senate Committee on Health, Education, Labor, and Pensions,
Washington, DC 20510.

Dear Senator Smith,

On behalf of the 43,000 working Minnesotans represented by AFSCME Council 5 and the 13,000 workers represented by AFSCME Council 65, we ask that this letter be part of the record of the February 1 hearing on Mental Health and Substance Use Disorders: Responding to the Growing Crisis. For too long behavioral health care has been an afterthought, leaving millions struggling to get the care they need for drug and opioid abuse, mental health, PTSD, and more. This hearing will help put this issue front and center.

AFSCME members who are certified peer recovery specialists, nurses, social workers, counselors, support staff, and other behavioral health care workers help individuals in a range of settings. It's not just a job for them; it's a calling. Our members see the services they provide can offer hope, change the trajectory of a person's life, and help repair fractured families. These workers are on the frontlines witnessing how the job loss, isolation, death, and illness from COVID have traumatized families and increased the risk for depression, anxiety, substance use disorder, and even suicidal ideation. These workers are building the resilience of our communities and healing families, one person at a time. They are ready to help our fellow Minnesotans begin that road to recovery, find their way back from a relapse, and support recovery. They are unsung heroes who deserve our respect.

As you consider developing legislation to improve our Nation's capacity to respond to the growing mental health and addiction crisis, we urge you to recognize that behavioral health staff are the foundation to any solution. Funds that are designed to increase the number of behavioral health care workers are important but not enough. Low pay, unsafe working conditions, and unacceptably high caseloads are factors that contribute to burnout and high staff turnover. Staff burnout and high staff turnover result in waiting lists for treatment, inconsistent care, wasted resources, and poor results. We need sustainable policies that ensure new funding is specifically targeted to rectify staff burnout and high turnover. This is how we can show our respect to this workforce and the clients they serve. We stand ready to work with you to remedy this dire situation.

Sincerely,
Julie Bleyhl,
Executive Director,
AFSCME Council 5.

Shannon Douvier,
Executive Director,
AFSCME Council 65.

Questions and Answers

Response by Mitch Prinstein to Questions of Senator Murphy, Senator Kaine, Senator Smith, Senator Luján, and Senator Murkowski

Senator Murphy

Question 1. How can we better prepare professionals in frequent contact with children and teens, such as teachers and pediatricians, to better deal with young people's unique behavioral health needs?

Answer 1. We need to rethink the ways in which we approach mental health care for all populations, including our youth, by moving away from a focus primarily on crisis management and instead investing more in prevention. Therefore, we must meet kids where they are. This means their schools and communities. Evidence-based comprehensive behavioral health systems in schools provide a full complement of supports and services that establish multi-tier interventions and promote positive school environments.

To help achieve this, teachers need increased training on embedding social and emotional learning in classroom curriculum. This would help build skills such as motivation and engagement, problem-solving, emotional intelligence, resiliency, agency, and relation- ship-building. To be successful, this must be done in partnership with parents, families, and caregivers.

Finally, it is important to remember that mental health is health. Maintaining siloes between physical and behavioral health makes little sense, hurts overall health care outcomes, and perpetuates stigma around mental health. Most people, children included, receive their health care from their primary health provider. Adopting flexible models of integrating mental health care with primary care—which starts in the way we train providers—is key to increasing access to services for all populations, including children and adolescents.

This also means increasing adoption of evidence-based models of integrated primary and behavioral healthcare. Children and teens routinely receive care in primary care settings, and identifying and addressing behavioral health issues could be made much easier if behavioral health specialists are embedded in those settings as part of the primary care team. Integrating psychologists into pediatric primary care practices through the Primary Care Behavioral Health (PCBH) model gives pediatricians a powerful ally in addressing the behavioral health needs of children, youth, and their families, and has a solid track record of success. Congress should support broader implementation of PCBH and other evidence-based integrated care models by providing stronger assistance and incentives for its adoption by primary care practices and behavioral health providers.

Question 2. How might additional training for these professionals improve supports for young people?

Answer 2. Additional training for these professionals can help bolster early detection and early interventions efforts, which are especially important for young people, as most mental health disorders begin between the ages of 14 and 24. Schools in particular are key to these efforts.

Leveraging partnerships between community and school-based entities can provide training to teachers, administrators, and support personnel, as well as families, students, and community members to recognize signs of emotional and psychological concerns and provide best practices for the delivery of mental health care in schools. To help promote the mental health of all students, educator preparation and professional development programs should also include training on mental health literacy, social-emotional learning competencies, and reducing mental health stigma.

Making training for integrated care service delivery broadly available to healthcare providers would help expand access to this treatment modality. Effective implementation of integrated primary and behavioral healthcare requires more than simply co-locating behavioral health and primary care providers. Research shows that training and technical assistance are frequently needed, since neither general medical providers nor behavioral health providers typically receive training in team-based care.

Question 3. Knowing that we have significant health care disparities stratified by income, race, and geography (e.g. rural areas), how do we ensure health equity in addressing the behavioral health needs of children and teens?

Answer 3. Despite the significant need for access to mental health services among young people, the mental health system remains largely geared toward adults. However, many of the same issues that plague the delivery of mental health care for adults, also arise in efforts to provide such services to children and adolescents: workforce shortages; a siloed healthcare system; and poor reimbursement rates for behavioral health services. These barriers disproportionately impact traditionally underserved and underrepresented populations.

One of the ways in which we can begin to build a more equitable mental health care system is invest in programs that educate psychologists and diversify the field, such as the Graduate Psychology Education and Minority Fellowship programs. Student loan debt, which is carried in significantly larger numbers by psychologists of color, also impedes workforce diversity efforts. Pathways to student loan forgiveness, which also incentivize service in communities with lack of access to care, is critical. Once these professionals are in the field, we must also adequately reimburse them for the care they provide by fully enforcing Federal parity law.

However, mental health does not exist in a vacuum and the psychological well-being of children is frequently tied to the overall health, safety, and stability of their surroundings, such as their communities, schools, and homes. COVID–19 has further strained individuals, families, and communities, with low-income and underrepresented minority populations being affected at even higher levels. Addressing the social determinants of health, including by investing in public education, affordable housing, and food security, is crucial to ensuring psychological health among all age populations, including children and adolescents.

Senator Kaine

Even before the COVID–19 pandemic, children across America faced mental health challenges. In 2019, suicide served as the second leading cause of death among adolescents. Further, over the course of the pandemic, nearly two in three young people expressed that they were feeling down, depressed, or hopeless. As we work to address the youth mental health crisis, we cannot forget about our military families and youth that receive services through Tricare.

Question 1. As we strengthen our investment in programs addressing youth mental health, how can we ensure that there is co- ordination and sharing among the agencies so that children and youth in military families, who rely on Tricare and often receive care in the military health systems, have access to the best practices and innovative solutions these programs provide?

Answer 1. APA strongly encourages the Congress and the DoD to take steps toward addressing DoD IG's recommendations in their August 2020 report, including creating a system-wide staffing plan for MHS for the Behavioral Health System of Care and requiring TRICARE to adhere to the same standardized psycho-therapy follow-up assessments currently in place in the Defense Health Agency (DHA).[74] Implementing these, as well as OIG's other recommendations would be a step in the right direction toward guaranteeing access to quality mental health care for our service members and their families.

Additionally, the current, unsustainably low reimbursement rate for mental health providers, including psychologists, through the TRICARE network is limiting the number of outside providers who would be able to serve our men and women in uniform. APA contacted DHA back in 2017 with our concerns[75] 2 but we are unaware of any action taken to rectify this issue. Additionally, the current pandemic has highlighted the disparity in reimbursement rates for telehealth compared to in-person care. Studies have shown that telehealth interventions are just as successful as face-to-face interventions[76,77] and during the pandemic and beyond, the telehealth reimbursement rate should be equal to the reimbursement rate for face-to-face visits. APA recommends adequately reimbursing psychologists in the TRICARE network and bringing parity to reimbursements for telehealth services. APA additionally recommends maintaining a strong in-house

---

[74] Department of Defense Office of the Inspector General, Evaluation of Access to Mental Health Care in the Department of Defense (Aug. 10, 2020) https://media.defense.gov/2020/Aug/12/2002475605/–1/–1/1/DODIG–2020–112—REDACTED.PDF.

[75] Letter from APA Practice Organization to Adm. Bono, Defense Health Agency. https://www.apaservices.org/practice/advocacy/humana-reimbursement-tricare.pdf.

[76] Greenbaum, Z. (July 1, 2020). How well is telepsychology working? Monitor on Psychology, Vol. 51, Issue.5, 46. Retrieved from https://www.apa.org/monitor/ 2020/07/cover-telepsychology.

[77] Bashshur, R. L., Shannon, G.W., Bashshur, N., Yellowlees, P. M. (Feb. 1, 2016). The empirical evidence for telemedicine interventions in mental disorders. Telemed J E Health, Vol. 22 Issue 2, 87–113. Retrieved from https://www.ncbi.nlm.nih.gov/pmc/articles/PMC4744872/.

Military Health System by continuing to fund the Uniformed Services University and maintaining medical billets.

Senator Smith

Question 1. What are specific examples of initiatives that you have seen in your work that have done a good job of incorporating mental health into the broader response to COVID–19? What should Congress learn from these successes?

Answer 1. The COVID–19 pandemic caused a seismic reevaluation of how patients are assessed for and receive mental health treatment. Expanded access to new modalities of treatment such as telehealth have extended access to communities that have traditionally struggled to access treatment. Increasing implementation of evidence-based integrated pediatric primary and behavioral healthcare could also significantly increase access to care, improve treatment outcomes, promote healthy development, and aid in addressing social determinants of health. A substantial percentage of patients visiting primary care practices are experiencing behavioral health issues affecting their well-being, including both mental health and substance use disorders or difficulties, and behavioral factors associated with physical conditions or chronic disease management.

More than a decade of research has documented the effectiveness of programs implementing the primary care behavioral health (PCBH) model, the collaborative care model (CoCM), and blended models of integrated care. One of the leading models of integrated care is the Primary Care Behavioral Health Model (PCBH), in which primary care providers, behavioral health consultants (BHCs), and care managers work as a team, sharing the same health record systems, administrative support staff, and waiting areas, and collaborate in monitoring and managing patient progress in order to improve the management of behavioral health problems and conditions.

Generally, the BHC strives to see patients on the same day the primary care provider (PCP) requests help and works with the PCP to implement clinical pathways for treatment. An integrated care psychologist's day may include meeting with a parent of a child exhibiting behavioral difficulties or hyperactivity, seeing a new mother experiencing symptoms of depression, helping another patient manage chronic pain or diabetes, and working with another patient who has recently discontinued using his psychotropic medication. Both patients and providers have reported high levels of satisfaction with PCBH model services. From the patient's perspective, behavioral health services are seamlessly interwoven with medical care, mitigating the stigma often associated with behavioral health services.

The PCBH model is particularly well-suited to use in pediatric care. Interventions and supports to promote children's physical, behavioral, and emotional health can positively influence the long-term trajectory of their health and well-being into adulthood. Almost all children are seen in primary care, and it is estimated that one in four pediatric primary care office visits involve behavioral or mental health problems. Psychologists can be especially helpful in pediatric care because assessing behavioral and emotional issues in children is generally more difficult than in adults, and pediatric education traditionally focuses on children's physical health. In addition to improving treatment in this area, early childhood behavioral health services can help mitigate the effect of adverse social determinants of health. Ideally, integrated pediatric primary care includes a whole-family approach to services that encompasses screening and services for perinatal and maternal depression, domestic violence, and adverse childhood experiences.

Adoption of PCBH and other integrated care models is often challenging for primary care providers, as they face barriers related to physical office space, the need for improved information technology systems, management procedures, clinical staffing and policies, health records and data tracking practices, and provider education and training. APA supports the provision of Federal financial and technical assistance to aid in the expansion of integrated care, whether provided through partnerships (including state agencies) or through direct aid to primary care providers. Initiatives and incentives to promote integrated care should support implementation of not just PCBH programs, but all evidence-based models of integrated care. Because of differences in providers' patient populations and access to behavioral health providers, there is no "one-size-fits-all" approach to effective integrated primary care. APA urges Congress to continue giving primary care practices the flexibility to choose the model of integrated care that works best for their community.

Question 2. What steps should Congress take to protect tele-mental health access, and what specific policies should be pursued for private federally regulated health plans, which fall under the jurisdiction of the HELP Committee?

Answer 1. As you know, expanded access to mental health services via telehealth is proving to be a literal lifeline to the many Americans who are struggling during the pandemic. This expansion is especially beneficial to individuals in geographic areas and communities that have long lacked access to these services. We know, however, that the pandemic will have a mental health impact that will last far longer than the pandemic itself. We appreciate the Administration's efforts to preserve the current pandemic-era flexibilities on telehealth coverage—for example, its recognition of audio- only telehealth as a vital modality of treatment. However, we also feel that Congress can further support expanded access to telehealth in two primary ways: first, by removing unnecessary barriers to mental health treatment, such as the statutory requirement for periodic in-person visits. To that end, APA asks that the Committee take up and pass the bill you co-sponsored with Senator Cassidy to repeal this requirement, the Telemental Health Care Access Act (S. 2061). Second, to ensure that providers continue to offer telehealth services to the same extent going forward, Members of this Committee can pass legislation requiring private insurance plans to cover mental health services furnished via telehealth on the same terms and at the same reimbursement rates as their in-person counterparts. Specifically, we ask that the Committee introduce and adopt a Senate counterpart to the Telehealth Coverage and Payment Parity Act (H.R. 4480).

Senator Luján

Question 1. The pandemic has exacerbated longstanding challenges patients and their loved ones have in seeking behavioral health services. This includes major workforce shortages, months-long waitlists for treatment, and entire regions of the country with no behavioral health providers. While these challenges are nationwide, barriers to care are amplified in largely rural states such as New Mexico. One solution that shows promise is the rise of peer support workers—behavioral health providers who have been successful in their recovery and work in their communities to help others. It is critical that we support these workers and give them re- sources to combat the burnout and high turnover that prevents us from building an experienced and consistent workforce. What can we do to not only recruit new substance use disorder workforce employees, but also retain those we already have?

Answer 1. APA shares your concern about provider burnout amidst increased demand for mental and behavioral health services. Indeed, the data shows that this phenomenon was clearly present long before the current pandemic. With added demand for services due to pandemic-related stressors, coupled with resurgent rates in abuse of opioids, stimulants, and other substances, we fear that, without prompt action, increased rates of provider burnout will impede providers' ability to provide quality evidence-based care.

One essential step to developing and maintaining an adequate substance use disorder workforce is ensuring that they are adequately paid. Reimbursement rates for substance use disorder staff and programs is notoriously low. In 2017 the State of Virginia implemented the Addiction and Recovery Treatment Services (ARTS) benefit for Medicaid beneficiaries with substance use disorders, with a goal of substantially increasing access to care. The initiative included increased provider reimbursement rates for many existing services, and the addition of coverage for a new office-based opioid treatment model. Since ARTS was implemented, Virginia has seen substantial increases in the number of participating addiction treatment providers and facilities, including a quadrupling of the number of practitioners billing for addiction treatment services above 2016 levels. Treatment rates for opioid use disorders and other substance use disorders have more than doubled with initiation of ARTS.

To increase the size and diversity of the behavioral health workforce, Congress can increase its support for key behavioral health workforce programs such as the Graduate Psychology Education (GPE) Program, the Minority Fellowship Program (MFP), and the Behavioral Health Workforce Education and Training (BHWET) Program. Additionally, to improve the pipeline of behavioral health providers, Congress can support efforts to allow psychology trainees—who receive 500–700 hours of direct patient experience through their training program—to bill for services they provide under the supervision of a licensed psychologist, similar to the flexibilities that medical school trainees currently enjoy. Finally, Congress can take steps to eliminate duplicative and unnecessary administrative burdens on independent practitioners; for example, while APA supported the policy goals of the No Surprises Act to provide a measure of cost transparency to patients, we are concerned that the way the Administration is implementing No Surprises Act imposes unnecessary burdens on behavioral health practitioners—such as the repetitive preparation "good faith estimates" of costs—that do not further the Act's purposes.

Question 2. We know that patients who are able to receive culturally sensitive behavioral health care and community centered care have improved outcomes. How can we better recruit and retain diverse behavioral health care providers who are able to provide high-quality care to their patients?

Answer 2. In order to better recruit and retain diverse healthcare providers, it would be useful to provide increased funding to programs such as the Minority Fellowship Program that have a proven success record of providing support to a qualified, diverse population of mental health providers. The program provides mentorship and guidance for those interested in serving culturally diverse populations. It may be useful to also offer incentives to those entering the workforce in a diverse community. Incentives could include higher pay, educational opportunities, student loan forgiveness or repayment programs specific to those working directly with diverse populations.

Question 3. In New Mexico, the COVID pandemic has overwhelmed an already strained behavioral health infrastructure. In some cases, patients experiencing substance use disorder or mental health crises wait months to be seen by a provider able to provide treatment. From your experience in the behavioral health space, can you speak to the importance of patients being able to access timely care?

Answer 3. The importance of early intervention—both in response to a short-term crisis and over the long-term trajectory over a child's life—cannot be overstated. Even relatively small investments in children's mental health early in their lives can have clear positive long-term effects. Most common mental health disorders, including those with the greatest morbidity, have onset in childhood or adolescence.[78] Childhood and adolescence provide critical periods for prevention, early detection, and intervention to promote lifetime well-being. Rather than activate resources only when a child experiences a crisis, which may inhibit the long-term effectiveness of treatment, our behavioral health system must focus resources earlier in a child's life and address the factors that led to the child experiencing a crisis in the first place.

Senator Murkowski

Military Suicides: The Army in Alaska has experienced numerous suicides from 2016 to 2021, most of them occurred at the remote location of Ft. Wainwright. Army leadership has taken steps to improve quality of life, but suicides continue. Furthermore, aspects of military culture that value toughness and resiliency discourage help-seeking behavior. Studies have shown that some service members perceive a stigma attached to seeking mental health care, and express concerns that seeking care will harm their career opportunities.

Question 1. What suggestions would you offer to military leadership to help combat this stigma and encourage military members to seek help when needed?

---

[78] Kessler, R.C. & Wang, P.S. (2008). The descriptive epidemiology of commonly occurring mental disorders in the United States. Annual Review of Public Health, 29, 115–129.

Answer 1. Improve Access to Direct Care and Purchased Care Systems to Ensure Access to Mental Health Care for our Servicemembers and their Families. The mental health of our Servicemembers and their Families is a critical readiness issue. A 2020 DoD Inspector General (IG) report that found that DoD did not consistently meet outpatient mental health access to care standards for active-duty Servicemembers and their Families.[79] APA has expressed serious concern multiple times in the past few years about network adequacy and cuts to reimbursement rates for psychologists.[80,81] The IG report shows that the TRICARE network is inadequate to meet the mental health care needs of our Servicemembers and their Families. APA encourages you to improve access to care across both direct and purchased care systems to include holding TRICARE contractors accountable when they fail to meet the needs of Servicemembers and their Families.

Maintain efforts to improve DoD's culture and climate. APA applauds previous efforts to end sexual harassment and assault, root out extremism, and make the DoD a safe place to work for all Servicemembers, regardless of gender, sexual orientation, gender identity, race, ethnicity, or religion. These quick-reaction efforts from the Task Forces to Stand Down must be accompanied by long-term policy changes. Members of the military must be able to rely on and trust their fellow Servicemembers. Any actions that undermine that trust, such as fearing sexual assault, racism, retaliation, or extremism, must be addressed directly at all levels of command. This is a critical readiness issue for the DoD, and we urge Congress to ensure DoD continues these efforts.

Continue to Focus on Suicide Prevention and Lethal Means Safety. As you know, the DoD has been focused on suicide prevention among Servicemembers for several years. Data from previous annual suicide reports and ongoing surveillance indicate that this continued emphasis is greatly

---

[79] Department of Defense Office of the Inspector General. (2020). Evaluation of Access to Mental Health Care in the Department of Defense. Retrieved from *https://media.defense.gov/2020/Aug/12/2002475605/-1/-1/1/DODIG-2020-112—REDACTED.PDF.*

[80] APA Practice Organization. (2017) Letter to Admiral Bono, Defense Health Agency. Retrieved from *https://www.apaservices.org/practice/advocacy/humana-reimbursement-tricare.pdf.*

[81] American Psychological Association. (2020). Letter to Secretary Esper, Department of Defense. Retrieved from *https://www.apa.org/news/press/releases/2020/10/letter-mental-health- access-tricare.pdf.*

needed.[82,83] DoD's Annual Suicide Report for Calendar Year 2019 found that the primary method of suicide was by firearm for Servicemembers and their Families, with rates ranging from 59.6 percent to 78.7 percent across military populations. Lethal means safety is critical to reducing suicide rates among these populations.

Increase Continuity for Separating Servicemembers as they Transition out of Service. Studies have shown that transitioning out of the military to civilian life increases risk for suicide, especially in certain populations.[84] The DoD's in Transition program, the Transition Assistance Program, and Yellow Ribbon Reintegration Program must be fully funded and continuously improved to meet the needs of Servicemembers across active and reserve components. It is also critical that Servicemembers are aware of, and have access to, Department of Veterans Affairs (VA) services. We encourage the DoD to devote more resources to data-sharing with VA and other agencies to ensure a smooth transition to civilian life. Support Basic and Applied Research. The basic and applied behavioral science research conducted by civilian and uniformed psychologists in the DoD is essential to modernize military personnel and talent management systems and to improve readiness, capacity, performance, and effectiveness at the individual, team, unit, and organizational levels. Basic and applied research is also needed to understand and address the stigma associated with mental health care and ways to ensure fairness toward and the full integration of women and minority groups. Moreover, psychologists should be involved in data analytics and artificial intelligence research to address how human cognitive biases have unintentionally been incorporated into various algorithms. Continued investment in the Minerva Research Initiative and social science research is essential to these efforts and must remain fully funded to strengthen the US national security apparatus. Finally, increased support for Minority Serving Institutions is critical in order to maintain a competitive advantage.

---

[82] Department of Defense, Under Secretary of Defense for Personnel and Readiness. (2020). Annual Suicide Report: Calendar Year 2019. Retrieved from *https://www.dspo.mil/Portals/113/Documents/CY2019 percent20Suicide percent20Report/DoD percent20Calendar percent20Year percent20CY percent202019 percent20Annual percent20Suicide percent20Report.pdf'ver—YOA4IZVcVA9mzwtsfdO5Ew percent3d.*

[83] Department of Defense, Defense Suicide Prevention Office. (2020). Department of Defense (DoD) Quarterly Suicide Report (QSR) 3d Quarter, CY2020. Retrieved from *https://www.dspo.mil/Portals/113/TAB percent20A—20201112—OFR—Rpt—Q3 percent20CY percent202020 percent20QSR—final—1.pdf.*

[84] Ravindran C, Morley SW, Stephens BM, Stanley IH, Reger MA. Association of Suicide Risk with Transition to Civilian Life Among US Military Service Members. JAMA Netw Open. 2020;3(9):e2016261. doi:10.1001/jamanetworkopen.2020.16261.

Question 2. What steps would you suggest for leadership to take in order to improve suicide prevention efforts in remote and isolated locations, like Interior Alaska?

Answer 2. Research is needed to better understand the contributors to regional differences in suicide mortality across the United States. Rural areas are highly diverse with respect to their landscapes, demographic composition, and socioeconomic conditions. Studies are needed to identify risk and protective factors for mental health outcomes within different types of rural communities and across the rural-urban continuum.

For rural populations, firearms and poisoning are the most common means of suicide, and those populations are at higher risk for suicide via firearms and pesticide ingestion because of greater familiarity and accessibility. Classification as a military veteran also confers risk; for example, in a study of over five million veterans in the United States, rural veterans were at 20 percent greater risk for suicide than urban veterans.[85] Research reviewing the effectiveness of lethal means safety interventions has shown that re- stricting access to handguns, pesticides or other lethal means for patients with suicidal ideation or training clinicians to recommend lethal means restriction can reduce rates of suicide by these means.[86]

Particularly striking are the suicide rates among adolescents and young adults in these communities. Suicide rates in 2014 for American Indian/Alaskan Native individuals between the age of 15 to 24 years old was 39.7 per 100,000, compared with the overall U.S. rate of 9.9 per 100,000. This rate is more than 3 and a half times the suicide rate for males of all races in the age group. The suicide rate for AI/AN females in the same age group was lower than males at 20.2 per 100,000. However, this rate was still nearly six times the rate for females of all races.[87]

As part of the coordinating role, the NIMH Office of Rural Mental Health Research should collaborate with other departments that are building networks to reach high risk rural populations, including veterans, farmer, ranchers and

[85] McCarthy, J. F., Blow, F. C., Ignacio, R. V., Ilgen, M. A., Austin, K. L., & Valenstein, M. (2012). Suicide among patients in the Veterans Affairs health system: rural-urban differences. in rates, risks, and methods. American journal of public health, 102 Suppl 1(Suppl 1), S111—S117. *https://doi.org/10.2105/AJPH.2011.300463.*

[86] Stewart, E.G. (2018). Mental Health in Rural America: A Field Guide (1st ed.). Routledge. *https://doi—org.ezproxy.lib.vt.edu/10.4324/9781315189857.*

[87] U.S. Department of Health and Human Services, Substance Abuse and Mental Health Services Administration, (2017). Suicide Clusters within American Indian and Alaska Native Communities: A review of the literature and recommendations. HHS Publication No. SMA17– 5050. Rockville, MD. Retrieved from: *https://store.samhsa.gov/sites/default/files/d7/priv/ sma17–5050.pdf.*

the agricultural community. The Department of Veterans' Affairs, the Department of Agriculture, the Substance Abuse and Mental Health Services Administration, Health Resources and Services Administration, Indian Health Service and others. Farmers, agricultural and migrant workers face unique stressors. The CDC results on deaths by suicide per capita (by occupation) reveal that these stressors can have tragic effects. Farmers, agricultural workers and their families likely would benefit from stress assistance programs tailored to the specific needs of this population. including such elements as a stress hotline and prescription drug abuse education for farmers, ranchers and agricultural workers.

To achieve health equity for rural and frontier populations, APA recommends taking a population health approach that also recognizes the cultural and geographic diversity of rural and frontier populations, including African Americans, Native American/American Indian, Latinx, Hispanic, veterans, women, farmers, LGBTQ populations, ranchers, migrants, individuals with disabilities and those living in resource-limited areas with declining population density. While the prevalence of mental health disorders is similar to populations in urban settings, rural and frontier communities face unique barriers to care that have been classified broadly in terms of accessibility, availability, acceptability, affordability and stigma, and a robust research agenda should seek to address each of these barriers.[88]

Access to psychologists in rural and frontier communities is of particular concern to APA, which has documented these workforce shortages. Of the 734 U.S. counties that were entirely rural, the vast majority (93.6 percent) had no records of licensed psychologists, about 2.4 percent had one to four licensed psychologists, and 4.0 percent had five or more licensed psychologists.[89] Research is needed on specific effective and innovative recruitment strategies for rural mental health providers, including a focus on cultural competence in rural populations.

The expansion of integrated care and telemental health holds promise for improving access to mental and behavioral health care and improving outcomes, but more research is needed to determine the essential components

---

[88] Juntunen, C.L., & Quincer, M.A. (2017). Underserved rural communities: Challenges and opportunities for improved practice. In. J.M. Casas, L.A. Suzuki, C.M. Alexander & M.A. Jackson (Eds) Handbook of Multicultural Counseling (4th edition) (pp. 447–456). Thousand Oaks, CA: Sage Publications.

[89] American Psychological Association. (2016). County-Level Analysis of U.S. Licensed Psychologists and Health Indicators. *https://www.apa.org/workforce/publications/15-county-anal-ysis.*

of integrated health care teams and ensure that workforce shortages do not undermine the ability to implement evidence-based interventions in these communities. Research is also needed to increase the availability of evidence-based behavioral health assessment, evaluation, prevention, and treatment within medical practices (in addition to primary care) in rural settings, including barriers to access.

Historically, research takes an urban-centered approach that has not focused on the unique needs of rural and frontier populations when developing or conducting research and implementing interventions. APA supports the greater recognition of the need to develop research programs that recognize the tremendous diversity of, and within, rural and frontier communities. To achieve health equity, community-based participatory research should include community engagement strategies that take into consideration these diverse cultures to increase the participation of rural communities in research and diversify the research workforce. As much of the research on rural health disparities examines disparities between rural and urban communities, additional research could focus on disparities within rural communities. Growing diversity increases the difficulty of fully understanding the psychological characteristics and needs of rural citizens. Culturally competent providers must also recognize the culture inherent in the geographic and social locations of rural citizens and be open to both the challenges and opportunities to supporting rural psychological health and well-being.[90]

In addition to the complexity of rurality itself, it is important to note that other vulnerable populations, including elders and people living in poverty, are over-represented in rural communities. Rural areas also include culturally diverse populations, although this is not consistently recognized. Racial and ethnic minorities in rural areas may live in even more isolated communities (such as American Indian reservation and tribal lands) and often are overlooked in diversity conversations, but that is also changing as rural demographics reflect more ethnic and racial diversity.[91] 18 Some tribes do not recognize traditional diagnoses like major depressive disorder.

---

[90] Juntunen, C.L., & Quincer, M.A. (2017). Underserved rural communities: Challenges and opportunities for improved practice. In. J.M. Casas, L.A. Suzuki, C.M. Alexander & M.A. Jackson (Eds) Handbook of Multicultural Counseling (4th edition) (pp. 447–456). Thousand Oaks, CA: Sage Publications.

[91] Lichter, D.T. (2012). Immigration and the new racial diversity in rural America. Rural Sociology, 77, 3–35. doi: 10. 0.1111/j.1549–0831.2012.00070.

American Indians and Alaska Natives have a much higher reported rate of distress (13 percent) in comparison to the general population (9 percent).[92]

Refugees and undocumented immigrants are a group which face a number of mental health issues such as PTSD and attachment issues (relevant to family separation both at the border and in general). When traveling to the United States, they face a number of traumatic events like abuse or torture, leading to social adjustment issues. These are very unique problems, which need to be treated with culturally competent care. There are also language and cultural barriers which need to be taken into account. Similar to Native Americans and Alaskan Natives, this group have different cultural understandings of what we would consider a diagnosis.[93]

Considering that much of the research on empirically supported treatments is conducted with urban populations, little is generalizable to rural residents' who often face unique challenges that may act as barriers to care, treatment engagement and retention, and treatment outcomes. Research is needed to more explicitly identify clinical and professional methods and strategies that engage and retain rural patients in behavioral health treatment.

To counter disparities in mental health care there has been a growing momentum to introduce technologies to deliver mental health care remotely. Tele-mental health enables effective care management, expands access to services, and promotes the integration of primary and mental healthcare services. The Veterans Affairs Health Administration has been a leading health care system in delivering these types of services with great success.[94] 21 More recently, due to the global pandemic, telemental health expansion across other health care systems has also shown great promise in offering adequate and timely mental health care.[95] These technologies have been found acceptable to older adult communities.[96] Despite the advantages of telehealth for care services, several barriers exist. For example, critical issues remain

---

[92] Stewart, E.G. (2018). Mental Health in Rural America: A Field Guide (1st ed.). Routledge. *https://doi—org.ezproxy.lib.vt.edu/10.4324/9781315189857.*

[93] Stewart, E.G. (2018). Mental Health in Rural America: A Field Guide (1st ed.). Routledge. https://doi-org.ezproxy.lib.vt.edu/10.4324/9781315189857.

[94] Caver, K. A., Shearer, E. M., Burks, D. J., Perry, K., De Paul, N. F., McGinn, M. M., & Felker, B. L. (2020). Telemental health training in the veterans administration puget sound health care system. Journal of clinical psychology, 76(6), 1108–1124.

[95] Patel, S. Y., Huskamp, H. A., Busch, A. B., & Mehrotra, A. (2020). Telemental Health and US Rural—Urban Differences in Specialty Mental Health Use, 2010—2017. American Journal of Public Health, 110(9), 1308–1314.

[96] Choi, N. G., Caamano, J., Vences, K., Marti, C. N., & Kunik, M. E. (2020). Acceptability and effects of tele-delivered behavioral activation for depression in low-income homebound older adults: in their own words. Aging & Mental Health, 1–8.

with coverage and reimbursement, licensure, broadband access and adequacy, privacy and policy barriers. There are also concerns related to shortages in the community-based geriatric healthcare workforce shortage in delivering care and using these technologies.

Research on the effectiveness of different modalities of telehealth care delivery in rural communities is needed. While video-based telehealth and telepsychiatry services provide clinicians the opportunity to observe important, non-verbal cues that may have clinical relevance, many rural and frontier residents lack adequate broadband infrastructure to support the delivery of video-based services (Graves et al., 2020; FCC, 2020).[97,98,99] Prioritizing the effectiveness of other telehealth delivery models to increase access to behavioral health care is warranted given this geographic digital divide.

Research addressing the impact of audio-only telehealth services on mental health treatment access in rural and remote regions is needed. The pandemic has demonstrated significant access related opportunities through audio-only services that have uniquely met rural patients' needs. Rural individuals are more likely to face internet service and technology-based barriers to telehealth services. Audio-only services that rely on phone access is typically more reliable and available in rural areas when compared to internet-based video telehealth services. APA recommends that NIMH invest in research to test multiple tele-mental health delivery systems (e.g., telephone, versus videoconference, or hybrid formats) to address optimal care in rural settings, including for older adults.

Increasing access to evidence-based integrated primary and behavioral healthcare could also aid in preventing suicide in rural areas, especially in conjunction with telehealth. In the primary care behavioral health (PCBH) model of integrated care, psychologists and other behavioral health providers work together with primary care providers in delivering team-based care. Congress should support broader implementation of PCBH and other evidence-based integrated care models by providing stronger assistance and

---

[97] Lindsay JA, Hogan JB, Ecker AH, Day SC, Chen P, Helm A. The Importance of Video Visits in the Time of COVID–19. J Rural Health. 2021 Jan;37(1):242–245. doi: 10.1111/jrh.12480. Epub 2020 Jun 30. PMID: 32506751; PMCID: PMC7300637.

[98] Graves JM, Mackelprang JL, Amiri S, Abshire DA. Barriers to Telemedicine Implementation in Southwest Tribal Communities During COVID–19. J Rural Health. 2021 Jan;37(1):239– 241—doi: 10.1111/jrh.12479. Epub 2020 Jun 30. PMID: 32506685; PMCID: PMC7300815.

[99] Federal Communications Commission. (2021). Bridging the Digital Divide for All Americans. *https://www.fcc.gov/about—fcc/fcc—initiatives/bridging-digital-divide-all—americans.*

incentives for its adoption by primary care practices and behavioral health providers. Integrated care is already in use by both the Veterans Health Administration and the Department of Defense to improve the identification and treatment of mental health and substance use disorders for their patients.

Schools are important settings for accessing mental health professionals, yet rural students are less likely to have access to school-based mental health services.[100] School-based mental health service is an ever-evolving and growing service that effectively meets the needs of rural and underserved children and adolescents. There are a number of successful school-based programs that have been established and tested by psychologists but relatively few have been specifically implemented or tested in rural schools. In many rural areas, the school bus is the most reliable form of transportation, making school-based settings the optimal setting to access children and families in need. This service presents diverse opportunities for screening, prevention, and treatment of some of our most at-risk rural individuals and families. APA recommends behavioral health services in schools to address rural-urban disparities in access to mental health care. Expanding research partnerships with schools and school-based health centers could demonstrate effectiveness in school-based interventions for children and adolescent mental health.

Question 3. On what aspects of military suicide prevention should future congressionally funded research efforts focus?

Answer 3. One of the biggest issues in the military community specifically is the ongoing stigma surrounding mental health and lack of access to resources that Veterans and active Servicemembers feel comfortable accessing. There is still a lot of concern out there that if a Servicemember seeks mental health treatment their career will be derailed, or they will lose security clearance. Research into the current state of this stigma is necessary to develop adequate solutions. Additionally, APA supports the Guarding Mental Health Act that helps to reduce this stigma specifically for U.S. Coast Guard Members.

APA also supports the use of high-quality, evidence based mental health care for the treatment of mental health conditions Veterans are experiencing. When considering non-traditional and innovative approaches in caring for Veterans, they should be done in conjunction with evidence-based care. This is exemplified by the VA's Whole Health approach to care, which focuses on

---

[100] Shelton AJ, Owens EW. Mental Health Services in the United States Public High Schools. J Sch Health. 2021 Jan;91(1):70–76. doi: 10.1111/josh.12976. Epub 2020 Nov 8. PMID: 33161576.

centering the Veteran and caring for them in a more holistic manner. In focusing on traditional and innovative approaches to care, the COVER (Creating Options for Veterans' Expedited Recovery) Commission report includes information about what types of therapies may be useful in caring for Veterans experiencing mental health issues.[101] Critically, the VA must ensure that therapies that do not have evidence are not funded. This funding could be better used for other therapies that have more research showing their efficacy, such as yoga, acupuncture, mindfulness and chiropractic care.

Suicide prevention and lethal means counseling tailored to veterans should be further encouraged, which would require education and training for VA providers and community care providers on lethal means safety and suicide prevention and would direct VA to create a veteran-specific lethal means counseling and suicide prevention session. Nearly 70 percent of suicide deaths were due to firearms, compared to less than 50 percent in the general population.[102] Additionally, APA recognizes the need for workforce development. Scholarship programs for psychologists who agree to work at Vet Centers after graduating are vital to ensuring the VA has the workforce necessary to support current demands.

We support the Access to Suicide Prevention Coordinators Act, which requires VA medical centers to have at least one suicide prevention coordinator on staff and calls for a study on the feasibility of reorganizing suicide prevention coordinators to report to the Office of Mental Health and Suicide Prevention. Suicide Prevention Coordinators are vital to VA's efforts to reduce veteran suicide and ensuring appropriate staffing and prioritization of these positions within VA is a crucial step toward lowering rates of veteran suicides.

Congress must also increase Continuity for Separating Servicemembers as they Transition out of Service. Studies have shown that transitioning out of the military to civilian life increases risk for suicide, especially in certain populations.[103] DoD's inTransition program is an excellent resource for servicemembers as they are separating from the service and throughout their

---

[101] Creating Options for Veterans' Expedited Recovery. United States Department of Veterans Affairs. 2020 Jan. *https://www.va.gov/COVER/docs/COVER-Commission-Final-Report–2020– 01–24.pdf.*

[102] 22019 National Veteran Suicide Prevention Annual Report. *https://www.mental health.va .gov/docs/data—sheets/2019/2019—National—Veteran—Suicide—Preven-tion—Annual—Report—508.pdf.*

[103] Ravindran C, Morley SW, Stephens BM, Stanley IH, Reger MA. Association of Suicide Risk with Transition to Civilian Life Among US Military Service Members. JAMA Netw Open. 2020;3(9):e2016261. doi:10.1001/jamanetworkopen.2020.16261.

career. It is critical that inTransition, the Transition Assistance Program, and the Yellow Ribbon Reintegration Program are fully funded to meet the needs of active duty servicemembers as well as the National Guard and Reserve. It is also critical that transitioning servicemembers know about and have access to Department of Veterans Affairs (VA) services.

DoD and VA-specific services and research must be complemented by suicide prevention programs directed at the broader population, but also available to current and former Servicemembers. Removing barriers to the provision of telehealth services in Medicare, Medicaid and commercial insurers, including allowing audio-only telehealth services, reimbursement parity, the ability providers to practice across state lines are important steps to increase access. Community mental and behavioral health infrastructures also need to be kept from collapse to ensure providers have resources to maintain operations and meet increasing needs of treatment. This includes Medicaid funded community mental and behavioral health centers, other nonprofit community mental health organizations and providers of mental health and addiction services.

Provider Burnout: Throughout the pandemic, I have been concerned about our health care workforce. Now, with a workforce shortage across the country, acute shortages in workers as infected staff isolate, and mounting burnout as we enter year three of this pandemic, I am more concerned than ever about the future of our health workforce.

Question 1. Specifically in the mental health care sector, what steps can we take to help support the mental health needs of health providers, and expand and improve retention in an already- depleted workforce?

Answer 1. APA shares your concern about provider burnout amidst increased demand for mental and behavioral health services. Indeed, the data shows that this phenomenon was clearly present long before the current pandemic. With added demand for services due to pandemic-related stressors, coupled with resurgent rates in abuse of opioids, stimulants, and other substances, we fear that, without prompt action, increased rates of provider burnout will impede providers' ability to provide quality evidence-based care. To increase the size and diversity of the behavioral health workforce, Congress can increase its support for key behavioral health workforce programs such as the Graduate Psychology Education (GPE) Program, the Minority Fellowship Program (MFP), and the Behavioral Health Workforce Education and Training (BHWET) Program. Additionally, to improve the pipeline of behavioral health providers, Congress can support efforts to allow psychology trainees—who receive 500–700 hours of direct patient experience through their training program—to bill for services they provide under the supervision of a licensed psychologist, similar to the flexibilities that medical school trainees currently enjoy. Finally, Congress can take steps to eliminate duplicative and unnecessary administrative burdens on independent practitioners; for example, while APA supported the policy goals of the No Surprises Act to provide a measure of cost transparency to patients, we are concerned that the way the Administration is implementing No Surprises Act imposes unnecessary burdens on behavioral health practitioners—such as the repetitive preparation "good faith estimates" of costs—that do not further the Act's purposes.

Suicide Prevention and Screening: A study from 2016 estimated that 11 percent of ED patients present with suicide ideation. However, only 3 percent of patients were being identified by screening. In addition, upwards of 70 percent of patients who leave the ED after a suicide attempt never attend their first outpatient appointment.

Question 1. I have sponsored a bill, S. 467, that provides direct assistance to hospital emergency departments so they can enhance their ability to screen for high-risk suicidal patients and improves the treatment they receive while in emergency rooms. Do you believe that hospital emergency departments can play important role in identifying and treating suicidal patients who otherwise would never be screened for possible suicide?

Answer 1. As you noted Senator, emergency rooms do provide crisis mental health care in almost every jurisdiction in the country and are often ill-equipped to manage that task. More than 500,000 people present to emergency departments each year with deliberate self-harm or suicidal ideation—both major risk factors for suicide. Up to 80 percent of suicide decedents visit healthcare settings in the year before death, and about a fifth of decedents are seen in healthcare within the week of death, making the delivery of effective interventions a top priority. Legislation such as yours can help improve training, staffing and procedures so that emergency rooms may better manage their mental health patients in crisis, improving the quality and consistency of the care those patients receive. It's critically important to ensure emergency departments have policies of consistent universal screening for suicide risk and resources to ensure their patients can receive follow-up care. Additional funding for research is also important, to understand how services can be targeted to the needs to different populations. Despite advances in treatments over the past several decades, and effective psychosocial interventions that reduce repeat suicide attempts, there remain few evidence-based interventions that have been tested for their rapid-onset benefits for reducing suicide risk.

Role of Social Media and Isolation: As Dr. Murthy highlighted last month, youth mental health and substance misuse has been on the rise even before the pandemic, meaning pre-global pandemic we were failing to address the factors that lead to mental health crisis and substance misuse in youth. Anecdotally we know that increased screen time and exposure to social media is having an impact on youth.

Question 2. What efforts are underway to research this impact and better understand the implications and recommendations for care?

Answer 2. There has never been a more important time to examine the impact of social media on children. Psychological scientists, in particular, are increasingly warning that the use of digital media platforms can exploit biological vulnerabilities among.[104,105] It has long been established that adolescence is associated with neurological changes that promote cravings for social attention, feedback, and status. Research demonstrates that digital media satisfies these cravings at a neural level, activating the same neural regions as drugs.[106,107,108] We know that there are ways to beneficially use social media platforms, especially for those individuals seeking to buffer the impacts of negative life events, decrease feelings of isolation, gain a sense of purpose, and experience feelings of acceptance or being understood.[109] 36 And early evidence of technology-based mental health interventions also show

---

[104] Crone, E.A., & Konijn, E.A. (2018). Media use and brain development during adolescence. Nature Communications, 9, 1—10. *https://doi.org/10.1038/s41467–018–03126-x.*

[105] Wilmer, H. H., & Chein, J. M. (2016). Mobile technology habits: Patterns of association among device usage, intertemporal preference, impulse control, and reward sensitivity. Psychonomic Bulletin and Review, 23(5), 1607—1614. *https://doi.org/10.3758/s13423–016– 1011-z.*

[106] De-Sola Gutierrez, J., Rodriguez De Fonseca, F., & Rubio, G. (2016). Cell-phone addiction: A review. Frontiers in Psychiatry, 7. *https://doi.org/10.3389/fpsyt.2016.00175.*

[107] Griffiths, M. D., Kuss, D. J., & Demetrovics, Z. (2014). Social networking addiction: An overview of preliminary findings. Behavioral Addictions: Criteria, Evidence, and Treatment, 119–141. *https://doi.org/10.1016/B978–0–12–407724–9.00006–9.*

[108] Kirby, B., Dapore, A., Ash, C., Malley, K., & West, R. (2020). Smartphone pathology, agency and reward processing. Lecture Notes in Information Systems and Organisation, 321–329. *https://doi.org/10.1007/978–3–030–60073–0–37.*

[109] Daine, K., Hawton, K., Singaravelu, V., Stewart, A., Simkin, S., & Montgomery, P. (2013). The Power of the Web: A systematic review of studies of the influence of the Internet on self- harm and suicide in young people. PLoS ONE, 8(10), e77555. *https://doi.org/10.1371/journal.pone.0077555.*

promise at treating a range of problems.[110,111,112] But users of social media platforms remain uninformed and biologically susceptible to negative outcomes.

Another area of concern among scientists is the heightened potential for peer influence facilitated by digital media platforms. This is exacerbated by the proliferation of misinformation and disinformation campaigns that gain traction specifically due to the accessibility of digital media. Psychological science demonstrates that digital media creates the illusion that expressed opinions represent many others' beliefs and not just the thinking of an isolated user.[113,114,115,116,117] Participation on digital media platforms changes how we think about what others think. Science demonstrates that this has

---

[110] Galla, B. M., Choukas—Bradley, S., Fiore, H. M., & Esposito, M. V. (2021). Values—alignment messaging boosts adolescents' motivation to control social media use. Child Development, 92(5), 1717–1734. *https://doi.org/10.1111/cdev.13553.*

[111] Myers, K. M., Valentine, J. M., Melzer, S. M. (2007, Nov). Feasibility, acceptability, and sustainability of telepsychiatry for children and adolescents. Psychiatric Services, 58(11), 1493– 1496. *https://doi.org/10.1176/ps.2007.58.11.1493.*

[112] Nelson, E. L., Cain, S., & Sharp, S. (2017, Jan). Considerations for conducting telemental health with children and adolescents. Child Adolescent Psychiatric Clinics of North America, 26(1), 77–91. *https://doi.org/10.1016/j.chc.2016.07.008.*

[113] Chen, J., Liang, Y., Mai, C., Zhong, X., & Qu, C. (2016). General deficit in inhibitory control of excessive smartphone users: Evidence from an event-related potential study. Frontiers in Psychology, 7, 511. *https://doi.org/10.3389/fpsyg.2016.00511.*

[114] Dong, G., Zhou, H., & Zhao, X. (2011). Male Internet addicts show impaired executive control ability: Evidence from a color-word Stroop task. Neuroscience Letters, 499(2), 114—118. *https://doi.org/10.1016/j.neulet.2011.05.047.*

[115] Gao, L., Zhang, J., Xie, H., Nie, Y., Zhao, Q., & Zhou, Z. (2020). Effect of the mobile phone related-background on inhibitory control of problematic mobile phone use: An event-related potentials study. Addictive Behaviors, 108, 106363. *https://doi.org/10.1016/j.addbeh.2020.106363.*

[116] Gao, Q., Jia, G., Zhao, J., & Zhang, D. (2019). Inhibitory control in excessive social networking users: Evidence from an ERP-based Go-Nogo task. Frontiers in Psychology, 10, 1810. *https://doi.org/10.3389/fpsyg.2019.01810.*

[117] Nesi, J.L., & Prinstein, M.J. (2015). Using social media for social comparison and feedback seeking: Gender and popularity moderate associations with depressive symptoms. Journal of Abnormal Child Psychology, 43(8), 1427—1438.

created a powerful link between young people's Instagram exposure and their offline risk-taking behavior, such as excessive alcohol use.[118,119,120,121]

Increased peer victimization and harassment, as well as more severe discrimination directed toward racial, ethnic, gender, and sexual minorities, represent another serious area of concern. Scientific findings have revealed more frequent and offensive forms of harassment directed toward youths online as compared with offline.[122,123] Brain scans of adults and youths reveal that these forms of harassment activate the same regions of the brain that respond to physical pain and trigger a cascade of reactions that replicate physical assault and create physical and mental health damage.[124] Finally, the lack of transparency into the inner workings, policies and measured impacts of these platforms must be addressed. The impact of social media algorithms on the user experience is woe-fully understudied due in large part to the lack of visibility by researchers into the data and how algorithms work.[125] Social media companies employing algorithms to

---

[118] Cabrera-Nguyen, E. P., Cavazos-Rehg, P., Krauss, M., Bierut, J., & Moreno, M. A. (2016). Young adults' exposure to alcohol-and marijuana-related content on Twitter. Journal of Studies on Alcohol and Drugs, 77(2), 349—353. *https://doi.org/10.15288/jsad.2016.77.349.*

[119] Curtis, B. L., Lookatch, S. J., Ramo, D. E., McKay, J. R., Feinn, R. S., & Kranzler, H.R. (2018). Meta-analysis of the association of alcohol-related social media use with alcohol consumption and alcohol-related problems in adolescents and young adults. Alcoholism: Clinical and Experimental Research, 42(6), 978—986. *https://doi.org/10.1111/acer.13642.*

[120] Pegg, K. J., O'Donnell, A. W., Lala, G., & Barber, B. L. (2018). The role of online social identity in the relationship between alcohol-related content on social networking sites and adolescent alcohol use. Cyberpsychology, Behavior, and Social Networking, 21(1), 50—55. *https:// doi.org/10.1089/cyber.2016.0665.*

[121] Moreno, M. A., Chassiakos, Y. R., Cross, C., Hill, D., Ameenuddin, N., Radesky, J., Hutchinson, J., Boyd, R., Mendelson, R., Smith, J., Swanson, W. S., & Media, C. C. (2016). Media use in school-aged children and adolescents. Pediatrics, 138(5). *https://doi.org/10.1542/peds.2016– 2592.*

[122] Tynes, B. M., Giang, M. T., Williams, D. R., & Thompson, G. N. (2008). Online racial discrimination and psychological adjustment among adolescents. Journal of Adolescent Health, 43(6), 565–569. *https://doi.org/10.1016/j—jadohealth.2008.08.021.*

[123] Cannon, D. S., Tiffany, S. T., Coon, H., Scholand, M. B., McMahon, W. M., & Leppert, M. F. (2007). The PHQ–9 as a brief assessment of lifetime major depression. Psychological Assess- ment, 19(2), 247–251. *https://doi.org/10.1037/1040–3590.19.2.247.*

[124] Epps-Darling, A., Bouyer, R. T., & Cramer, H. (2020, October). Artist gender representation in music streaming. In Proceedings of the 21st International Society for Music Information Retrieval Conference (Montreal, Canada) (ISMIR 2020). ISMIR (pp. 248–254).

[125] Bravo, D. Y., Jefferies, J., Epps, A., & Hill, N. E. (2019). When things go viral: Youth's discrimination exposure in the world of social media. In Handbook of Children and Prejudice (pp. 269–287). Springer, Cham. *https://doi.org/10.1007/978–3–030–12228–7—15.* Press Release: *https://www.bmc.org/news/press-releases/2020/09/09/boston-medical-center-and-proof-alliance-collaborate-reduce-prenatal.*

display content to users should provide explanations on how these technologies work and how they might drive or reward certain types of posts or behavior. Data from algorithms, along with internal research should also be made public to allow researchers and policymakers to achieve a greater understanding of the impacts of social media on users, particularly children. Federal agencies should prioritize research into the impacts of social media and providing private researchers with grants and other support to ensure findings relating to these platforms are made broadly available.

For a more comprehensive summary of the currently available research in this area, I am attaching a summary of a forthcoming research handbook I coedited. The Handbook of Adolescent Digital Media Use and Mental Health is scheduled for release by Cambridge University Press in 2022.

Question 3. What methods should we focus on to prevent the onset of substance misuse and mental health disorders in America's youth?

Early detection and early intervention are critical to preventing the onset of mental health and substance misuse disorder among children and adolescents, however a focus on prevention rather than crisis management continues to be rare. As most young people spend a majority of their time in school, school-based mental health care is an essential tool for prevention purposes. Such services can build resiliency and mental health literacy among youth, to both address needs and destigmatize mental health. Leveraging partnerships between community and school-based entities can provide training to teachers, administrators, and support personnel, as well as families, students, and community members to recognize signs of emotional and psychological concerns and provide best practices for the delivery of mental health care in schools.

Furthermore, increased adoption of evidence-based models of integrating primary and behavioral health care is another way to help increase prevention, early detection, and early intervention, while also reducing stigma around mental health, which prevents many ethnic and racial minority populations, including Black, Hispanic, Asian/Pacific Islander, and Tribal, from seeking needed care.

Response by Michelle P. Durham to Questions of Senator Murphy, Senator Kaine, Senator Smith, Senator Luján, Senator Collins, and Senator Murkowski

Senator Murphy

Question 1. How can we better prepare professionals in frequent contact with children and teens, such as teachers and pediatricians, to better deal with young people's unique behavioral health needs?

Answer 1. As the Director of Clinical Training at TEAM UP for Children, a pediatric integrated model in federally qualified health centers (FQHCs) in Massachusetts, I see firsthand the impact that targeted staff training and supports can have on quality of care and child health. The TEAM UP for Children model, co-developed by Boston Medical Center (BMC) and partner FQHCs, is based on the National Academy of Medicine's Promotion Framework and focuses on promotion, prevention, early identification of emerging behavioral health issues, and swift access to behavioral health services that are delivered by a multidisciplinary team. TEAM UP for Children enables pediatric primary care providers to better manage common behavioral health diagnoses in the primary care setting through clinical training, quality improvement support, and a team-based model that includes embedded behavioral health clinicians and community health workers. This type of model could be scaled up to serve additional clinical sites and adapted to suit other settings, such as schools, to increase the ability for frontline staff to identify and address children's behavioral health needs, while also making mental health services available in the places where children are.

Question 2. How might additional training for these professionals improve supports for young people?

Answer 2. The goal of this type of approach is really about prevention. In other words, reaching young people before they are in crisis. Bolstering mental health resources and supports in the places where children are—in schools and other community settings—allows for children to be able to access help at the time that they need it. Oftentimes this requires intervening before there is an actual behavioral health diagnosis, which conventional health insurance plans typically don't permit. In July 2021, Massachusetts' combined Medicaid and Children's Health Insurance Program (CHIP) or "MassHealth" added a new integrated behavioral health code to allow mental health clinicians to receive reimbursement for seeing a pediatric patient up to six times without needing a mental health diagnosis *https://www.mass.gov/doc/physician-bulletin—103—integrated—behavioral—health—service—code—description—and—billing—requirements—download.* This type of flexibility shows great promise and could serve as a prevention model other states could emulate.

Question 3. Knowing that we have significant health care disparities stratified by income, race, and geography (e.g. rural areas), how do we ensure health equity in addressing the behavioral health needs of children and teens?

Answer 3. The TEAM UP for Children model is designed to disrupt health care disparities. By strengthening the ability of FQHCs to recognize emerging child behavioral health issues and intervene early with appropriate treatment, TEAM UP for Children aims to improve life outcomes for tens of thousands of low-income children across Massachusetts. Ensuring that mild and moderate cases of common mental disorders (depression, anxiety, ADHD, etc.) can be managed in the pediatric primary care setting, and at FQHCs in particular, which disproportionately serve as the site of care for low-income children and children of color, opens up access to mental health care to a population that historically has high needs but faces the highest barriers to care. Investing in community health workers (CHWs), which play a central role in the TEAM UP for Children model, would also serve to advance health equity. CHWs serve as a bridge to the community as they are often members of the community and are trained to work with families to address basic needs, provide mental health education, and offer school support in culturally and linguistically appropriate ways.

Senator Kaine

Even before the pandemic, underserved, rural, and minority communities faced too many barriers in accessing health care, and mental health services are not exempt. This has only been exacerbated by nationwide physician shortages. And, while the number of mental health providers of color has grown in recent years, they still only account for 17 percent of the workforce according to the American Psychological Association. It is clear that we need more mental health professionals. We know that mental health services are delivered by a wide array of professionals, and that primary care providers are often at the forefront of mental health care.

One way we can address this issue is by diversifying and expanding our physician pipeline, as medical students of color and those from rural areas are more likely to practice in the communities they are from. This Congress, I reintroduced important legislation, the Expanding Medical School Education

Act, to help us get one step closer to ensuring communities have access to the medical professionals they need. This bill supports the creation or expansion of medical schools in medically underserved communities and at minority-serving institutions, including Historically Black Colleges and Universities.

Question 1. Could you speak to the importance of having cultural and linguistic diversity among mental health providers?

Answer 1. Senator Kaine, thank you for your question and for supporting this important bill. Increasing ethnic, cultural and linguistic diversity in the mental health workforce is critical to engaging diverse communities in treatment. There is great stigma around mental illness and seeking treatment. It is well known that those that do make the first step to treatment, do not feel heard or understood during clinical encounters. At times their symptoms are dismissed, overlooked, or misdiagnosed. We know that racism and discrimination create an unequal system of care for diverse populations. By increasing the diversity in the physician workforce, people can engage in treatment with folks who look like them, share the same faith, understand the language, and understand the person's culture to better inform care.

Senator Smith

Question 1. What steps should we be taking at the Federal level to address the immediate shortage of pediatric mental health beds?

Answer 1. A regional approach to expand the full continuum of care services, not just crisis services, including an emphasis on prevention and moving upstream to address health-related social needs, behavioral health integration in primary care settings, and other means of enabling individuals to access outpatient mental health services when they need it, could lead to reduced reliance on emergency services and inpatient mental health services for children and adults. Timely response is key and can potentially avoid requiring emergency or inpatient-level care.

Massachusetts has several models for investing in prevention that are ripe for replication:

- The Boston Emergency Services Team (BEST)—led by Boston Medical Center—provides a comprehensive and highly integrated system of crisis evaluation, intervention, and treatment services to residents of the Bostonarea, including mental health urgent care centers, mobile crisis intervention for youth, community crisis stabilization program for adults, and a jail diversion program.

- Children's Behavioral Health Initiative (CBHI), which initially focused on youth covered by MassHealth (Medicaid/CHIP) and has since expanded to include commercial health insurance, provides coverage for an enhanced continuum of home-and community-based behavioral health services and requires primary care providers to screen for behavioral health conditions as a routine part of care.

Question 2. What are specific examples of initiatives that you have seen in your work that have done a good job of incorporating mental health into the broader response to COVID–19? What should Congress learn from these successes?

Answer 2. Telehealth profoundly expanded access to mental health services during the COVID–19 pandemic. Telehealth enabled BMC to maintain and exceed our pre-pandemic volume of mental health services, with over 90 percent of our outpatient psychiatric visits conducted via telehealth at peak. In addition, show rates to telehealth visits (video and audio-only combined), which todate hover around 75–85 percent, have exceeded show rates to in-person behavioral health visits pre-COVID–19 by roughly 10 percentage points, suggesting that telehealth has significantly reduced barriers and enhanced timely access to care for our patients.

Even as in-person volume has steadily returned at BMC, audio- only services continue to account for a significantly greater percentage of our ambulatory visit volume compared to video. BMC data demonstrate that a higher proportion of White and English-speaking patients scheduled and completed ambulatory visits via video compared to non-White (particularly Black and Latinx) and non- English-speaking patients. This trend of differential utilization of video care by race/ethnicity and language has been shown to be consistent across diverse medical systems.

We urge Congress to pass the *"Telemental Health Care Access Act of 2021"* to remove the requirement for Medicare beneficiaries to have an in-person visit for mental health services in order to access telehealth for mental health services, and instead allow providers to rely on clinical discretion and patient preference to determine the appropriate treatment modality (audio, video, or in-person).

Question 3. What steps should Congress take to protect tele-mental health access, and what specific policies should be pursued for private federally regulated health plans, which fall under the jurisdiction of the HELP Committee?

Answer 3. In 2021, the BMC integrated behavioral health program launched a pilot telehealth hub for behavioral health counseling visits to take place in community in partnership with a local church. By providing access to video capable technology, high- speed, reliable internet, and a private space in a convenient, trusted location, the pilot seeks to reduce barriers for people to utilize telehealth. The Federal Government could play a role in helping accelerate the development of community telehealth hubs by providing grants to health systems, hospitals, federally qualified health centers, schools, and community-based organizations to purchase equipment, retrofit space, hire staff, and receive or provide technical assistance.

Question 4. Do existing systems of care recognize a developmental disorder such as fetal alcohol spectrum disorders (FASD), or do you believe that a lack of identification could be a significant gap in treating these individuals for their mental health disorders? What are the barriers in integrating FASD-informed identification and care into existing systems?

Answer 4. In September 2020, BMC was awarded a 3-year, $2.9 million Health Resources and Services Association (HRSA) grant to fund the SAFEST Choice Learning Collaborative, a program aimed at reducing the incidence of prenatal alcohol exposure and improving outcomes in children with suspected or diagnosed fetal alcohol spectrum disorders (FASD). The program—which is a joint effort between BMC, Boston University Schools of Medicine and Public Health, and Minnesota-based Proof Alliance—uses the Extension for Community Healthcare Outcomes (ECHO) virtual education platform to provide primary care providers at community health centers in New England and the Upper Midwest with training and support from experts about FASD and how to screen for and counsel women about the risks of alcohol use during pregnancy, as well as train pediatric providers on identifying and caring for children and adolescents with suspected or diagnosed FASD.[126] More information on the program is available on our website: https:// www.bmc.org/addiction/training-education/safest-choice.

Senator Luján

Question 1. Health care worker burnout is devastating given the great debt of gratitude we owe them. That is why I was pleased to support the American Rescue Plan that dedicated $103 million to reduce burnout and promote

[126] Epps-Darling, A., Bouyer, R. T., & Cramer, H. (2020, October). Artist gender representation in music streaming. In Proceedings of the 21st International Society for Music Information Retrieval Conference (Montreal, Canada) (ISMIR 2020). ISMIR (pp. 248–254).

mental health and wellness of health care workers, which over $1 million went to the University of New Mexico Hospital to support the frontline workers who are sacrificing so much while caring for others. How can burnout be prevented or reduced among existing behavioral health providers?

Answer 1. I prefer the term "moral injury or moral distress" to "burnout" as I believe it better describes the reality facing our Nation's frontline healthcare workers. Both terms point to system failures whereas burnout places the onus on individuals, e.g. the clinicians with symptoms of exhaustion and low productivity. Systems have responded to calls to address healthcare worker burnout with "resilience training" yoga or other individually centered interventions without changing the system. This kind of misaligned ap- proach is problematic and unlikely to yield the intended results. Moral injury is more than just being overworked—it's the inability for providers to be able to do their jobs, confronting systemic issues that don't change, frequent barriers, and lack of supports.

> "Moral injury describes the challenge of simultaneously knowing what care patients need but being unable to provide it due to constraints that are beyond our control."[127,128]

Potential solutions to address moral injury include:

- decreasing administrative burden such as prior authorizations;
- increasing the amount of time clinicians spend with patients especially those that have co-occuring illness and/ or need additional support due to housing, financial, and/or food needs;
- parity in payment for physical and mental health treatments.

Senator Collins

I have heard firsthand from parents and caregivers in Maine who are gravely concerned about a greater incidence of speech development delays in children. Compounding their concerns is the fact that increased absences and continued

[127] Dean W, Talbot S, Dean A (2019). Reframing Clinician Distress: Moral Injury Not Burnout. Federal practitioner: for the health care professionals of the VA, DoD, and PHS, 36(9), 400— 402.

[128] Epstein EG, Whitehead PB, Prompahakul C, Thacker LR & Hamric AB (2019). Enhancing Understanding of Moral Distress: The Measure of Moral Distress for Health Care Professionals, AJOB Empirical Bioethics, 10:2, 113–124, DOI: 10.1080/23294515.2019. 1586008.

daycare and preschool closures are still widespread across the country. Parents and teachers have anecdotally raised concerns that this may be related to mask use. Actually, seeing people talk is foundational to phonetic development for all children, and especially those with disabilities or learning disorders.

Harvard's Center on the Developing Child explains that, "As early experiences shape the architecture of the developing brain, they also lay the foundations of sound mental health. Disruptions to this developmental process can impair a child's capacities for learning and relating to others—with lifelong implications."

Question 1. Dr. Durham, are children with speech delays at a greater risk of developing mental health problems compared to other children? If so, what are clinicians doing now to prepare for the pandemic's secondary mental health consequences on children?

Answer 1. Children of all ages have the potential to be impacted by the pandemic. Many of the families we serve at BMC have had to work outside of the home throughout the pandemic to continue providing for their families. This meant families living in multigenerational homes often were exposed to the virus. We have seen recent data indicating many children have lost parents and/ or caregivers due to COVID–19 (linked below). Grief from death of loves ones, loss of school connections, loss of activities once enjoyed and/or the inability to stay fully connected to friends and family will impact many across all ages. The Federal Government could ensure that mental health services in schools and in communities are well equipped to support children and their families. In schools, in particular, supports should be in place not only for children, but for staff as well. It is imperative the adults caring for children at schools have the supports they need to continue to be mentally prepared to also be a source of support for children in schools.[129] 4

Senator Murkowski

Mental Health Workforce: I am deeply concerned by the worsening, widespread shortage of mental health professionals, which has only been exacerbated by the COVID–19 pandemic. Over half of Alaska's population, three hundred and eighty thousand Alaskans, live in a designated Mental Health Professional shortage area. Workforce shortages create another serious barrier to accessing mental health care services, especially for those living in rural communities, like many Alaskans. Last May, I joined Senator

[129] Reference: https://www.thelancet—com/infographics/COVID-0919—associated—care giver— deaths.

Smith in introducing the Mental Health Professionals Workforce Shortage Loan Repayment Act. This bill establishes a student loan repayment program for mental health professionals who work in these shortage areas. My hope is that this legislation will help expand the mental health workforce and incentivize professionals to provide much-needed mental health care to those living in rural communities and other underserved areas.

Question 1. What other steps do you recommend taking to address mental health workforce shortages, specifically with regard to the shortages facing Americans in underserved and rural areas?

Answer 1. Congress should consider expanding the list of eligible sites that qualify for the National Health Service Corps (NHSC) loan repayment program as a means to entice more clinicians to enter the mental health field. A promising example of this is the Health Resources and Services Administration (HRSA) Substance Use Disorder Treatment and Recovery Loan Repayment Program (STAR-LRP)—authorized by the SUPPORT for Patients and Communities Act of 2018—which allows certain clinical roles providing substance use disorder treatment to receive up to $250,000 in loan repayment after 6 years. BMC recently became a STAR-LRP approved facility and expects this will be a significant asset to our recruitment efforts. Conversely, BMC, despite being an urban safety-net hospital that provides a continuum of mental health services to historically marginalized communities, does not qualify as a NHSC-approved site, meaning our mental health providers are not eligible to receive loan repayment.

Beyond the shortage of providers, the mental health workforce is not representative or reflective of the U.S. population—for instance, only 2 percent of Psychiatrists identify as Black. In addition to expanding the NHSC loan repayment program for the mental health workforce to include urban safety-net providers, efforts should be directed toward providing greater investment in a racially and ethnically diverse mental health workforce, such as proposed in the *"Pursuing Equity in Mental Health Act" (S. 1795).*

Question 2. What can and should be done to grow the employee pipeline in this field?

Answer 2. In order to grow the mental health employee pipeline, we must understand that the issue at its root is a pipeline issue that requires holistic solutions. Just as we say in medicine, that a person's zip code is more influential than their genetic code in determining life trajectory and long-term health, where a person lives, the color of their skin, and language they speak is highly determinative of the quality of education and resources available, the level of exposure to the mental health field, and stigma associated with mental illness.

Substance Use: During COVID, we have seen a sharp rise in substance misuse specifically alcohol, the most widely used and misused substance. Unfortunately, a landmark NIH study in 2018 established that 1 in 20 school-aged children are affected by fetal alcohol spectrum disorders—FASD. Because of its significance and its status as an overlooked disability that includes debilitating stigma, I introduced S. 2238, the FASD Respect Act. My legislation establishes common standards of care and increases the capacity to manage FASD in medical and mental health settings.

Question 3. Do you believe pediatricians, psychiatrists, and other professionals need to be better informed about FASD—is knowledge of FASD sufficient in your department? If more education and training is needed, how can that be achieved? How can stigma be lessened for individuals living with scorned behavioral health conditions, like FASD?

Answer 3. In September 2020, BMC was awarded a 3-year, $2.9 million Health Resources and Services Association (HRSA) grant to fund the SAFEST Choice Learning Collaborative, a program aimed at reducing the incidence of prenatal alcohol exposure and improving outcomes in children with suspected or diagnosed fetal alcohol spectrum disorders (FASD). The program—which is a joint effort between BMC, Boston University Schools of Medicine and Public Health, and Minnesota-based Proof Alliance—uses the Extension for Community Healthcare Outcomes (ECHO) virtual education platform to provide primary care providers at community health centers in New England and the Upper Midwest with training and support from experts about FASD and how to screen for and counsel women about the risks of alcohol use during pregnancy, as well as train pediatric providers on identifying and caring for children and adolescents with suspected or diagnosed FASD.[130] [5] More information on the program is available on our website: https:// www.bmc.org/addiction/training-education/safest-choice.

Suicide Screening in the Emergency Department: A recent CDC report on emergency department visits for people age 12–25 found an over 50 percent increase visits for suspected suicide attempts during early 2021. This not only underscores the devastating mental health impact of the pandemic on our youth, but highlights yet another way that COVID–19 has strained our hospitals and medical staff.

---

[130] Press Release: https://www.bmc.org/news/press-releases/2020/09/09/boston-medical-center-and-proof-alliance-collaborate-reduce-prenatal.

I introduced a bill, the Effective Suicide Screening and Assessment in the Emergency Department Act, to improve the screening and treatment of patients in hospital emergency departments who are at high risk for suicide. It will make sure that we can better identify our most vulnerable mental health patients so they do not slip through the cracks when they are treated in hospitals, and make sure hospitals have the resources they need to provide these critical services.

Question 4. Can you talk about the need for improved suicide screening protocols in the Nation's emergency rooms and, second, do you support efforts to bolster the resources available to emergency rooms so they can enhance their screening for high-risk suicide patients?

Answer 4. Boston Medical Center has a Psychiatric Emergency Department and is the lead agency for the Boston Emergency Services Team (BEST), which provides a comprehensive and highly integrated system of crisis evaluation, intervention, and treatment services. However, I'm fully aware that this is not typical of emergency departments everywhere. While I support screening for high-risk suicide patients in emergency departments, it's absolutely essential that a positive screen result in an appropriate response with access to appropriate resources for follow-up.

Response by Sara Goldsby to Questions of Senator Murphy, Senator Smith, Senate Luján, Senator Murkowski, Senator Braun, and Senator Scott

Senator Murphy

Question 1. How can we better prepare professionals in frequent contact with children and teens, such as teachers and pediatricians, to better deal with young people's unique behavioral health needs?

Answer 1. More education and training can always be done for all professionals to understand that all behaviors have meaning.

Schools are well positioned to provide mental health and substance use programming and services to youth. In particular, school-based student assistance programs can be effective in providing substance use prevention, mental health promotion, early intervention, referral to treatment and guided support programming and services. As described by the Substance Abuse and Mental health Services Administration (SAMHSA), student assistance programs "integrate trained personnel into schools to support and enhance the work of school faculty, as well as provide direct intervention services to students (Student Assistance: A Guide for School Administrators, SAMHSA, 2019).

For health care professionals, more must be done to integrate training related to mental health and youth into medical education curricula. This includes screening, early identification and referral processes. In addition, more must be done to recruit and train more people interested in serving youth and young adults. Our nation faces a severe workforce shortage—including a shortage of those serving children and teens.

We can also support professionals to be healthy models of emotion and behavior regulation, which implicitly reinforces positive feedback loops, helps children and teens connect with emotions, regulate behaviors, and improve decision-making.

Professionals could also be supported to increase overall comfort addressing difficult conversations with children and parents and caregivers.

Question 2. How might additional training for these professionals improve supports for young people?

Answer 2. Additional training for professionals and increasing pediatric time with young people stands to improve treatment outcomes. As an example, trauma, depression and ADHD present in similar ways. When professionals can get at a distinct and accurate diagnosis young people have improved outcomes.

When professionals feel more confident in their capabilities and practices with unique and difficult behavioral needs young people will be better helped earlier.

Question 3. Knowing that we have significant health care disparities stratified by income, race, and geography (e.g. rural areas), how do we ensure health equity in addressing the behavioral health needs of children and teens?

Answer 3. Focusing more resources, programs, and services on the populations experiencing worse outcomes and less access due to income, race, and location will help ensure better health equity. Moreover, the most significant long-term impact on disparities will occur when the resources, programs, and services are aimed at improving the social determinants well-being overall. Finally, we know the therapeutic relationships for youth and young adults are incredibly important. More work can be done to recruit and train people of color to work in the mental health and substance use fields.

Senator Smith

Question 1. What are specific examples of initiatives that you have seen in your work that have done a good job of incorporating mental health into the broader response to COVID–19? What should Congress learn from these successes?

Answer 1. Rapid implementation of telehealth during COVID–19 isolation measures to deliver mental health and substance use services was an instant solution to many who had challenges with access due to transportation and childcare before the pandemic. Implementing the policy and finance mechanisms that enabled telehealth was done quickly out of necessity. And we are still evidencing the successes of patient engagement and retention to services having eliminated those long-standing barriers. We can learn that a universal and coordinated response for a probable solution or promising practice can advance our goals overall even without urgent circumstances.

Additionally, phone and text availability to mental health and addictions counselors that were implemented during COVID–19 continue to be a utilized connection to care. As the 988-crisis line is implemented nation-wide we hope to see continued success and development of a service array that meets the needs of all callers.

Senator Luján

Question 1. Access to MAT improves patient survival, but some estimate that only 10 percent of those with opioid use disorder can access MAT. I applaud the Department of Health and Human Services under Secretary Becerra's leadership for working to remove barriers that were keeping qualified practitioners from treating opioid use disorder with MAT. As someone working to combat substance use disorder at the state level, what policy recommendations would you make to ensure that there's a broad provider network that's adequately trained in medically assisted treatment?

Answer 1. We are very grateful for the recent policy changes that have given more practitioners greater flexibility to provide MAT. In South Carolina, we have thousands of qualified prescribers who have taken the training allowing them to do office-based buprenorphine treatment. Despite their training and DATA 2000 Waiver approval, most of the practitioners are still not actively treating patients with addiction. Through our years of work with the healthcare community and providers across our state, we believe that earlier experiential practice and training in MAT services will break down the biases that some professionals hold toward people with addiction.

Additionally, practical and supported experience earlier in training helps providers feel more confidence in the service delivery.

Question 2. In addition to increasing the workforce, what other barriers are keeping those with substance use disorder from accessing MAT?

Answer 2. There are still strong philosophies among care providers, decisionmakers, and the public that medications for opioid use disorder are simply a substitution for the substances people use illicitly. Many people believe that the only successful recovery is recovery without medications of any kind. This lack of understanding of the science and uniformed narrative drives a bias against evidence-based services, hindering the implementation of the medical services, and deterring people from them.

Question 3. What additional barriers to treatment impact communities of color?

Answer 3. The stigma of substance use disorders and their treatments, the costs of treatment, and stigmatizing attitudes of healthcare workers can all be unique barriers to communities of color. Early intervention programs, prevention services, and education about evidence-based treatment that is developed by local community leaders in trusted community organizations helps ensure cultural and language preferences are addressed. This can lead to improving earlier access to treatment and recovery support. In South Carolina, we work with our faith-based organizations to do this kind of work. Additionally, punitive responses to substance use have disproportionately impacted communities of color. There are higher arrest rates for drug-related offenses for black individuals than white individuals. However, criminal justice systems can evolve to become a point of entry to treatment with diversion and deflection programs that adhere to standards, and support evidence-based treatment.

Question 4. The first year of the COVID–19 pandemic saw the highest number of overdose deaths on record. Now that Pandora's Box has been opened and opioids are readily available in every corner of our country, we must use every tool at our disposal to save lives. As with MAT, there is growing evidence that harm reduction programs prevent death and connect those experiencing substance use disorder with the resources they need to move toward recovery. Dr. Goldsby, what more can the Federal Government do to support states hoping to expand harm reduction resources?

Answer 4. In December 2021, SAMHSA released a grant funding opportunity for harm reduction programming that was included in the American Rescue Plan Act (ARPA). While only 25 awards are anticipated for the 3-year projects, hundreds of people across the states and territories attended the SAMHSA-supported webinars for the prospective applicants. At least six entities from South Carolina alone applied for the funds to begin and expand their harm reduction programs. DAODAS assisted many of the applicants in their planning conversations with local municipal leaders and community stakeholders. The result of the conversations that stemmed from the funding opportunity is a better understanding of harm reduction activities, and more acceptance of harm reduction as prevention and intervention strategy on the continuum of care. More support for the education of the evidence-based approach, and the implementation of the programs and services will help the harm reduction expand to undoubtedly save more lives.

Senator Murkowski

SUD Treatment and Recovery: While treatment receives the bulk of attention and investment from Congress, and prevention has dedicated funding via the Substance Abuse Prevention and Treatment Block Grant (SABG), there are no comparable dedicated funding streams for recovery support services. Once consumers receive treatment, they require a variety of services to help them get their lives on track. These can include housing, job training, the benefits of fellowship, and the services of peer professionals. SUD prevention, treatment, and recovery is a continuum of care and services.

Question 1. Congress has proposed a 10-percent set aside in the SABG so that states may invest in recovery. How do you believe this money would best be spent?

Answer 1. As the Single State Authority (SSA) managing the SAPT Block Grant in South Carolina, we have used existing funds, including SAPT Block Grant funds, to support a number of initiatives along the recovery continuum. For example, we support the development of collegiate recovery programs at our colleges and universities, and the development and growth of several independent recovery community organizations (RCOs) around the state.

From 2018 to 2021 we supported the training and certification of 344 Peer Support Specialists. Many of these peers are now employed by are treatment services providers and recovery community organizations. Because Medicaid and private insurance coverage of the peer services is so little, we also support the salaries for most of these positions. Additionally, DAODAS has had a long-time partnership with Oxford House Inc. to ensure recovery housing is available across the state. A 10-percent set aside in the SABG, with a corresponding increase in this program, would enable us to build on, expand, and sustain these kinds of programs and services.

Question 2. Ms. Goldsby, are you seeing increased usage of alcohol and other harmful substances among pregnant and parenting women due to COVID–19 and other factors? If so, how is your department responding, and what measures have proven effective in educating the public, training primary care professionals, and increasing access to therapeutic recovery services for women?

Answer 2. In South Carolina we began to worry about pregnant and parenting women specifically in March 2020. As soon as isolation measures due to COVID–19 were put in place we began seeing social media messages reinforcing increased alcohol use and medication misuse for women who were working from home and managing childcare and homeschooling simultaneously. In May 2020, our agency began pushing messages on social media platforms to counter the messages and reinforce healthier coping behaviors and less consumption.

Knowing that some women were drinking more, earlier in the day, and possibly using other substances leads us to believe that many who otherwise would never have had a substance use disorder might have developed one during the last 2 years.

We continue to work with the South Carolina Birth Outcomes Initiative with many partners to include health systems and women's services providers as we advocate for screening brief intervention and referrals to treatment for pregnant and parenting women at medical visits, which is not consistently done currently.

With the December COVID–19 Supplement and the March COVID–19 Supplement to the SAPT Block Grant, we developed and are supporting a statewide call line, and telehealth services as a supplement to our Plan of Safe Care effort follow-up for pregnant and postpartum women identified with substance use issues. It is modeled after the Massachusetts Child Psychiatry Access Program for Moms that promotes maternal/infant/child health for 1 year after delivery. Our program will train and educate healthcare providers in South Carolina on substance use disorders and mental disorders for pregnant and postpartum women. It will provide real-time psychiatric consultation via telehealth, and access to a care coordinator who will provide resources and referrals to women during the 12 months postpartum. This will be transformative for our families and our providers and our state. It is wholly supported by short-term COVID–19 relief funds. We will be looking at ways to sustain this programming to stay on track with non-punitive interventions and care for families that could otherwise have social service intervention.

In South Carolina, we support four Family Care Centers which are residential programs for pregnant and postpartum women specifically designed to deliver family centered services where women receive clinical substance use treatment while living with their baby or young children and receiving therapeutic services to healing as a family unit. The SAPT Block Grant and Medicaid reimbursement helps supports these Centers.

Finally, we appreciate the funds provided in the Pregnant and Postpartum Women's (PPW) Residential Services Grant Program within SAMHSA's Center for Substance Abuse Treatment (CSAT). This program allocates grants to programs that support family centered services in residential settings. In 2016, the Comprehensive Addiction and Recovery Act (CARA) re-authorized the PPW Residential Services Grant Program, and authorized a pilot program to enhance flexibility in the use of funds to provide family centered substance use services to pregnant and postpartum women in non-residential service settings. We sincerely appreciate both the residential program and the pilot initiative. We hope Congress will continue to support these initiatives.

Question 3. What is your state doing to improve recovery support services, and what lessons can the Federal Government take from your efforts? We are interested in hearing about your progress in both urban and rural areas, and amongst all demographics.

Answer 3. With State Opioid Response funds, we have funded recovery community organizations (RCOs) across the state. While only a couple of RCOs have been established longer than 5 years, we aim to meet the needs of their growth to address urban needs while also meeting the needs of RCOs that are emerging, (or have been established fewer than 5 years) and those RCOs that are new and just establishing themselves as service delivery organizations.

Our funds and technical assistance support implementation and continuation of recovery-based initiatives and programs for persons and families affected by substance use disorders in an effort to reduce the consequences of opioid and stimulant misuse in our state. Our approved strategies that RCOs implement, and allowable use of the funds guide organizations to engage with specific populations and encourage service delivery and outreach to rural areas or locations that bring access to the people in need of services. Examples of this include providing mutual aid groups outside of the organization's walls and immediate geographic area, and providing Certified Peer Support Specialist services in specific locations such as detention centers, hospitals, and to faith-based groups.

In our field we say you should 'meet the person where they are' literally and figuratively. As administrators, we do this with recovery community organizations with the aim of being supportive and collaborative for the best possible outcomes.

We are also currently working with the National Alliance of Recovery Residences (NARR) to support independent recovery residences as they work toward national standards and certification. The South Carolina legislature is considering a bill that would require recovery residences to be certified and adhering to national standards in order to received state funds or referrals. This stands to improve our awareness of the many recovery residences around our state, and ensure adherence to ethical practices and conditions for residents.

Senator Braun

CDC recently published a report finding that two drugs—para-fluorofentanyl and metonitazene—are being seen more often by medical examiners looking into overdose deaths. They often are taken with—or mixed with—illicit fentanyl, the drug mainly responsible for the more than 100,000 U.S. overdose deaths in the last year. A news report in the Indiana Gazette last Friday stated that U.S. overdose deaths have been rising for more than two decades, but they accelerated in the past 2 years—jumping more than 20 percent in the latest year alone, according to the most recently available CDC data, through June 2021.

Yet, even as the crisis escalates, the Substance Abuse and Mental Health Services Administration (SAMHSA) found that in 2020, only 11.2 percent (nearly 300,000) of people aged 12 or older with a past year opioid use disorder received medication treatment, which reduces the risk for overdose. This data demonstrates a shocking gap between the need for service and access and availability.

Question 1. As a cosponsor of the Mainstreaming Addiction Treatment Act, I'd like to hear from you how we can further increase access to life-saving medication. What other policies are needed to ensure those suffering from opioid use disorder can get the treatment they need?

Answer 1. The recent policy changes that have given more practitioners greater flexibility to practice medication-assisted treatment have helped. Still in South Carolina, we have thousands of prescribers who can treat addiction, but they do not. Many healthcare professionals still do not screen patients for substance use disorders. This obstructs access to care when most people may only ever encounter an opportunity for intervention and treatment with a primary care or hospital experience.

There is still a need for primary care and hospital service practice transformation to include screening, brief interventions, and referral to specialty addiction treatment (SBIRT), as well as the practice of medical treatment for substance use disorders in those settings. This could develop with strong technical assistance, supported practice implementation, and perhaps even with financial incentives. Until our healthcare providers understand and realize the reward and benefit to addressing addiction like they do other chronic diseases, bias and stigma will remain inside of healthcare. Training and practical application stands to change hearts and minds to create access. Still, without local policymakers' understanding of evidence-based treatment, feasibility of more integrated care remains varied. An example of this is local regulation that prohibiting Opioid Treatment Programs or other specialty addiction treatment services to be integrated into other healthcare settings or commercially zoned to convenient and safe geographic locations.

Senator Scott

SUDs and Treatment Access: Sadly, we are all too familiar with the ongoing addiction crisis in this country, which has been exacerbated by the pandemic. South Carolina, like many other states, is experiencing high rates of alcohol abuse, opioid abuse, stimulant abuse, and broad polysubstance use. During the pandemic, we saw dangerous substance abuse behavior promoted on social media platforms. For instance, memes, hashtags, and other references normalized day drinking to address the effects of lockdowns, unemployment, and other pandemic-fueled stressors. Sadly, what may have started as a casual way to pass the time, changed consumption habits, and spiraled Americans into addiction.

Question 1. Director Goldsby—Can you discuss the work being done to address these issues in South Carolina, specifically how you're utilizing Federal support to combat not just opioid abuse, but also alcohol and stimulant abuse?

Answer 1. In May 2020 as we began to see social media normalizing drinking to cope with the stressors of the pandemic. We launched our own social media effort creating memes to counter the messages and show support for healthier relationships with alcohol. The messages carried links to the Alcohol Use Disorder Identification Test, quick self-test on our website to help determine risk of alcohol problems.

In June 2020, with the support of a $1.9 million SAMHSA grant award for COVID–19 Crisis Response, we partnered with the South Carolina Department of Mental Health to launch the SC Hopes Mental Health and Addictions Support Line, offering 24/7 telephonic connection to mental health and addictions counselors, and certified peer support specialists. The addictions counselors and peer specialists we engaged to rotate on the call line are all primarily serve in our public system supported by the SAPT Block Grant. Strong TV, social media, and billboard marketing around the state, and the inclusion of Spanish and hearing impaired services has driven use of the line to more than 5,640 calls since June 1st, 2020.

Question 2. Following up here, Director Goldsby—Can you describe some of the difficulties you have encountered in the limitation on what certain programs can be used to treat and whether or not additional flexibility would be helpful to give you additional tools and resources to better combat the broader epidemic?

Answer 2. We were able to use the State Opioid Response (SOR) funds that we had on hand in March 2020 to immediately, almost proactively respond when we knew isolation was going to occur and impact people with substance use issues. While we support a robust public education and prevention campaign about the dangers of and the resources for opioid and stimulant use issues, we were limited in what we could leverage for messaging on problematic alcohol, and problematic substance use more broadly, and had to rely on a limited amount of state funds we had on hand for those efforts.

We have used SOR funds to purchase transportation vouchers for patients to get to and from treatment. This has been helpful short term especially in rural counties when patients would otherwise not access care.

The SOR dollars limit resources to patients who have opioid and stimulant use disorders. As we roll out programs and services like the transportation vouchers, these Federal spending limitations generate the appearance that to our addiction service providers or our programs favor certain people with certain types of addiction issues. We have relied on a limited amount of state funds we have on hand for transportation vouchers to support people with other substance use diagnoses.

Furthermore, the substance specific funding requires the service providers and the state administration to track dollars to specific diagnoses which adds heavy administrative burden all around that could be alleviated if funds were intended for any substance use disorder diagnosis.

Until the December 2020 and March 2021 COVID relief supplements came to South Carolina, none of the Federal funds we had on hand allowed the purchase of important technology such as phones, laptops, and broadband to support the transition to telehealth services. Luckily, we had a limited amount of state funds on hand to support those needs in early 2020 when the transition occurred.

Rural Access to Opioid Treatment: On January 3, 2022, HHS Secretary Becerra renewed the public health emergency for opioids. The opioid epidemic doesn't discriminate and has touched every community in America. Throughout rural America, including most of South Carolina, access to evidence-based treatment for substance use disorders has always been a challenge. In 2018, the U.S. Department of Health and Human Services' Office of Inspector General released a report that showed 40 percent of all counties in the country didn't have a single medical practitioner able to prescribe buprenorphine, 1 of only 3 FDA-approved medications for treating opioid use disorder. This includes almost a quarter of my own state and disproportionately impacts rural counties across the country.

Question 3. Director Goldsby—Your department has worked with the National Institute on Drug Abuse and the South Carolina Department of Health and Human Services to improve access to treatment for opioid use disorder in rural emergency rooms across our state. What has worked well in bringing treatment for opioid use disorder to rural residents of our state and what can Congress and the Federal Government do to help?

Answer 3. The SUPPORT Act gave practitioners greater flexibility to practice medication-assisted treatment (MAT) extending the privilege of prescribing buprenorphine in office-based settings to other qualifying practitioners like nurses and Physician Assistants. In addition, Federal policy allowing certain practitioners to treat up to 100 patients is a change that helped. Still in South Carolina, we have thousands of prescribers who can treat addiction, but do not. This dynamic is creating an access barrier in rural areas. There is still a need for primary care and hospital service practice transformation to include screening and medical treatment of substance use disorders. This could be developed with strong technical assistance, supported practical change implementation, and perhaps even with financial incentives. Until our healthcare providers understand and realize the reward and benefit to addressing addiction like they do other chronic diseases, bias and stigma will remain inside of healthcare. Training and practical application stands to change hearts and minds to create access.

Response by Jennifer D. Lockman to Questions of Senator Murphy, Senator Smith, Senator Murkowski, and Senator Scott

Senator Murphy

Question 1. How can we better prepare professionals in frequent contact with children and teens, such as teachers and pediatricians, to better deal with young people's unique behavioral health needs?

Question 2. How might additional training for these professionals improve supports for young people?

Answer 1. Pediatricians should all be taught in universal screening practices utilizing universal screeners such as the Pediatric Screening Checklist and suicide-specific screeners such as the Columbia Suicide Severity Rating Scale.

Answer 2. Pediatricians and Teachers could benefit from effective, tailored trainings in brief engagement and intervention strategies:

- Pediatricians who utilize motivational interviewing, a brief (10–15 minute) intervention focused on increasing client engagement in their goals, can increase engagement in mental health care for clients (Desai, 2019; Reinauer et al., 2021)
- For pediatricians who identify a patient that is at risk of harm to themselves or others; safety planning and lethal means counseling are a necessary step to engage in with clients prior to discharge to increase probability the client's crisis is allayed prior to entry in mental health care (Schwartzman et al, 2021; Sisler et al., 2020). Those clients—who are screened, have developed a safety plan/ blocked access to lethal means, and have a referral to follow-up care—have a significantly higher chance of getting to their appointment with tools to help them through crises that may present prior to engagement in specialty behavioral health care.
- Effective tailored trainings include those that have a simulation based learning or immersive trainings. These types of trainings are intrinsic to other high stakes environments (i.e., pilots, surgeons, etc.); however, despite strong evidence suggesting high efficacy of simulation-trainings—there is little uptake in behavioral health settings of these types of trainings. Given the high risk nature of suicide and the need for consistent practice—simulation based training may increase mastery and decrease length of booster

trainings (Matterson et al, 2018; Carter et al, 2018). In addition, simulation trainings are effective at increasing confidence and preparedness in talking to students about mental health (Green et al., 2020). Therefore, increasing the effectiveness of interventions while increasing systemic feasibility of training. Funding that includes time for institutions to offset revenue as well as pay pediatricians, teachers, and other relevant staff to participate in simulated training experiences is needed.

This is an area where our Research Institute can offer significant subject matter expertise. As such, should you or any of your staff have any specific questions about simulation training for suicide intervention/prevention—please do not hesitate to reach out to our team.

Both teachers and pediatricians should have support from their superiors to devote the time and space necessary for mental health—this requires cultural and institutional shifts to ensure time and resources are allocated.

- There should be support (either physically or tele-located) for students screened/identified as being at risk for suicide. Pediatricians and teachers could be trained in identification tools and brief motivational enhancement strategies—as mentioned above—then refer to more highly trained specialists and school-based liaisons.
- Specialists and school-based liaisons trained in crisis assessment/triage/intervention could then take on the key roles of suicide risk assessment and triage. Individualized education plans (IEPs) for those students identified at higher risk should include weekly treatment team meetings between counselors/teachers/families/pediatri-cians/specialists/liaisons. Using this model, pediatricians and teachers could have a key, but minimal role, which would allow for them to focus on the primary jobs that they have been trained to do.
- Ultimately, expanded and consistent funding or reimbursement/coverage for school-based and emergency-room based mental health liaisons, as well funding for the necessary training in crisis strategies, would greatly improve continuity of care between identification of students at risk and engagement with these students.

Quicker and prolonged engagement in treatment. Research suggests that children that engage in care as fast as possible after identified and those that receive more consistent care get better faster than those who have lag times between identification and treatment (see samhsa.gov at https://ncsacw.samhsa.gov/files/ rpg-ta-brief-referral-engagement.pdf).

Finally, we can have all the best evidence and training in the world, but without the workforce—our response to the current (and projected growing) need will be woefully insufficient. Above all other policy measures, we urge that Congress prioritize policy solutions to address the mental health staff shortages.

To this end, we strongly urge that Congress consider both short-term emergency and long term policy solutions to address the current gap in the workforce. Following we outline one short term measure Congress can immediately take as well as longer term policy solutions to address the behavioral health workforce crisis in America.

With regard to short-term solutions to the behavioral health workforce crisis, we urge Senate HELP and Finance to consider short/medium-term, emergency measures to ensure providers have tools to better recruit and retain their workforce. According to Centerstone's own internal exit interview data, staff leaving cite salary as the No. 1 reason they are leaving. As such we suggest the introduction of the following new, emergency grant program:

- Introduce an Emergency Workforce Funding Bill
- Create a new grant program, that community/safety net provides could apply to request funding to support retention bonuses, wage increases, and more to incentive workforce recruitment and retention for front line staff
- Eligible Provide Types
- Psychiatrists
- Physicians with a buprenorphine waiver
- Psychologists
- Nurse practitioners with a buprenorphine waiver
- Physician assistants with a buprenorphine waiver
- Clinical social workers
- Licensed mental health counselors
- Licensed marriage & family therapists
- Case managers
- Peer support specialists

Use of Funds. The eligible entities described below are permitted to use the funds toward:

- Retention bonuses
- Hazard pay
- Overtime
- Shift deferential pay (wage increases)
- Other additional compensation and employee benefits deemed by the Secretary as necessary to retain clinical staff

In terms of long term solutions to address the behavioral health workforce crisis, we suggest the following legislative vehicles which we believe get at longer term, systemic barriers that restrict workforce and access to evidence-based behavioral health services:

- Pass the Excellence in Mental Health and Addiction Treatment Act of 2021 (S. 2069).
- We see this legislation as the single most critical piece of legislation that Congress can pass to increase training for evidence-based practices, elevate the quality/standard of care in community mental health settings, and address long standing workforce barriers through the Prospective Payment System (PPS) payment methodology that allows providers to offer more competitive wages to their frontline staff. Furthermore, Certified Community Behavioral Health Clinics (CCBHCs) are required to serve patients regardless of payer type and offer a wide area of required services, including mobile crisis and crisis stabilization.
- Full implementation of this model can take a couple years; thus, we recommend that Congress take shorter term measures—as noted above. That being said, in the long term—this legislation is probably the most critical piece of behavioral health legislation Congress can pass in 2022 to transform the community mental health system.
- Pass the Behavioral Health Services Crisis Expansion Act (S. 1902).
- Coverage is a key component toward ensuring that services are sustainable and available to consumers in a time of crisis. Ensuring that both public and private payers cover crisis services can drastically increase availability and access for consumers when they need it most.

- Ensure that any telehealth extensions include a delay of the in-person requirement on telemental health services, as outlined in The Telemental Health Care Access Act (S. 2061).
- This in-person requirement of telemental health services—if implemented—will further encumber already overworked providers to arbitrarily delineate between their patients on "who gets what type of service" based on diagnosis, rather than clinical presentation and best practice. This approach is counter to the gold standard of providing the "right care at the right time" to improve patient and population health outcomes. Passage of S. 2061 would address this barrier.

Finally we urge passage of the Mental Health Access Improvement Act of 2021 (S. 828).

- This legislation would add other master's level therapists (i.e., Marriage & Family Therapists, etc.) to eligible providers under Medicare (which is currently restricted to only Licensed Clinical Social Workers). Passage of this legislation would allow our behavioral health workforce to work with the full scope of their training and education.

In conclusion, in order to better prepare professionals in frequent contact with children and teens, we need mental health professionals to refer them to. Employees are leaving the mental health workforce at a rapid pace due to low wages and high stress. To address the behavioral health workforce crisis—that is particularly elevated in community, not-for-profit mental health settings—we need Congress to pass legislation that ensures providers have the tools they need to not only recruit and retain staff, but to elevate the quality of care—while increasing access.

Question 3. Knowing that we have significant health care disparities stratified by income, race, and geography (e.g. rural areas), how do we ensure health equity in addressing the behavioral health needs of children and teens?

Telehealth

Answer 3. We know that telehealth has increased access to care for clients that otherwise have difficulty with transportation or scheduling. In fact, we also know that treatment for depressive symptoms using telehealth services is equivalent to face-to-face services in reduction of depressive symptoms based on evaluation data from our CCBHC during the COVID–19 pandemic (unpublished data, 2022).

988 and Crisis Services

- As we look toward addressing health disparities in addressing the behavioral health needs of children and teens—there is tremendous opportunity to ensure the Nation's new 988 three-digit dialing code for the National Suicide Prevention Lifeline (set to launch July 16, 2022) and corresponding services through the crisis continuum are culturally competent and meets the needs of vulnerable, marginalized populations. Specifically:
- Crisis teams, ideally, should reflect the diversity of the communities served and ensure community response and stabilization services meets the needs of everyone in the community; and
- Congress can urge SAMHSA to develop child-focused crisis engagement guidelines to emphasize both evidence- based strategies specific to child and adolescent populations as well as provide further guidelines toward ensuring services address long-standing health disparities.

Senator Smith

Question 1. What are specific examples of initiatives that you have seen in your work that have done a good job of incorporating mental health into the broader response to COVID–19? What should Congress learn from these successes?

Telehealth Expansion

Answer 1. We know that telehealth flexibilities availed through the COVID–19 Public Health Emergency has increased access to care for clients that otherwise have difficulty with transportation or scheduling. In fact, we also know that treatment for depressive symptoms using telehealth services is equivalent to face-to-face services in reduction of depressive symptoms based on evaluation data from our Certified Community Behavioral Health Clinic (CCBHC) during the COVID–19 pandemic (unpublished data, 2022). Additionally, initial findings indicated that a cohort of clients receiving telehealth medication assisted treatment (MAT) experienced a 9 percent reduction in average days using any substance, a 29 percent reduction in average days depressed or anxious, and a 9 percent increase in treatment satisfaction at 6 months relative to face-to-face clients (Hanauer, M., Moore, J. T., & Lockman, J, 2020).

- To that end we thank you and Senator Cassidy for your leadership on Telemental Health Care Access Act—S. 2061. The Telemental Health Care Access Act would provide continuity in behavioral health care access by removing the statutory requirement that Medicare beneficiaries be seen in person within 6 months of being treated for a mental health service via telehealth. We strongly urge that this provision be included with any extension of telehealth flexibilities—as is currently being considered for the fiscal year 2022 omnibus spending bill.

Increasing Engagement

Utilizing funding from our SAMHSA Emergency Response for Suicide Prevention grants, we were able to form a team of clinicians to deploy suicide prevention strategies in novel ways that increase engagement and decrease resources. In Indiana, our staff utilized a weekly suicide screen/safety plan review approach with bachelor's level unlicensed staff. Those staff would then refer onto master's level counselors for further assessment if the client screened positive for increasing suicide risk. In addition, these clients could be seen biweekly for suicide-specific treatment, which allowed for decreased resourcing (as opposed to weekly visits for screening/safety plan review with a bachelor's-level staff person).

- To ensure on-going engagement for those in a mental health crisis, we strongly urge that Congress consider passage of the Behavioral Health Services Crisis Expansion Act (S. 1902) as a crucial component to financing the crisis care continuum via ensuring coverage as well as the Excellence in Mental Health and Addiction Treatment Act of 2021 (S. 2069) which advances the CCBHC model—a model in which care coordination, access, and crisis services are required components of the care delivery model.

Senator Murkowski

Suicide Screening in the Emergency Department: A recent CDC report on emergency department visits for people age 12–25 found an over 50 percent increase visits for suspected suicide attempts during early 2021. This not only underscores the devastating mental health impact of the pandemic on our youth, but highlights yet another way that COVID–19 has strained our hospitals and medical staff.

I introduced a bill, the Effective Suicide Screening and Assessment in the Emergency Department Act, to improve the screening and treatment of patients in hospital emergency departments who are at high risk for suicide. It will make sure that we can better identify our most vulnerable mental health patients so they do not slip through the cracks when they are treated in hospitals, and make sure hospitals have the resources they need to provide these critical services.

Question 1. Can you talk about the need for improved suicide screening protocols in the Nation's emergency rooms and, second, do you support efforts to bolster the resources available to emergency rooms so they can enhance their screening for high-risk suicide patients?

Suicide Screening

Answer 1. It is admirable and vital to increase suicide screening protocols to better catch high risk patients. To do so comprehensively, two specific actions are required.

First, funding is needed to study and administer adaptive screening measures (see King et al., 2021) that have been found to be best at predicting future suicide attempts and to study upstream screening measures (such as measures of interpersonal drivers of suicide) to better understand why people are driven to suicide and treat these drivers upstream so fewer people are thinking about suicide. Both of these types of measures would be exceptional in an emergency department screening.

Second, to match the increased need for suicide screening and supports in emergency rooms we need to answer the following question: what happens to those individuals after the emergency room? How do we improve continuity of care post-screening? If a person is coming into the emergency room for suicidal thoughts or a suicide attempt, they are in a vulnerable space and needed to be treated with respect, transparency, honesty, and be given the hope that things will change. We support resources dedicated to screening and assessment in hospitals with a caveat; that these changes also support triage and engagement practices with follow-up care. Post hospitalization is the most critical risk period for suicide known to researchers, with rates of suicide 100x higher than the global suicide rate in the 3 months following hospital discharge (Chung et al., 2017). Screenings and assessments are only good for hospital emergency rooms if they can quickly triage and transport patients. Screenings and assessments in hospital emergency rooms are only good for the behavioral health of our clients if they are respected and cared for enough to be connected with immediate follow-up care. Therefore, funding for resources not only for screening and assessment practices but also triage, transportation, and engagement with intensive outpatient or outpatient mental health treatment is necessary. Continuity of care to the crisis continuum is key for comprehensive suicide prevention.

To that end, we applaud and thank your and Senator King's leadership in advancing the Effective Suicide Screening and Assessment in the Emergency Department Act of 2021 (S. 467). We support the passage of this bill, and appreciate that the legislative text specifically emphasizes "enhancing the coordination of care for such individuals after discharge" as well as the provision which requires grantees "to establish and implement policies and procedures with respect to care coordination, integrated care models, or referral to evidence-based treatment to be used upon the discharge from the emergency department of patients who are at risk of suicide." Thank you for your leadership for this highly vulnerable population.

Senator Scott

Question 1. According to the U.S. Department of Health and Human Services, 20 percent of children and adolescents experience some type of mental health issue during their school years and a 2019 report by the Substance Abuse and Mental Health Services Administration stated that "Among the 3.8 million adolescents ages 12–17 who reported a major depressive episode in the past year, nearly 60 percent did not receive any treatment." Can you speak to the role of telehealth in expanding access to mental and behavioral health services for children in school-based settings and opportunities for public-private partnerships?

Answer 1. Telehealth allows the opportunity for more children in school-based settings to connect with psychiatrists, nurse practitioners, psychologists, and more who cannot be physically integrated into the school setting due to lack of resourcing. Centerstone does not have any public-private partnerships in school-based settings, but we have partnered in adult crisis diversion settings with private funders (e.g., Cook Medical Group in Indiana) to match funds raised by Centerstone and their partners in the Bloomington, Indiana community.

With regard to our public-private partnership in Indiana, the Stride Center fulfills a community-wide need for people experiencing substance use or mental health crisis who need a connection to care and a place to go rather than hospitalization or imprisonment (this is often referred to as crisis receiving or stabilization). Many times the options for an individual in a moment of crisis are hospitalization or jail, both of which are more costly and do not treat presenting symptoms or diagnosis. The goal of the Stride Center is to deescalate the situation and connect the guest with appropriate treatment resources (i.e., the right care at the right time). To date, the average amount of time for law enforcement to complete a drop off at the Stride Center is under 5 minutes; whereas processing for jail or the emergency department is 2 hours—saving both time and money through allowing law enforcement to spend their time addressing criminal activity and individuals in need of mental health or addiction treatment care—to receive the care they need. From our experience, public-private partnerships can add immense value to community-based services and the associated outcomes.

[Whereupon, at 12:08 p.m., the hearing was adjourned.]

Chapter 3

Substance Abuse and Mental Health Services Administration (SAMHSA): Overview of the Agency and Major Programs*

Johnathan H. Duff

Summary

The Substance Abuse and Mental Health Services Administration (SAMHSA) is the federal agency primarily responsible for supporting community-based mental health and substance abuse treatment and prevention services. Located within the Department of Health and Human Services (HHS), SAMHSA provides federal funding to states, local communities, and private entities by administering block grants and other formula and discretionary grants. Through such grants, SAMHSA supports activities that include education and training, prevention programs, early intervention activities, treatment services, and technical assistance. SAMHSA does not provide mental health or substance abuse treatment. Rather, the agency supports states' efforts in providing community-based behavioral health services. SAMHSA also conducts surveillance and data collection of national behavioral health issues, provides statistical and analytic support to grantees, and administers other agency-wide initiatives. SAMHSA derives most of its statutory authority from the Public Health Service Act (PHSA). More specifically, Title V and Title XIX of the PHSA contain most authorities for SAMHSA programs and activities.

SAMHSA's two largest programs are the Substance Abuse Prevention and Treatment Block Grant (SABG) and the Community Mental Health

* This is an edited, reformatted and augmented version of Congressional Research Service Publication No. R46426, dated June 23, 2020.

In: Mental Health and Substance Use Disorders: A Growing Crisis
Editor: Darren D. Stewart
ISBN: 979-8-89530-699-4

Services Block Grant (MHBG). Both block grant programs distribute funds to states (including the District of Columbia and territories) according to a formula specified in statute. The states, in turn, may distribute funds to local government entities and nonprofit organizations in accordance with a plan the state submits to SAMHSA.

SAMHSA also operates several discretionary programs, known as Programs of Regional and National Significance (PRNS). The PRNS encompass numerous grants and activities in the areas of substance abuse treatment, substance abuse prevention, and mental health. Typically, PRNS consist of programs for specific populations or areas of concern (e.g., children, suicide, opioid abuse). Some PRNS are explicitly authorized in statute while others are carried out under SAMHSA's general authorities. In addition, SAMHSA conducts surveillance and data collection, statistical and analytic support, and other agency-wide initiatives. SAMHSA provides resources for providers on treatment, prevention, and recovery for mental and substance use disorders and administers technical assistance to grantees.

SAMHSA's main source of funding is the discretionary budget authority it receives through the annual appropriations process. SAMHSAis funded through the annual Departments of Labor, Health and Human Services, and Education, and Related Agencies (Labor-HHS-ED) appropriations bill. SAMHSA's budget and appropriations fall under four categories: (1) substance abuse treatment, (2) substance abuse prevention, (3) mental health, and (4) health surveillance and program support. These categories roughly correspond with SAMHSA's four centers: (1) the Center for Substance Abuse Treatment; (2) the Center for Substance Abuse Prevention; (3) the Center for Mental Health Services; and (4) the Center for Behavioral Health Statistics and Quality.

Since its inception in 1992, SAMHSA and many of its programs have been reauthorized through legislation. While programs have been added or removed over the years, SAMHSA's primary responsibilities—including administering block grants to the states supporting mental health and substance abuse treatment services—have remained relatively consistent.

Background and Role

The Substance Abuse and Mental Health Services Administration (SAMHSA) is the federal agency primarily responsible for supporting community-based mental health and substance abuse treatment and prevention services. Located within the Department of Health and Human Services (HHS), SAMHSA provides federal funding for these services by administering two large formula-based block grant programs (one for substance abuse prevention and treatment services, the other for mental health services) and other formula and discretionary grants to local communities, states, and private entities.[1]

SAMHSA does not directly deliver treatment services. Rather, it supports state and local efforts in providing mental health and substance abuse (collectively known as behavioral health) services, primarily through funding and technical assistance. Behavioral health prevention and treatment activities have historically been the responsibilities of states. The federal government contributes supplementary support by providing funding and some direction for activities.[2] SAMHSA is the primary agency responsible for supporting state efforts in providing behavioral health treatment services. SAMHSA funds a wide range of activities including education and training for the behavioral health workforce, prevention and early intervention programs, and treatment services.

SAMHSA administers its larger grant programs directly to states, and some smaller grants to localities or directly to services providers. SAMHSAalso conducts surveillance and data collection, provides statistical and analytic support, maintains performance and quality information systems, and administers other agency-wide initiatives. SAMHSA derives most of its statutory authority from the Public Health Service Act (PHSA). More specifically, Title V and Title XIX of the PHSA contain most authorities for SAMHSA programs and activities.

Strategic Plan

SAMHSA's mission is to reduce the impact of substance misuse and mental illness on America's communities.[3] SAMHSA is required to develop a strategic plan every four years.[4] In its Strategic Plan FY2019-FY2023, SAMHSAarticulates its mission, vision, and five core principles which

[1] SAMHSA awards discretionary funds to substance abuse and mental health programs through its authorities in Title V of the Public Health Service Act (PHSA) and provides the formula-based Substance Abuse Prevention and Treatment Block Grant and Community Mental Health Services Block Grant through its authorities in Title XIX of the PHSA.

[2] Medicaid—a joint federal-state program—also plays a significant role in funding behavioral health treatment. For more information, see CRS Report R43357, *Medicaid: An Overview* and CRS In Focus IF10222, *Medicaid's Institutions for Mental Disease (IMD) Exclusion.*

[3] HHS, SAMHSA, *SAMHSA Strategic Plan FY2019-FY2023*, Rockville, MD, 2018, https://www.samhsa.gov/about-us/ strategic-plan.

[4] PHSA §501(l) (42 U.S.C. §290aa(l)).

include (1) supporting the adoption of evidence-based practices; (2) increasing access to the full continuum of services for mental and substance use disorders; (3) engaging in outreach to clinicians, grantees, patients, and the American public; (4) collecting, analyzing, and disseminating data to inform policies, programs, and practices; and (5) recognizing that the availability of mental and substance use disorder services is integral to everyone's health.[5]

SAMHSA also outlines five priority areas for FY2019-FY2023:

1) Combating the opioid crisis through the expansion of prevention, treatment, and recovery support services.
2) Addressing serious mental illness and serious emotional disturbance.
3) Advancing prevention, treatment, and recovery support services for substance use.
4) Improving data collection, analysis, dissemination, and program and policy evaluation.
5) Strengthening health practitioners training and education.

For each area, SAMHSA sets an overarching goal and identifies a series of measurable objectives. Additionally, SAMHSA describes examples of key performance and outcome measures to track progress in each area.

History of SAMHSA

SAMHSA was formed in 1992 following reorganization of the Alcohol, Drug Abuse and Mental Health Administration (ADAMHA). Prior to 1992, ADAMHA supported treatment service delivery and scientific research related to mental health and addiction. The ADAMHA Reorganization Act of 1992 (P.L. 102-321) moved the three existing research institutes within ADAMHA—the National Institute of Mental Health (NIMH), the National Institute on Drug Abuse (NIDA), and the National Institute on Alcohol Abuse and Alcoholism (NIAAA)—to the National Institutes of Health. ADAMHA was then renamed SAMHSA to reflect its primary focus on funding community-based treatment services.

[5] SAMHSA, *Strategic Plan FY2019-FY2023*.

Community-Based Treatment Services

The early U.S. health care system offered little treatment for mental illness. By the mid-19th century, state psychiatric hospitals had begun to grow in number and size; this institutional mental health care was seen as a state responsibility and was not funded by the federal government. Due to poor conditions and largely ineffective treatment practices in institutional facilities, a movement to shift mental health treatment into community-based settings began in the 1960s. This community mental health movement advocated for treatment to take place where individuals could also receive support from their community, without the disruption of being removed from the community to receive care. The community mental health movement corresponded with the evolution of more effective, evidence-based treatments for mental health conditions: treatments that could be delivered in outpatient settings. Over time, outpatient community mental health centers replaced inpatient and residential treatment facilities. In some instances, this change was directly supported by the federal government, through grant programs and laws such as The Community Mental Health Act of 1963 (P.L. 88-164). Today, most individuals receiving mental health care receive it in community-based outpatient settings. Some short-term inpatient and residential facilities also provide care to individuals in crises or those requiring treatment for serious mental illnesses.

For more information, see CRS In Focus IF10870, Psychiatric Institutionalization and Deinstitutionalization.

Behavioral health services in the United States—which include substance abuse treatment and mental health care—have historically been the responsibility of states. The federal role has typically involved supporting state efforts through grant funding. This financial support has often consisted of block grants, with minimal direction to states regarding how to use these funds.

Federal support for behavioral health activities was not designed for the federal government to be the primary payer, nor did the federal government intend to be the primary architect of these programs. While the federal government had nearly always played a more robust role in biomedical and health research—through the National Institutes of Health (NIH)—it did not make substantial investments in behavioral health services until the latter half of the 20th century. During the 1960s, congressional interest in mental health shifted toward a greater emphasis on service development and provision.[6] At that time, Congress enacted grant programs to establish community-based psychiatric services, improve state hospitals, and develop centers for substance abuse treatment.[7]

The Alcohol, Drug Abuse and Mental Health Administration was created in 1973 to support states in administering substance abuse and mental health treatment services. ADAMHA provided federal funding to bolster state efforts in behavioral health care services. ADAMHA also served as the parent agency for the three research agencies covering substance use and mental health: NIMH, NIDA, and NIAAA.[8] NIDA and NIAAA were also created in the early 1970s following increased awareness of substance abuse and alcoholism as public health problems. NIMH had been established in 1946, in recognition of the burden that brain and behavioral disorders place on national health resources. Congress, determining that a strong program of research and research training would contribute to improving mental health and to treating mental illness, alcoholism, and drug abuse, established NIMH as one of the original components of the National Institutes of Health (NIH).

In addition to research, the original NIMH's mission included educating and training clinical personnel and providing grants to states to establish clinical treatment centers. This role changed with the creation of SAMHSA. As part of a reorganization of the Public Health Service agencies[9] in 1992, SAMHSA took on responsibility for education and training of providers, and for administering treatment services—activities it continues today.[10] NIMH, NIDA, and NIAAA—all now within NIH—remain the agencies primarily responsible for advancing mental health and addiction research.

Since its inception in 1992, SAMHSA and many of its programs have undergone multiple reauthorizations through legislation. Two laws—the Children's' Health Act of 2000 (P.L. 106-310) and the Helping Families in Mental Health Crisis Reform Act (Division B of P.L. 114-255, The 21st Century Cures Act)—provided comprehensive reauthorization of multiple

---

[6] Institute of Medicine (IOM), *Research and Service Programs in the PHS: Challenges in Organization*, Washington, DC, 1991, pp. 27-42, https://doi.org/10.17226/1871.

[7] Ibid.

[8] Ibid.

[9] The Public Health Service agencies represent eight of the eleven operating divisions of the Department of Health and Human Services focused on public health. For more information, see CRS Report R44916, *Public Health Service Agencies: Overview and Funding (FY2016 -FY2018)*.

[10] SAMHSA shares responsibility for training behavioral health providers with the Health Services and Research Administration (HRSA) within HHS.

SAMHSA programs. Most of the other reauthorizing laws established or reauthorized specific SAMHSA activities, such as individual grant programs. While many programs have been added or repealed over the years, SAMHSA's primary responsibilities—including administering block grants to the states supporting mental health and substance abuse treatment services—have remained consistent with few significant changes.

- **1992** ADAMHA Reorganization Act (P.L. 102-321)
- **2000** Children's Health Act (P.L. 106-310)[a]
- **2002** No Child Left Behind Act (P.L. 107-110)[b]
- **2004** Garrett Lee Smith Memorial Act (P.L. 108-355)[c]
- **2005** Sober Truth on Preventing Underage Drinking Act (P.L. 109-422)[d]
- **2010** Affordable Care Act (P.L. 111-148)[e]
- **2016** Comprehensive Addiction and Recovery Act (P.L. 114-198)[f]
- **2016** 21st Century Cures Act/Helping Families in Mental Health Crisis Reform Act (P.L. 114-255)[g]
- **2018** SUPPORT for Patients and Communities Act (P.L. 115-271)[h]

Source: Figure prepared by the Congressional Research Service (CRS) based on analysis of relevant legislation. Acts were included here if they established multiple new authorizations or made amendments to multiple existing SAMHSA authorities.

Notes: Most of these laws authorized or reauthorized several select SAMHSA activities rather than the entirety of programs or the agency as a whole. Of note, the Omnibus Budget Reconciliation Act 1981 (P.L. 97-35) provided the initial authorization for the block grant that would eventually become the mental health and substance abuse block grants administered by SAMHSA. *ADAMHA* stands for the Alcohol, Drug Abuse and Mental Health Administration. *SAMHSA* stands for the Substance Abuse and Mental Health Services Administration.

[a] The Children's Health Act amended SAMHSA's existing authorities under Title V, added several new authorities, and authorized appropriations through FY2003. The 2000 reauthorization legislation also incorporated the Drug Addiction Treatment Act (DATA) of 2000 (P.L. 106-310, Title XXXV) which expanded opioid use disorder treatment using buprenorphine.[11]

[b] The No Child Left Behind Act of 2001 (P.L. 107-110, Sec. 4129; enacted January 8, 2002) required SAMHSA to provide consultation to the Secretary of Education in awarding grants to local educational agencies for reducing alcohol abuse in secondary schools.

---

[11] For more information, see CRS Report R45279, Buprenorphine and the Opioid Crisis: *A Primer for Congress.*

[c] The Garrett Lee Smith Memorial Act of 2004 (P.L. 108-355) authorized three suicide prevention programs at SAMHSA—two grant programs and a resource center.

[d] The 2005 Sober Truth on Preventing Underage Drinking (STOP) Act (P.L. 109-422) authorized SAMHSA to award grants for reducing underage drinking.

[e] The Patient Protection and Affordable Care Act of 2010 (ACA; P.L. 111-148) contained several provisions relating to mental health and substance abuse services, including new SAMHSA authorities.

[f] The Comprehensive Addiction and Recovery Act (P.L. 114-198) of 2016 established new—or reauthorized existing—substance abuse treatment-related activities.

[g] The Helping Families in Mental Health Crisis Reform Act (Division B of the 21st Century Cures Act; P.L. 114-255) made changes to the organization of the agency and amended a number of programs.

[h] The SUPPORT for Patients and Communities Act (P.L. 115-271) of 2018 primarily established new—or reauthorized existing—substance abuse treatment-related activities.

Figure 1. Timeline of Major Legislation Authorizing Programs and Activities Administered by SAMHSA.

Authority and Organization

SAMHSA and most of its programs and activities are authorized under Title V of the Public Health Service Act (PHSA). The substance abuse block grant (SABG) and community mental health block grant (MHBG) are separately authorized under PHSA Title XIX Part B. PHSA Title V provides the authorities for an Assistant Secretary of Mental Health and Substance Use (Assistant Secretary)[12] and four centers: the Center for Substance Abuse Treatment, the Center for Substance Abuse Prevention, the Center for Mental Health Services, and the Center for Behavioral Health Statistics and Quality. SAMHSA's four centers and main offices are depicted in Figure 2. Each of the four centers has a director who reports to the Assistant Secretary.

In addition to administering SAMHSA's major block grant programs, each center has general authority to fund states and communities to address priority substance abuse and mental health needs. This authority, called Programs of Regional and National Significance (PRNS), authorizes

[12] Subtitle A (§6001 and §6002) of the 21st Century Cures Act (P.L. 114-255) replaced the position of SAMHSA Administrator with a newly established Assistant Secretary for Mental Health and Substance Use (Assistant Secretary), to be appointed by the President and subject to Senate confirmation (as was the case with the Administrator). It also expanded and revised the list of responsibilities to be carried out by the HHS Secretary, acting through the newly established Assistant Secretary.

SAMHSA to fund projects that (1) translate promising new research findings to community-based prevention and treatment services; (2) provide training and technical assistance; and (3) target resources to increase service capacity where it is most needed.[13] SAMHSA conducts several programs under PRNS authorities, some of which are explicitly authorized in statute while others exist at the discretion of SAMHSA, the Secretary of HHS, or elsewhere within HHS or the Administration. SAMHSA determines its funding priorities in consultation with states and other stakeholders.

The PHSA also directs SAMHSA to conduct data collection and analysis activities related to mental health and substance abuse. These activities are centrally coordinated in the Center for Behavioral Health Statistics and Quality.

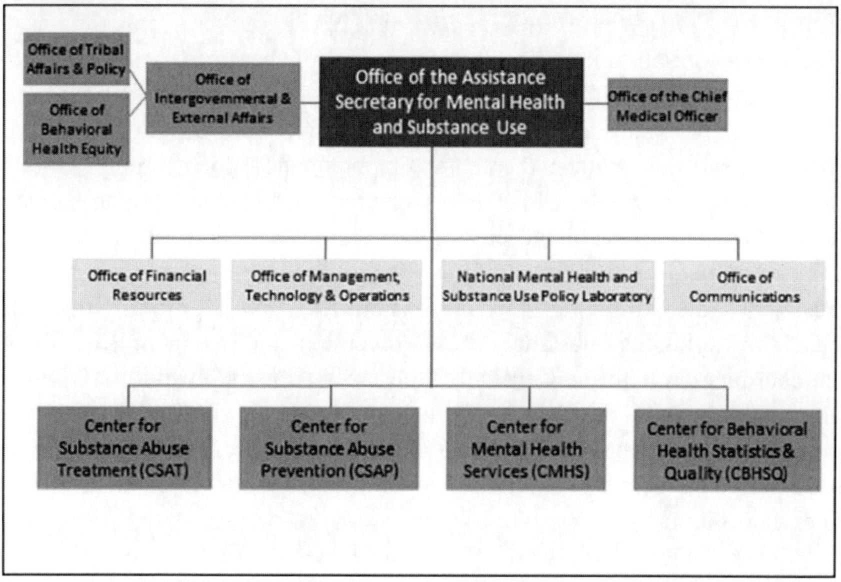

Source: CRS figure based on U.S. Department of Health and Human Services, SAMHSA, Justification of Estimates for Appropriations Committees for FY2020 and SAMHSA, About Us; Who We Are; SAMHSA Headquarters Offices and Centers, available at https://www.samhsa.gov/about-us/who-we-are/offices-centers/.

Figure 2. SAMHSA Organizational Chart.Major Offices and Centers at the Substance Abuse and Mental Health Services Administration.

[13] See, for instance, PHSA §509, §516, and §520A.

For a list of specific program authorities within each of SAMHSA's centers, see Table 1 describing the "Substance Abuse Treatment PRNS" Table 2 describing "Substance Abuse Prevention PRNS", and Table 3 describing "Mental Health PRNS" later in this report.

Centers

SAMHSA carries out most of its programs and activities through four statutorily established centers focusing on substance abuse treatment, substance abuse prevention, mental health services, and health surveillance and program support.

Center for Substance Abuse Treatment (CSAT)

The Center for Substance Abuse Treatment (CSAT) has primary responsibility for promoting community-based treatment and recovery services for individuals with substance use disorders.[14] CSAT does not directly deliver treatment services. Rather, the center supports state efforts through funding and technical assistance. CSAT is responsible for leading efforts to increase access to effective treatment; closing the gap between demand and capacity for treatment; promoting evidence-based practices; and strengthening treatment systems (among other responsibilities). CSAT primarily does this by administering the Substance Abuse Prevention and Treatment Block Grant (in coordination with the Center for Substance Abuse Prevention). CSAT is also authorized to develop, evaluate, and implement effective treatment programs; and enable improvement of service quality and access. For an example of the center's activities, see "Substance Abuse Treatment PRNS" later in this report.

PHSA Title V, Part B, Subpart 1 establishes CSAT, lists the Director's duties, and authorizes various programs.[15] The CSAT Director's duties include administering the Substance Abuse Prevention and Treatment Block Grant (SABG).[16] Except for the SABG, all of CSAT's programs and activities fall under the category of substance abuse treatment PRNS (for more details,

[14] HHS, SAMHSA, *Center for Substance Abuse Treatment*, http://www.samhsa.gov/about-us/who-we-are/offices- centers/csat.

[15] PHSA Title V, Part B, Subpart 1 (42 U.S.C. §290bb et seq.).

[16] PHSA §507(b)(1) (42 U.S.C. §290bb(b)(1)).

see Table 1 in the "Substance Abuse Treatment PRNS" section later in this report).[17]

Center for Substance Abuse Prevention (CSAP)

The Center for Substance Abuse Prevention (CSAP) has primary responsibility for preventing misuse (and underage use) of alcohol, tobacco, prescription drugs, and illegal drugs.[18] CSAP is responsible for leading the development of effective prevention policies, programs, and services, and enabling states, local communities, and organizations to adopt such policies, programs, and services (among other responsibilities). CSAP is authorized to prevent substance abuse through public education, training, technical assistance, and dissemination of research findings. The center primarily executes this through workforce training programs and technical assistance to grantees. The center also provides states with grants to support their strategic planning activities and for demonstration programs. For an example of the center's activities, see "Substance Abuse Prevention PRNS" later in this report.

PHSA Title V, Part B, Subpart 2 establishes CSAP, lists the Director's duties, and authorizes various programs.[19] Currently all of CSAP's programs and activities fall under the category of substance abuse prevention PRNS (for more details, see Table 2 later in this report). CSAP works with CSAT to administer the Substance Abuse Prevention and Treatment Block Grant. The block grant includes a 20% set-aside for prevention.[20]

Center for Mental Health Services (CMHS)

The Center for Mental Health Services (CMHS) leads federal efforts supporting the prevention and treatment of mental disorders.[21] The goals of CMHS include preventing mental illness and promoting mental health.[22] CMHS is responsible for leading efforts to increase access to mental health

---

[17] The CSAT also plays a role in administering two opioid-specific grant programs authorized to HHS generally, but operated by SAMHSA. See " Additional Opioid Grant Programs" later in this report.

[18] SAMHSA, *Center for Substance Abuse Prevention*, http://www.samhsa.gov/about-us/who-we-are/offices-centers/ csap.

[19] PHSA Title V, Part B, Subpart 2 (42 U.S.C. §290bb-21 et seq.).

[20] HHS, SAMHSA, *FY2019 Justification of Estimates for Appropriations Committees.* The 20% prevention set -aside is specified at PHSA §1922(a)(1) (42 U.S.C. §300x-22(a)(1)).

[21] SAMHSA, *Center for Mental Health Services*, http://www.samhsa.gov/about-us/who-we-are/offices-centers/cmhs.

[22] PHSA §520(b)(1) (42 U.S.C. §290bb-31(b)(1)).

services and improve their quality. CMHS is authorized to help prevent mental illness and promote mental health by providing funds to evaluate, improve and implement effective treatment practices; provide technical assistance to state and local mental health agencies; and collect data. CMHS supports mental health services provided by states and local governments through its mental health block grant and discretionary grant programs. For an example of the center's activities, see "Mental Health PRNS" later in this report.

PHSA Title V, Part B, Subpart 3 establishes CMHS, lists the Director's duties, and authorizes various programs.[23] The CMHS Director's duties include administering the Community Mental Health Services Block Grant (MHBG)[24] and other funding programs that target specific populations or activities such as the Projects for Assistance in Transition from Homelessness (PATH) program[25] and the Protection and Advocacy for Individuals with Mental Illness (PAIMI) program.[26] PHSASection 561 requires the HHS Secretary, acting through the CMHS Director, to award grants under the Children's Mental Health Services program.[27] CMHS is also responsible for administering the Certified Community Behavioral Health Clinics grant program.[28] All other CMHS programs fall under the category of mental health PRNS (for more details, see Table 3 later in this report).

Center for Behavioral Health Statistics and Quality (CBHSQ)

The Center for Behavioral Health Statistics and Quality (CBHSQ) has primary responsibility for collecting and analyzing behavioral health statistics. As the federal government's lead agency for behavioral health statistics, CBHSQ designs and implements data collection and analysis projects, advises the HHS Secretary and SAMHSA Assistant Secretary on behavioral health epidemiology, and partners with other agencies to develop federal health statistics policy (among other responsibilities).[29] CBHSQ was explicitly

[23] PHSA Title V, Part B, Subpart 3 (42 U.S.C. §290bb-31 et seq.).
[24] PHSA §520(b)(7) (42 U.S.C. §290bb-31(b)(7)).
[25] PHSA §520(b)(9) (42 U.S.C. §290bb-31(b)(9)).
[26] PHSA §520(b)(8) (42 U.S.C. §290bb-31(b)(8)).
[27] PHSA §561(a)(1) (42 U.S.C. §290ff(a)(1)).
[28] Established by §223 of the Protecting Access to Medicare Act of 2014 (P.L. 113-93; 42 U.S.C. §1936(a) footnote entitled "Demonstration Programs To Improve Community Mental Health Services").
[29] HHS, SAMHSA, Center for Behavioral Health Statistics and Quality, http://www.samhsa.gov/about-us/who-we-are/offices-centers/cbhsq. Of note, other federal agencies also collect data related to behavioral health, such as the Centers for Disease Control and Prevention (CDC), the Health Resources and Services Administration (HRSA), the Agency for Healthcare Research and Quality (AHRQ), and the National Institute of Mental Health

established in statute in 2016, though the center conducted many of its activities under other authorizations prior to its formal codification.[30]

CBHSQ's data collection programs include the National Survey on Drug Use and Health (NSDUH) and the Behavioral Health Services Information System (BHSIS), which includes the National Mental Health Services Survey (N-MHSS), the Treatment Episode Data Set (TEDS), and the National Survey of Substance Abuse Treatment Services (N-SSATS), among others.[31] One element of the BHSIS is the Inventory of Behavioral Health Services, which provides a listing of all known mental health and substance use treatment facilities used to inform SAMHSA's Behavioral Health Treatment Services Locator webpage.[32] CBHSQ also maintains the Evidence-Based Practices Resource Center.[33]

CBHSQ maintains a data archive and conducts research on behavioral health access, cost, quality, outcomes, policy, and practices.[34] The center disseminates information through articles, short reports, and data spotlights. Through the Substance Abuse and Mental Health Data Archive (SAMHDA), CBHSQ provides public access to much of the data they collect for research analysis.[35] CBHSQ is also responsible for agency-wide initiatives such as efforts to develop the behavioral health workforce. Most CBHSQ activities are integrated with the other centers and cross over multiple funding lines.[36]

PHSA Title V, Section 505 establishes CBHSQ, lists the Director's duties, and authorizes various programs.[37] The CBHSQ Director's duties include coordinating SAMHSA's integrated data strategy, which includes collecting data on the incidence and prevalence of mental illness and substance abuse (the NSDUH survey), the number of individuals seeking treatment for mental illness and substance abuse issues, and the number of individuals admitted to

---

(NIMH) and National Institute for Drug Abuse (NIDA) within the National Institutes of Health (NIH).

[30] PHSA §505 (42 U.S.C. §290aa-4).

[31] HHS, SAMHSA, FY2019 Justification of Estimates for Appropriations Committees, http://www.hhs.gov/budget.

[32] SAMHSA, Behavioral Health Treatment Services Locator, https://findtreatment.samhsa.gov/.

[33] SAMHSA, Evidence-Based Practices Resource Center, https://www.samhsa.gov/ebp-resource-center. The Evidence-Based Practice Resource Center replaced the National Registry of Evidence-based Programs and Practices (NREPP) in2018.

[34] HHS, SAMHSA, Center for Behavioral Health Statistics and Quality.

[35] SAMHSA, Substance Abuse & Mental Health Data Archive, What is SAMHDA?, https://www.datafiles.samhsa.gov/faq/what-samhda-nid23. SAMHDA data are available at https://www.datafiles.samhsa.gov/.

[36] HHS, SAMHSA, Justification of Estimates for Appropriations Committees for FY2020, http://www.hhs.gov/budget.

[37] PHSA Title V, Section 505 (42 U.S.C. §290aa-4).

emergency rooms as a result of substances (the Drug Abuse Warning Network [DAWN] surveillance system).

Duties of the Director also include collecting data on mental health and substance abuse treatment programs (the N-SSATS survey) and making recommendations for performance metrics to evaluate SAMHSA activities. PHSA Section 505 specifies that summaries and analyses of data collected shall be made available to the public.

Headquarters Offices

Key offices within SAMHSA's headquarters are described briefly below.[38]

The Office of the Assistant Secretary for Mental Health and Substance Use is responsible for managing and directing the agency, leading policy and program development, and working with the Office of the Secretary in HHS (among other responsibilities). Within the Office of the Assistant Secretary is the Office of Intergovernmental and External Affairs and several other offices:

- The Office of Behavioral Health Equity is responsible for coordinating SAMHSA's efforts to ensure equitable access to high-quality behavioral health care and reduce disparities in health outcomes (among other responsibilities).[39]
- The Office of Tribal Affairs and Policy is responsible for supporting agency efforts to implement the Tribal Law and Order Act of 2010 (Title II of P.L. 111- 211) and address behavioral health issues affecting tribal communities in collaboration with tribal governments and tribal organizations (among other responsibilities).[40]
- The Office of the Chief Medical Officer (OCMO) is responsible for ensuring that medically researched and clinically approved practices are incorporated in SAMHSA programs and activities. The Chief

[38] Unless otherwise noted, information in this section is drawn from HHS, SAMHSA, *Offices and Centers: SAMHSA Headquarters Offices*, http://www.samhsa.gov/about-us/who-we-are/offices-centers.

[39] SAMHSA, Justification of Estimates for Appropriations Committees for FY2020 and SAMHSA, Organizational Structure: Substance Abuse and mental Health Services Administration (SAMHSA), available at https://www.samhsa.gov/sites/default/files/508_samhsa-org-chart04032019.pdf.

[40] SAMHSA, "New SAMHSA Office of Tribal Affairs and Policy," SAMHSA News, vol. 22, no. 4 (Fall 2014).

Medical Officer also advises the Assistant Secretary on appropriate performance metrics and evaluation designs.[41]

The *Office of Communications* is responsible for guiding the agency's strategic communications plan, managing its online presence, disseminating products through the SAMHSAstore (among other responsibilities).

The *Office of Financial Resources* is responsible for all functions of the Chief Financial Officer, including advising the Assistant Secretary on the agency's budget, assisting with financial management, and reducing waste, fraud, and abuse (among other responsibilities).

The *Office of Management, Technology, and Operations* is responsible for administrative services, human resources management, and information technology (among other responsibilities).

The *National Mental Health and Substance Use Policy Laboratory* is responsible for promoting evidence-based practices, evaluating service delivery models of treatment and facilitating adoption of data-driven policies (among other responsibilities).[42]

Regional Administrators

HHS has 10 regional offices to ensure that "the Department maintains close contact with state, local, and tribal partners and addresses the needs of communities and individuals served through HHS programs and policies."[43] SAMHSA's regional administrators represent SAMHSAwithin these areas; promote behavioral health initiatives; collaborate with other federal agencies;

---

[41] SAMHSA, *About Us; Who We Are; Leadership*, https://www.samhsa.gov/about-us/who-we-are/leadershipPHSA §501(g). This office was established by §6003 of The 21st Century Cures Act of 2016 (P.L. 114-255).

[42] Prior to enactment of the 21st Century Cures Act (P.L. 114-255) in 2016, SAMHSA's Office of Policy, Planning, and Innovation, which was not explicitly authorized in statute, facilitated the adoption of evidence-based policies and practices to improve behavioral health services outcomes. Title VII of the Cures Act added a new PHSA §501A which established within SAMHSA a "National Mental Health and Substance Use Policy Laboratory" (the "Laboratory"). The law requires the Laboratory to carry out "the authorities and activities that were in effect for the Office of Policy, Planning, and Innovation" before enactment of the Cures Act. The Laboratory was established by §7001 of the Cures Act.

[43] HHS, *Regional Offices*, http://www.hhs.gov/about/agencies/regional-offices/.

provide support (e.g., technical assistance) to stakeholders; and periodically report on relevant trends, issues, and policies.[44]

Advisory Councils and Committees

To help draw advice from mental health and substance abuse professionals and members of the public, SAMHSA has several advisory councils and committees:[45]

- SAMHSA National Advisory Council,
- CSAT National Advisory Council,
- CSAP National Advisory Council,
- CMHS National Advisory Council,
- Advisory Committee for Women's Services,
- Drug Testing Advisory Board (DTAB),
- Tribal Technical Advisory Committee,
- Interdepartmental Serious Mental Illness Coordinating Committee, and
- Interdepartmental Substance Use Disorders Coordinating Committee.

PHSA Sections 501 and 222 (respectively) require the Assistant Secretary to "establish such peer review groups and program advisory committees as are needed."[46] Some advisory councils and committees are established under SAMHSA's general authorities, while others are explicitly required in statute. For example, PHSA Section 502 requires the HHS Secretary to appoint an advisory council for SAMHSA and three of its statutorily established centers (CMHS, CSAT, and CSAP).[47] PHSA Section 501 requires the Assistant Secretary to appoint an Associate Administrator for Women's Services, who must establish an Advisory Committee for Women's Services.[48] SAMHSA

[44] HHS, SAMHSA, *SAMHSA Regional Administrators*, http://www.samhsa.gov/about-us/who-we-are/regional-administrators.
[45] SAMHSA, *Advisory Councils*, http://www.samhsa.gov/about-us/advisory-councils.
[46] PHSA §501(i) (42 U.S.C. §290aa(i)).
[47] 42 U.S.C. §290aa-1.
[48] PHSA §501(f)(2)(C) (42 U.S.C. §290aa(f)(2)(C)).

also has a Tribal Technical Advisory Committee consistent HHS's Tribal Consultation Policy.[49]

Interagency Activities

SAMHSA is not the sole federal agency responsible for behavioral health-related activities. SAMHSA participates in interagency efforts to coordinate programs, share knowledge, and advance behavioral health.[50] While SAMHSA primarily supports direct behavioral health prevention and treatment services, other agencies conduct behavioral health research, provide workforce development resources, and operate other behavioral health-related programs. Other federal agencies may support other behavioral health activities—including direct services in some instances—as well.

SAMHSA is statutorily required to collaborate with other agencies—such as the Department of Veterans Affairs, the Department of Justice, and other HHS agencies like NIH and the Agency for Health Care Research and Quality (AHRQ)—to coordinate behavioral health activities and translate research findings into services.[51] For example, SAMHSA cooperated, along with the Health Resources and Services Administration (HRSA), the SAMHSA-HRSA Center for Integrated Solutions. This body promoted the integration of primary care and behavioral health services through training and technical assistance for treatment organizations.[52] The Behavioral Health Coordinating Council and the Interagency Coordinating Committee on the Prevention of Underage Drinking are other examples of formal collaborations with other agencies.

---

[49] HHS, *Tribal Consultation*, http://www.hhs.gov/about/agencies/iea/tribal-affairs/consultation/index.html. This committee is also consistent with several recent presidential policies including Executive Order 13175, " Consultation and Coordination with Indian Tribal Governments," *Public Papers of the Presidents of the United States: William J. Clinton* (Washington: GPO, 2000), U.S. President (G.W. Bush), " Memorandum on Government -to-Government Relationship with Tribal Governments," September 23, 2004, and U.S. President (Obama), " A Renewed Era of Federal-Tribal Relations," *2016 White House Tribal Nations Conference Progress Report*, January 2017.

[50] SAMHSA, *About Us; Interagency Activities*, https://www.samhsa.gov/about-us/interagency, accessed March 2019.

[51] See, for example, PHSA §501(d), PHSA §507(b), PHSA §515(b), and PHSA §520(b).

[52] HHS, SAMHSA, HRSA, *SAMHSA-HRSA Center for Integrated Health Solutions*, https://www.integration.samhsa.gov/. Beginning in 2020, the center is operated by the National Council for Behavioral Health through a contract with SAMHSA. It was renamed the Center of Excellence for Integrated Health Solutions. More information can be found at https://www.thenationalcouncil.org/integrated-health-coe/.

The 21st Century Cures Act of 2016 (Cures; P.L. 114-255) established the Interdepartmental Serious Mental Illness Coordinating Committee (ISMICC). The committee is tasked with making recommendations to improve the coordination and administration of services for adults with serious mental illness and children with serious emotional disturbance. The committee provided recommendations in the first of two statutorily required reports to Congress submitted in December 2017.[53] According to statute, the ISMICC will sunset in 2023.[54]

Budget and Funding

The total amount of funding available to SAMHSA (i.e., total program level) traditionally includes discretionary budget authority provided in annual appropriations acts, Public Health Service (PHS) Program Evaluation Set-Aside funds,[55] Prevention and Public Health Fund (PPHF) transfers,[56] and data request and publications user fees.[57] The main source of funding for SAMHSA

---

[53] HHS, *Interdepartmental Serious Mental Illness Coordinating Committee Releases its First Report to Congress*, News, Washington, DC, December 14, 2017, https://www.hhs.gov/about/news/2017/12/14/ismicc-releases-its-first-report-to-congress.html and ISMICC, *The Way Forward: Federal Action for a System That Works for All People Living With SMI and SED and Their Families and Caregivers*, Report to Congress, December 13, 2017, https://www.samhsa.gov/sites/default/ files/ programs_campaigns/ismicc_2017_report_to_congress.pdf.

[54] §6031 of Cures required the HHS Secretary, upon submission of the committee's second report, to make a recommendation to Congress as to whether operation of the committee should be extended beyond the six-year sunset.

[55] The PHS Evaluation Tap allows the HHS Secretary to redistribute a portion of eligible PHS agency appropriations for program evaluation across HHS. In the annual Labor-HHS-ED appropriations acts, Congress specifies the maximum percentage for the set -aside and directs specific amounts of funding from the tap to a number of HHS programs. See the "Public Health Service Evaluation Tap" section in CRS Report R45869, *Labor, Health and Human Services, and Education: FY2019 Appropriations*.

[56] The Patient Protection and Affordable Care Act (ACA) established the Prevention and Public Health Fund (PPHF) and provided it with a permanent annual mandatory appropriation. PPHF funds are to be transferred by the HHS Secretary for prevention, wellness, and public health activities. PPHF funds are available to the HHS Secretary on October 1 of each year, when the new fiscal year begins. The Administration's annual budget proposal for the PPHF reflects its intended distribution and use of the funds. For more information see CRS Report R44796, *The ACA Prevention and Public Health Fund: In Brief*.

[57] The Consolidated Appropriations Act, 2014 (P.L. 113-76) authorized SAMHSA to collect fees "for the costs of publications, data, data tabulations, and data analysis completed under [PHSA Title V] and provided to a public or private entity upon request, which

is the discretionary budget authority it receives through the annual appropriations process.[58] SAMHSAis funded through the Departments of Labor, Health and Human Services, and Education, and Related Agencies (Labor-HHS-ED) appropriations act.[59]

SAMHSA's budget and appropriations fall under four categories: (1) mental health, (2) substance abuse treatment, (3) substance abuse prevention, and (4) health surveillance and program support. These categories roughly correspond with SAMHSA's four centers. CBHSQ activities, however, are integrated throughout the other centers and cross over multiple funding lines. CBHSQ receives much of its funding from the health surveillance and program support category in addition to a set-aside in the SABG.[60]

Table 1. SAMHSA budget, by fiscal year FY2016-FY2020 discretionary budget authority, by budget category (dollars in millions)

Category	FY2016	FY2017	FY2018	FY2019	FY2020
Mental Health	1,133	1,145	1,454	1,519	1,645
Substance Abuse Treatment	2,111	2,627	3,676	3,735	3,757
Substance Abuse Prevention	211	222	248	205	206
Health Surveillance and Program Support	175	117	129	129	129
Total Discretionary Budget Authority	3,630	4,111	5,507	5,588	5,737

Source: SAMHSA, Operating Plan, FY2016-2020, available at https://www.samhsa.gov/about-us/budget.

shall be credited to this appropriation and shall remain available until expended for such purposes."

58 Budget authority is the "authority provided by federal law to enter into financial obligations that will result in ... outlays involving federal funds." Discretionary budget authority "refers to outlays from budget authority that is provided in and controlled by appropriation acts." U.S. Government Accountability Office (GAO), A Glossary of Terms Used in the Federal Budget Process, GAO-05-734SP, September 1, 2005, http://www.gao.gov/products/GAO- 05-734SP. SAMHSA receives more than 97% of its budget through discretionary budget authority in annual appropriations acts.

59 Sometimes referred to as the *Labor-HHS* appropriations bill or simply the *Labor-H* bill.

60 SAMHSA, *Justification of Estimates for Appropriations Committees for FY2021*, pp. 274-279. Historically, the CBHSQ has received funding from transfers from the PHSEvaluation Tap and transfers from the Prevention and Public Health Fund (see, for example, the SAMHSA *Justification of Estimates for Appropriations Committees* for FY2017, pp. 293-294).

In FY2020, SAMHSA had a program level budget of $5.89 billion ($5.74 billion in discretionary budget authority).[61] SAMHSA supported 494 full-time employee equivalents in FY2019.[62]62 More detailed descriptions and funding levels for SAMHSA's programs and activities are available in SAMHSA's annual budget request.[63]63 For a list of SAMHSA authorizations and their funding levels, see Table 1, Table 2, and Table 3.

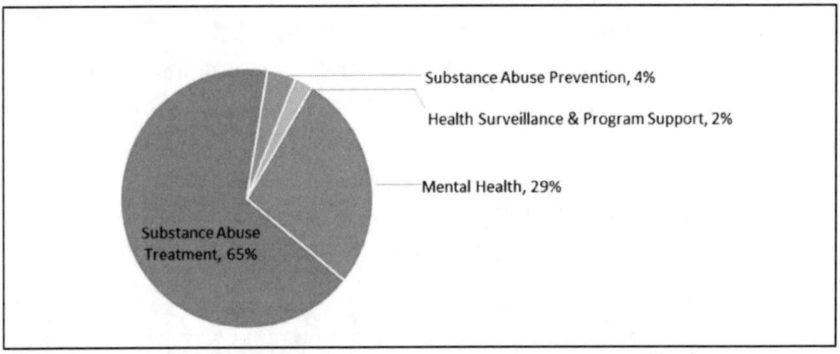

Source: CRS analysis based on SAMHSA, Operating Plan for FY2020.

Figure 3. SAMHSA Budget at a Glance. Percent of Budget by Category, FY2020.

Major Programs and Activities

SAMHSA's major programs and activities include two block grant programs, numerous activities known as Programs of Regional and National Significance (PRNS), several other grant programs, technical assistance to grantees, data collection and other related activities.

The majority of SAMHSA's programming consists of grants to support mental health and substance abuse treatment and prevention activities, including direct treatment services. The largest grants are awarded to states via a designated Single State Agency. The state may then distribute funds—often in the form of subgrants and contracts—to localities for redistribution or

[61] The difference between the discretionary budget authority and total program level is attributed to the Public Health Evaluation Set-Aside Funds and funds from the Prevention and Public Health Fund and user fees. For more information, see CRS Report R45869, *Labor, Health and Human Services, and Education: FY2019 Appropriations*.

[62] SAMHSA, *FY2021 Justification of Estimates for Appropriations Committees*, p. 290.

[63] SAMHSA, *FY2021 Justification of Estimates for Appropriations Committees.*

directly to treatment providers. Similarly, SAMHSA may award some grants directly to mental health and substance abuse service providers. For other grants, SAMHSA distributes the funds to local government entities, organizations, Indian tribes, or local educational agencies, for instance, who in turn support entities providing direct treatment or prevention activities (see Figure 4).

Some of SAMHSA's programs are directed through statute. Most of SAMHSA's activities are carried out under general authorities, though they may target specific substances of abuse, particular mental health issues, specified populations, or certain prevention or treatment activities.

SAMHSA's general PRNS authority gives the agency, in consultation with states, flexibility to determine the specific problem the funds will be used to address, such as unique or emerging substance abuse issues in a particular state. This practice may also make it easier to provide coordinated care for those in need of multiple substance abuse treatment services. The dynamic nature of SAMHSA's PRNS authorities and the flexible uses of block grant funding, however, can make tracking activities and determining spending on specific issues challenging.[64]

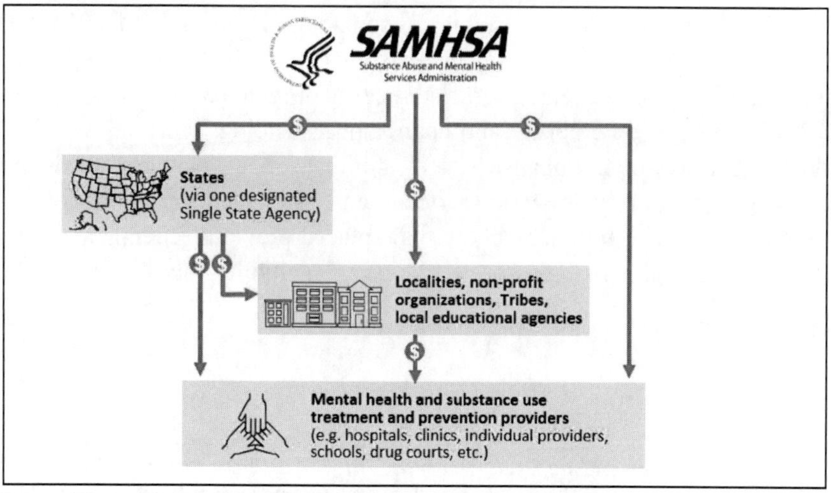

Source: Figure prepared by the Congressional Research Service.

Figure 4. Distribution of SAMHSA Grants. Course of grant funding from SAMHSA to prevention and treatment providers.

---

[64] See textbox "Tracking SAMHSA Grants and Spending" later in this report for more information.

Block Grants

SAMHSA's two biggest programs are block grant programs. One block grant supports substance abuse prevention and treatment services (the SABG) and the other supports mental health services (the MHBG). SAMHSA has estimated that the Substance Abuse Prevention and Treatment Block Grant (SABG) accounts for nearly a third of the expenses of state agencies responsible for substance abuse.[65] By comparison, SAMHSA's Community Mental Health Services Block Grant (MHBG) funds an average of 1% of the expenses for state mental health agencies.[66] The difference reflects the historical role federal and state governments have played in funding services in these two areas.[67] As behavioral health services have primarily been the responsibilities of states, the block grant programs administered by SAMHSA were designed to supplement these activities, not provide the primary source of financial support.

History

A predecessor to the current block grant programs, the Alcohol, Drug, and Mental Health Services (ADMS) block grant was one of seven block grants established by the Omnibus Budget Reconciliation Act of 1981 (OBRA).[68] This block grant consolidated several existing categorical grants for substance abuse and community mental health services in order to provide state and local governments more flexibility and control over funding. Shifting to a single block grant sought to enhance states' ability to meet localized needs, end duplication of effort in delivering services, and enable better coordination. The flexibility provided by the block grants replaced previous federal categorical grant authorizations that specified uses, including authorizations for

---

[65] SAMHSA, *Funding and Characteristics of Single State Agencies for Substance Abuse Services and State Mental Health Agencies, 2015*, HHS Publication No. (SMA) SMA-17-5029, Rockville, MD, 2017, https://store.samhsa.gov/ system/files/sma17-5029.pdf and SAMHSA, *Substance Abuse Prevention and Treatment Block Grant*, Fact Sheet, nd, https://www.samhsa.gov/sites/default/files/sabg_fact_sheet_rev.pdf. The Substance Abuse Prevention and Treatment Block Grant is sometimes referred to by the acronym " SAPT."

[66] SAMHSA, *Funding and Characteristics of Single State Agencies*, 2017.

[67] For more information, see CRS In Focus IF10870, *Psychiatric Institutionalization and Deinstitutionalization.*

[68] P.L. 97-35.

establishing community mental health centers.[69] OBRA authorized ADMS block grant funds for FY1982 through FY1984 in proportion to the historical funding patterns of the original categorical grants. Due to the resulting inequities among states in per capita funding for substance abuse and mental health services, OBRA directed HHS to conduct a study that would produce a formula, considering population and state fiscal capacity, to more equitably distribute funds among states.

The 1984 ADAMHA Amendments renewed the block grants for three years with a new formula, while striving to maintain minimum existing levels for states.[70] The amendments included a "minor equity adjustment" that would hold harmless states that would have otherwise received decreased funding under the new calculation. Funds above the FY1984 hold-harmless level were to be allocated using a formula based equally on state population and relative per capita income.[71] The Amendments also required a nongovernmental entity to provide recommendations on the formula proposed by HHS. The resulting recommendations, from the Institute for Health and Aging (IHA), included phasing out the hold-harmless provisions, allocating funds based on populations at risk, and incorporating a state fiscal capacity measure.[72]

The Anti-Drug Abuse Act of 1988 revised the formula, based on the IHA recommendations, to phase out the hold-harmless provision, use total taxable resources as the measure of state fiscal capacity, and incorporate weighted age cohorts as a measure of population at risk.[73] The high-risk age cohorts, determined using an IHA study, were 25-64 years for alcohol abuse, 18-24 years for other drug abuse, and 25-44 for selected mental disorders. Later studies indicated that inequities in block grant distribution to states (regarding need for financial support for behavioral health services) persisted even after the recommendations were implemented.[74]

---

[69] Richard G. Frank and Sherry A. Glied, *Better But Not Well: Mental Health Policy in the United States Since 1950* (Baltimore, MD: The Johns Hopkins University Press, 2006), p. 60.

[70] P.L. 98-509.

[71] This hold-harmless provision assured that each state's block grant funding would not be less than the amount it received in FY1984.

[72] Dorothy Rice, Sander Kelman, and Leonard Miller, et al., *Economic Costs of Alcohol and Drug Abuse and Mental Illness: 1985*, U.S. Department of Health and Human Services, National Institute on Drug Abuse, Bethesda, MD, 1990. The Institute for Health and Aging is an institute within the University of California, San Francisco.

[73] P.L. 100-690.

[74] General Accounting Office (now Government Accountability Office), T -HRD-91-38, *Substance Abuse Funding: Not Justified by Urban-Rural Differences in Need*, 1991.

The 1992 ADAMHA Reorganization Act split the ADMS block grant into two separate block grants, one for mental health services (now the MHBG) and another for substance abuse services (the SABG).[75] The formulas for the two block grants were adjusted, in Sections 1918 and 1933 of the PHSA, to reflect the differences in the population in need of mental health and substance abuse services.[76] Hold-harmless provisions, state minimums, and maintenance of effort requirements were reestablished.[77] The current block grant formulas have undergone minimal amendment since their formulation in 1992.

The Cures Act reauthorized the block grants in 2016. The law amended the stated purposes of the programs and application and expenditure requirements, though the formulas remained unchanged. Among the adjustments was a provision permitting states to combine their applications for the MHBG and SABG.[78] This change acknowledged that behavioral health treatment often includes both types of care, particularly for individuals with co-occurring mental health and substance use disorders.

Community Mental Health Services Block Grant (MHBG)

The Community Mental Health Services Block Grant (MHBG) supports community mental health services for adults with *serious mental illness* (SMI) and children with *serious emotional disturbance* (SED).[79] SAMHSA distributes MHBG funds to states (including the District of Columbia and specified territories)[80] according to a formula specified in statute.

Each state may distribute MHBG funds to local government entities and nongovernmental organizations to provide community mental health services for adults with SMI and children with SED in accordance with the state's plan. States have flexibility in the use of MHBG funds within the framework of the state plan and federal requirements. The state must designate a Single State

---

75 P.L. 102-321.

76 General Accounting Office (now Government Accountability Office), T -HRD-91-32, *Mental Health Grants: Funding Not Distributed in Accordance with State Needs*, 1991.

77 Currently, the hold-harmless provision is set at the level received by the state in FY1998 for the mental health block grant, and the previous fiscal year for the substance abuse block grant. If there is a decrease in appropriation for the substance abuse block grant, states can get a proportionate decrease in their block grant amount. There is no similar provision for the mental health block grant.

78 PHSA §1958 (42 C.F.R. 300x-68).

79 SAMHSA's definitions of adults with SMI and children with SED were provided in a 1993 *Federal Register* notice (May 20, 1993; 58 FR 29422). See textbox on this page.

80 Puerto Rico, the U.S. Virgin Islands, American Samoa, Guam, Northern Mariana Islands, Palau, the Marshall Islands, and Micronesia. See 42 C.F.R. §300x-64(b)(3).

Agency responsible for administering the grant and submit the state plan to the HHS Secretary every two years.

Definitions of Adults with SMI and Children with SED

The Alcohol, Drug Abuse and Mental Health Services Administration (ADAMHA) Reorganization Act of 1992 (P.L. 102-321), which established SAMHSA, did not define adults with SMI and children with SED. Instead it required SAMHSA to establish definitions through rulemaking, which SAMHSA did in 1993. The definitions are as follows:

Adults with Serious Mental Illness (SMI): "persons age 18 and over, who currently or at any time during the past year, have had a diagnosable mental, behavioral, or emotional disorder of sufficient duration to meet diagnostic criteria ... that has resulted in functional impairment which substantially interferes with or limits one or more major life activities."

Children with Serious Emotional Disturbance (SED): "persons from birth up to age 18, who currently or at any time during the past year, have had a diagnosable mental, behavioral, or emotional disorder of sufficient duration to meet diagnostic criteria ... that resulted in functional impairment which substantially interferes with or limits the child's role or functioning in family, school, or community activities."

Source: Federal Register Volume 58, No 96, p. 29422 (May 20, 1993).

Each MHBG grantee must support a mental health planning council, which provides input on the state's plan for providing comprehensive community mental health services. Amajority of members of the mental health planning council must be mental health service consumers or family members (of children with SED); other members represent relevant state agencies (e.g., mental health, education, and social services). States may opt to have behavioral health planning councils, which are responsible for both mental health and substance abuse services.[81]

While use of funds is generally determined by the states, each state must expend at least 10% of its block grant funds each fiscal year (or at least 20% by the end of the succeeding fiscal year) to support evidence-based programs to address early serious mental illness (see above textbox). No more than 5% of the grant funding can be used for administrative expenses. For each of the

---

[81] SAMHSA, *Grants; Block Grants; Community Mental Health Services Block Grant*, https://www.samhsa.gov/grants/block-grants/mhbg.

50 states and the District of Columbia, the MHBG allotment formula is based on the population at risk (weighted), cost of services, and available resources.[82] The MHBG allotment for each territory is proportional to the civilian population of the territory.[83] All states (including the District of Columbia) and territories have minimum allotments. While states do not technically need to provide matching funds, they are statutorily required to maintain spending on community mental health services.[84]

Public Health Service Act Title XIX, Part B, Subpart I authorizes the MHBG program. Provisions in PHSA Title XIX, Part B, Subpart III also apply to the MHBG. PHSA Section 1920 explicitly authorizes to be appropriated $533 million (rounded) annually for each of FY2018–FY2022 for the MHBG.[85]

Substance Abuse Prevention and Treatment Block Grant (SABG)

The Substance Abuse Prevention and Treatment Block Grant (SABG) supports services to prevent and treat substance use disorders. SAMHSA distributes SABG funds to states (including the District of Columbia and specified territories[86]) and one tribal entity according to a formula specified in statute.

Each state may distribute SABG funds to local government entities, administrative service organizations, and prevention and treatment service providers (among others) in accordance with the state's plan for expending SABG funds.[87] States have flexibility in the use of SABG funds within the framework of the state plan and federal requirements. The state must designate a Single State Agency responsible for administering the grant and submit an application containing the state plan to the HHS Secretary by the first of October preceding the fiscal year.[88]

---

[82] PHSA §1918(a) (42 U.S.C. §300x-7(a)).

[83] PHSA §1918(c) (42 U.S.C. §300x-7(c)).

[84] Per Title VIII (§8001) of the 21st Century Cures Act—which amended PHSA §1915(b)—states may receive a waiver from the HHS Secretary for this requirement under certain circumstances.

[85] From 2003 when the authorization expired until reauthorization in 2016 under the Cures Act, the grant program operated under general authorities and continued to receive funding through the annual appropriations process.

[86] See footnote 80.

[87] PHSA §1932(b) (42 U.S.C. §300x-32(b)).

[88] PHSA §1932 (42 U.S.C. §300x-32). Of note, PHSA Section 1958 allows the Assistant Secretary to permit a joint application for the MHBG and SABG.

Block Grant Formula

The formula for calculating the grant amounts, for both the SABG and MHBG, is located in Sections 1918 and 1933 of the PHSA. The formula takes into account three measures: (1) the population in need of services, (2) costs of services in the state, and (3) fiscal capacity of the state. The first factor is intended to be a proxy for the extent of need for services in a state. The metric is based on the population of adults age 18-64 in the state. The second factor, which is the cost of services, is derived from the 1990 report of Health and Economics Research, Inc., and ranges from 0.9 to 1.1.[89] The third factor, which is the fiscal capacity of the state, is intended to adjust for differences in state capacity to pay for these services. This factor uses the three-year mean of the total taxable revenue of the state.

The three factors mentioned above are multiplied to produce a score for the state. To calculate the grant amount for a given state, that state's score is multiplied by the total available grant amount and divided by the sum of all the states' (and District of Columbia's) scores. The formula can be written as:

$Gi = A\ (Xi / \Sigma Xi)$ where

Gi = grant amount for the ith state,

A = total funds appropriated for distribution among the states, and Xi = score for the ith state.

There is a hold-harmless provision and a state minimum provision for both grants.

While the use of funds is generally determined by states, each SABG grantee must expend at least 20% of its SABG allotment on primary prevention strategies.[90] In addition, each SABG grantee must enact laws that prohibit the sale or distribution of tobacco products to minors; enforce such laws; inspect tobacco outlets; and report annually to the HHS Secretary on past-year enforcement activities (and the extent of success achieved), as well as enforcement strategies for the coming grant year.[91]

[89] G.C. Pope, Adjusting the Alcohol, Drug Abuse, and Mental Health Services Block Grant Allocations for Poverty Population and Cost-of-Service, Health Economics Research, Inc., Needham, MA, March 30, 1990.

[90] PHSA §1922(a)(1) (42 U.S.C. §300x-22(a)(1)). Primary prevention strategies refer to interventions designed to avoid manifestations of a disease before the health condition occurs or, in the case of the SABG authorization, "for individuals who do not require treatment for substance abuse."

[91] PHSA §1926 (42 U.S.C. §300x-26).

For each of the 50 states and the District of Columbia, the SABG allotment formula is based on the MHBG formula and takes into account the population at risk (unweighted), cost of services, and available resources.[92] The SABG allotment for each territory is proportional to the civilian population of the territory.[93] All states (including the District of Columbia) and territories have minimum allotments. For Indian tribes and tribal organizations that request SABG funds directly (and that the HHS Secretary determines would be better served by means of direct grants), the grant amount is reserved from the state's SABG allotment based on the ratio of the state's allotment expended for the tribal entity in FY1991.[94] While states do not technically need to provide matching funds, they are statutorily required to maintain spending on substance use disorder services.[95]

PHSA Title XIX, Part B, Subpart II authorizes the SABG. Provisions in PHSA Title XIX, Part B, Subpart III also apply to the SABG. PHSA Section 1935 explicitly authorizes to be appropriated $1.86 billion (rounded) annually for each of FY2018–FY2022 for the SABG.

Issues Regarding Block Grant Formulas and Distribution

Determinations of block grant distribution—in the form of the funding formula—have been critiqued since the program's inception. The block grants represent the majority of funding SAMHSA provides to states. Despite their prominent role in SAMHSA operations, the formula determining funding levels has undergone little change since 1992. A number of issues have been raised regarding the current formulas. Economists and health policy experts have raised concerns about the appropriateness of this formula for ensuring equitable distribution of block grant funds between the states. The variables in the formula may not aptly represent state need for funding or for support for behavioral health activities for instance. Other critiques have questioned the formulas' adequacy in responding to public health needs surrounding substance abuse and mental illness. While demands on the behavioral health

---

[92] PHSA §1933 (42 U.S.C. §300x-33). Population at risk means the population of adults between the ages of 18 and 64. Population at risk in the SABG formula includes the number of individuals age 18 to 24 *and* the number of individuals age 18 to 24 living in urban areas (in addition to the number of individuals age 25 to 64 in the state).

[93] PHSA §1933(c) (42 U.S.C. §300x-33(c)).

[94] PHSA §1933(d) (42 U.S.C. §300x-33(d)).

[95] Per Title VIII (§§8001-8002) of the 21st Century Cures Act—which amended PHSA §1915(b) and §1930—states may receive a waiver from the HHS Secretary for this requirement under certain circumstances and request a negotiated agreement to prevent a reduced SABG allotment if they do not meet these requirements.

infrastructure may shift with drug epidemics for example, block grant levels remain relatively constant.

After the reauthorization of the block grants in 1992, the RAND Corporation evaluated the equity of the formula used in the SABG and MHBG.[96] The formula considers three factors: (1) the size of the population needing services, (2) the cost of services in the state, and (3) the fiscal capacity of the state. RAND concluded that the measures for two of the three components in the formula could be improved. Specifically, the population in need and the costs of services would be better indicated by different metrics. For example, RAND explained that the number of young adults in urban areas—which is double counted in the SABG formula—is not as indicative of substance abuse treatment need in a state as other empirically supported variables, such as high school graduation rate and residence in rural areas.[97] Cost estimates—the second variable in the formula—could also be improved by changing the current equation which is based on wages, rents, and average fees of practicing physicians. These variables are not sensitive to the specific labor needs of substance abuse services (since physicians do not provide most substance use treatment services) or to cost differences in rural and urban settings. RAND recommended changes in the block grant formula that would make allocations more equitable and also result in "big shifts in funding" compared to the current approach.

Pursuant to a provision in the Cures Act of 2016, SAMHSA and the HHS Office of the Assistant Secretary for Planning and Evaluation (ASPE) again partnered with RAND to study the appropriateness of the current SAMHSAblock grant formulas.[98] In their 2019 report, RAND again concluded that the formulas for the block grants could be revised to improve their accuracy.[99] More specifically, they noted that the population need and the cost of service indicators could both be updated to incorporate the best data available, such as state-level prevalence of adults with serious mental illness. They also recommended removing the current minimum allotment rules. No

---

[96] M. Audrey Burnam, Peter Reuter, John L. Adams, et al., *Review and Evaluation of Substance Abuse and Mental Health Services Block Grant Allotment Formula*, RAND Corporation, Santa Monica, CA, 1997.

[97] See footnote 92.

[98] SAMHSA, "Agency Information Collection Activities: Proposed Collection; Comment Request," 83 *Federal Register* 53492, October 23, 2018.

[99] J. Scott Ashwood Karen Chan Osilla, and Maria DeYoreo, et al., *Review and Evaluation of the Substance Abuse, Mental Health, and Homelessness Grant Formulas*, RAND, RR-2454-ASPEC, Santa Monica, CA, 2019, https://www.rand.org/pubs/research_reports/RR2454.html.

changes have been made since the release of this congressionally mandated report.

Tracking SAMHSA Grants and Spending

SAMHSA typically publishes information on grants through Funding Opportunity Announcements (FOAs). While much of the information on grants is available on SAMHSA's website, the agency does not provide a centralized database for searching and tracking grants. Starting in 2017, SAMHSA operates a map providing broad information on grant funding by State by fiscal year: https://www.samhsa.gov/grants-awards-by-state). Other sites useful in tracking grants include http://www.grants.gov, http://www. usaspending.gov, and https://taggs.hhs.gov/.

Congress is often interested in determining how much the U.S. government is spending on treating or preventing particular substance abuse and mental health disorders. This is not usually possible to calculate because of the manner in which SAMHSA receives its appropriations and distributes its grants. SAMHSA's block grants, for example, allow for significant flexibility in use by states. SAMHSA does not systematically collect data on how block grant funds are used and the agency does not make the state plans describing activities publicly available.

SAMHSA has also invested significant resources in addressing the current opioid epidemic in the United Stated. In FY2019 the SAMHSA-administered State Opioid Response grants provided $1.5 billion to specifically address the opioid epidemic. This was in addition to three other opioid-specific programs that totaled over $100 million. Many states also used block grant funds, Targeted Capacity Expansion funds, and other grant funds for opioid-related activities making quantifying a total of funding expended on opioid-related activities difficult.

Other critiques have made similar recommendations regarding the block grant formulas. Some experts have recommended using data from major national epidemiological surveillance datasets that measure levels of mental illness and substance abuse in a state (rather than general population age distribution) to determine the population in need of services.[100] These may include data from the National Comorbidity Survey-Replication[101] for mental

[100] Burnam, et al., Review and Evaluation of Block Grant Formula, RAND, 1997.

[101] SAMHSA, The National Comorbidity Survey (NCS-1) studied the prevalence and correlates of mental disorders from 1990 to 1992. The NCS Replication (NCS-R) was carried out with

health needs, for example, or the National Survey on Drug Use and Health (NSDUH)[102] for mental health and substance abuse needs. Research also indicates that the cost-of-services measure currently used does not adequately represent interstate wage variations in occupations related to substance abuse and mental health.[103] The formula also does not consider variations in numbers of uninsured individuals across the states, and other federal funding (e.g., Medicare and Medicaid) that a state may also receive for mental health and substance abuse services.[104]

There are also questions as to whether a formula is the ideal approach to distributing substance abuse and mental health treatment funds. In their 2001 report Choosing the Right Formula, the National Academies of Science, Engineering, and Medicine (NASEM) described a tradeoff between providing stability in funding from one year to the next and flexibility to redirect funds to different jurisdictions as true needs change. Substance abuse needs may have significant regional differences and epidemics may shift over time, sometimes rapidly. Static funding may not adequately respond to fluctuating public health needs. At the same time, states may rely on federal funding to support essential behavioral health infrastructure. Consistent and reliable funding streams may be necessary to maintain needed substance use and mental health services. Predictable funding may also be essential in establishing prospective public health strategies and achieving long-term behavioral health goals.

There have also been questions about whether the block grants supplement or supplant state funding for substance abuse and mental health initiatives.[105] While the block grants have historically represented a small

---

a new national sample from 2001 to 2003 to study trends in a wide range of variables assessed in the baseline NCS-1.

[102] SAMHSA, NSDUH, which was formerly known as the National Household Survey on Drug Abuse (NHSDA), is designed to produce drug and alcohol use incidence and prevalence estimates and report the consequences and patterns of use and abuse in the general U.S. civilian population age 12 and older.

[103] RAND, Review of Block Grant Formula, 1997.

[104] Albert Woodward, The Substance Abuse and Treatment Block Grant is Still Important Even with the Expansion of Medicaid, Substance Abuse and Mental Health Services Administration, Center for Behavioral Health Statistics and Quality, CBHSQ Report, Rockville, MD, January 7, 2016.

[105] See, for example, Alexander Cowell, Dennis McCarty, and Albert Woodward, " Impact of Federal Substance Abuse Block Grants on State Substance Abuse Spending: Literature and Data Review," *The Journal of Mental Health Policy and Economics*, vol. 6 (2003), pp. 173-179 and U.S. Government Accountability Office, *Federal Grants: Design Improvements Could Help Federal Resources Go Further*, FAO/AIMD-97-7, December 1996.

percentage of state spending on behavioral health activities, there are no state matching requirements for these programs. Some have questioned whether increased federal funding results in a subsequent decrease in state spending on behavioral health initiatives. Research has demonstrated that state substance abuse spending is positively associated with substance abuse block grant allocation, however. One study found that for every $1.00 increase in state SABG funding, for example, state administered spending on alcohol treatment also increased by $0.80.[106] Other reports have found similar results; state investments in mental health and substance use treatment services increase in tandem with federal grant funding.[107] This suggests that federal block grant funding appears to have a positive correlation with state substance abuse treatment and prevention efforts and block grants may largely be used to supplement, not supplant, state funding.[108]

Other issues concern block grant funding not keeping up with health care inflation. The National Association of State Alcohol and Drug Abuse Directors (NASADAD) estimated that the inflation-adjusted value—the actual purchasing power—of the SABG block grant funding decreased 24% between 2009 and 2019.[109]

SAMHSA Charitable Choice Provisions

In 2000, the Children's Health Act of 2000 (P.L. 106-310) and the Consolidated Appropriations Act, 2001 (P.L. 106-554) added several provisions related to services provided through religious organizations to SAMHSA's authorities in the PHSA.[110] These provisions were part of several

---

106 Cowell et al., "Impact of Federal Substance Abuse Block Grants on State Substance Abuse Spending," 2003.

107 Tami Mark, Katharine Levit, and Rita Vandivort -Warren, et al., "Changes in US Spending on Mental Health and Substance Abuse Treatment, 1986-2005, And Implications for Policy," *Health Affairs*, vol. 30, no. 2 (February 2011).

108 Substance use and mental health treatment services are supported through a number of funders and payers, including through federal grants, state accounts, Medicaid, Medicare, private health insurance, and patients. A discussion of the interplay between these entities is beyond the scope of this report. For more information on patterns of U.S. spending for these services across funders, see for example, Mark et al., "Changes in US Spending," *Health Affairs*, 2011 from footnote 107.

109 National Association of State Alcohol and Drug Abuse Directors, Inc. (NASADAD), *Substance Abuse Prevention and Treatment (SAPT) Block Grant*, Washington, DC, March 2019, https://nasadad.org/wp-content/uploads/2019/03/SAPT-Block-Grant-Fact-Sheet-March-2019.pdf.

110 PHSA §581-584 (Part Gof Title V) and §1955. Of note, there are two Title V parts G and two sections 581 and 582. The SAMHSA Charitable Choice rules pertain to the

pieces of legislation enacted beginning in 1996 that sought to ensure that faith-based organizations could participate in federally funded social service programs on the same basis as other nongovernmental providers. These Charitable Choice rules make clear that religious organizations may receive public funding to offer social services without abandoning their religious character. The rules also outline certain qualifications involved in participation, such as restrictions on the use of public funds for religious activities and protections on the religious freedom of program beneficiaries.[111]

The SAMHSA Charitable Choice provisions enacted in 2000 —later clarified through HHS rulemaking in 2003[112]— apply to SAMHSA's discretionary grants and certain block grants such as the SABG and Projects for Assistance in Transition from Homelessness (PATH) program.[113] Collectively, these Charitable Choice rules prohibit discrimination in awarding funds to potential grantees based on that organization's religious character; prohibit the government from requiring an organization to alter its internal governance or remove religious symbols as a condition of eligibility; and prohibit the use of public funds received directly by religious organizations for explicitly religious activities. The rules also specify that receipt of public funds does not alter the exemption that religious organizations have under Title VII of the Civil Rights Act of 1964, which

---

provisions entitled Part G—Services Provided Through Religious Organizations" in Title V of the PHSA.

111 SAMHSA's Charitable Choice regulations are found in 42 C.F.R. Part 54 (discretionary grants) and Part 54a (SABG and PATH grants). Of note, these regulations may not apply to all grant programs that SAMHSA administers, such as the Community Mental Health Block Grant (MHBG), for instance. The MHBG is, however, governed by genera l HHS Charitable Choice regulations found in 45 C.F.R. Part 87.

112 Department of Health and Human Services, "Charitable Choice Regulations Applicable to States Receiving Substance Abuse Prevention and Treatment Block Grants, Projects for Assistance in Tran sition From Homelessness Formula Grants, and to Public and Private Providers Receiving Discretionary Grant Funding from SAMHSA for the Provision of Substance Abuse Services Providing for Equal Treatment of SAMHSA Program Participants," 68 *Federal Register* 56429-56449, September 30, 2003. See also, 42 C.F.R. Part 54; 42 C.F.R. Part 54a; 45 C.F.R. Part 87; and C.F.R. Part 96.

113 Additionally, all of SAMHSA's programs are covered under the following executive orders (and associated rules amending or establishing regulations to implement those executive orders): Executive Order 13279, " Equal Protection of the Laws for Faith-Based and Community Organizations," 67 *Federal Register* 77139-77144, December 12, 2002 (for final rule, see footnote 112); Executive Order 13559, " Fundamental Principles and Policymaking Criteria for Partnerships With Faith-Based and Other Neighborhood Organizations (final rule published in 81 *Federal Register* 19353-19430, May 4, 2016); Executive Order 13831, " Establishment of a White House Faith and Opportunity Initiative," 83 *Federal Register* 20718-20717 (proposed rule published in 85 *Federal Register* 2974-2987, January 17, 2020).

allows such organizations to discriminate based on religion in certain employment decisions. The Charitable Choice provisions also prohibit religious organizations receiving public funds from discriminating against beneficiaries on the basis of religion. SAMHSA Charitable Choice provisions declare that if a service program beneficiary objects to the religious character of the service program participant, the program beneficiary must be referred to an alternative provider capable of providing the same service(s).[114]

Some controversy surrounding these programs has centered on the constitutionality of the federal government funding faith-based social service programs. On one hand, providing federal funding for religious activities may, under some circumstances, violate the Establishment Clause of the U.S. Constitution's First Amendment. The Establishment Clause of the First Amendment prohibits the government from providing certain types of support to religion and religious entities. On the other hand, denying generally available benefits to organizations based solely on their religious affiliation may violate the First Amendment's Free Exercise, which prohibits the government from unlawfully discriminating against religious exercise. Charitable Choice rules have sought to ensure that religious organizations are eligible on an equal basis for public funds while also ensuring those funds are not used for explicitly religious activities.

Finally, a 2015 investigation by the Government Accountability Office (GAO) found variations in how SAMHSA oversees grants and documents grant-related activities.[115] While states are required to discuss the manner in which they use block grant funds in their application or plan, it is unclear how SAMHSA surveys this information and whether they audit states for accuracy.

SAMSHA does not publish this information publicly. An HHS OIG publication in 2017 noted that SAMHSA's reporting has improved since that GAO study.[116] While some concerns regarding SAMHSA's supervision of block grant activities remain, investigations into block grant spending largely

---

[114] PHSA §582(f) (42 USC 290kk–1(f)). The responsibility for providing the alternative service rests with the appropriate federal, state, or local government that administers the program or is a program participant.

[115] U.S. Government Accountability Office, *Mental Health: Better Documentation Needed to Oversee Substance Abuse and Mental Health Services Administration Grantees*, GAO-15-405, May 2015, http://www.gao.gov/products/GAP-15- 405.

[116] Suzanne Murrin, *SAMHSA Has Improved Outcome Reporting for the Substance Abuse Prevention and Treatment Block Grant*, U.S. Department of Health and Human Services, Office of Inspector General, Memorandum Report, OEI - 04-12-00160, Washington, DC, June 26, 2015, https://oig.hhs.gov/oei/reports/oei-04-12-00160.pdf.

demonstrate that states use the block grant funding as intended, despite historically little oversight.[117]

Programs of Regional and National Significance (PRNS)

In addition to the block grant programs, SAMHSAadministers other programs supporting mental health and substance use treatment and prevention activities. PHSATitle V Part B requires the HHS Secretary to "address priority ... needs of regional and national significance" in mental health, substance abuse treatment, and substance abuse prevention. The statute instructs the HHS Secretary to do so "directly or through grants or cooperative agreements with States, political subdivisions of States, Indian tribes and tribal organizations, other public or private nonprofit entities."[118] SAMHSA administers grants and activities under these authorities commonly known as Programs of Regional and National Significance (PRNS).

SAMHSA's Programs of Regional and National Significance encompass numerous grants and activities within each of three areas: (1) substance abuse treatment, (2) substance abuse prevention, and (3) mental health. PRNS activities may include competitive grants, contracts, and cooperative agreements. PRNS programs are either determined by HHS and SAMHSA (sometimes at direction of the presidential administration) or by Congress through statutory authorizations/requirements or appropriations language. Some of the PRNS grants and activities have explicit authorizations in statute; at some point Congress enacted a law explicitly authorizing the PRNS program. Other PRNS initiatives have never had explicit authorizations and operate under SAMHSA's general PRNS authorities for mental health, substance abuse treatment, or substance abuse prevention. Commonly, Congress will codify existing programs without explicit authorizations through legislation. PRNS programs themselves may vary from year to year as existing programs are terminated or new programs are created, either at SAMHSA's discretion or at the direction of Congress.

PRNS grants and activities within each area fall into two categories, called "Capacity" and "Science and Service." Most PRNS programs are in the

---

[117] Cowell et al., "Impact of Federal Substance Abuse Block Grants on State Substance Abuse Spending," 2003.

[118] Mental health PRNS: PHSA §520A(a) (42 U.S.C. §290bb-32(a)). Substance abuse treatment PRNS: PHSA §509(a) (42 U.S.C. §290bb-2(a)). Substance abuse prevention PRNS: PHSA §516(a) (42 U.S.C. §290bb-22(a)).

Capacity category. Capacity grants emphasize expanding service system activities. Those in the Science and Service category tend to focus on training and technical assistance. For example, within mental health PRNS, primary and behavioral health care integration activities appear under both categories: grants to community mental health centers for treatment services appear under Capacity, and a competitive cooperative agreement for a training and technical assistance center appears under Science and Service.

Substance Abuse Treatment PRNS

The substance abuse treatment PRNS support states and communities in carrying out activities related to substance use treatment services. PHSASection 509 authorizes the substance abuse treatment PRNS generally. Subsequent PHSA sections authorize specific substance abuse treatment PRNS programs. PHSASection 509(f) authorizes to be appropriated $334 million (rounded) annually for each of FY2018–FY2022 to carry out the substance abuse treatment PRNS. Table 1 lists FY2020 grant programs and activities categorized as substance abuse treatment PRNS; additional details (e.g., program descriptions and funding levels) are available in SAMHSA's FY2021 budget request.[119]

Table 1. FY2020 substance abuse treatment PRNS

Program or Activity	Authorizing Law	Authorization of Appropriations
Substance Abuse Treatment PRNS General Authority	PHSA §509	$333,806,000 for each of FY2018-FY2022
Substance Abuse Treatment PRNS Capacity		
Opioid Treatment Programs/Regulatory Activities	—	—
Screening, Brief Intervention and Referral to Treatment	—	—
Targeted Capacity Expansion	—	—
Grants to Prevent Prescription Drug/Opioid Overdose[a]	PHSA §516 &§546	$36,000,000 for each of FY2019-FY2023
First Responder Training	PHSA §546	$36,000,000 for each of FY2019-FY2023
Improving Access to Overdose Treatment	PHSA §545	$5,000,000 for the period of FY2017-FY2019
Pregnant and Postpartum Women	PHSA §508	$29,931,000 for each of FY2019-FY2023

[119] SAMHSA, FY2021 Justification of Estimates for Appropriations Committees.

Program or Activity	Authorizing Law	Authorization of Appropriations
Building Communities of Recovery	PHSA §547	$5,000,000 for each of FY2019-FY2023
Recovery Community Services Program	—	—
Children and Families	PHSA §514	$29,605,000 for each of FY2018-FY2022
Treatment Systems for Homeless	PHSA §506	$41,304,000 for each of FY2018-FY2022
Minority AIDS	—	—
Criminal Justice Activities	—	—
Substance Abuse Treatment PRNS Science and Service		
Addiction Technology Transfer Centers	—	—
Minority Fellowship Program	PHSA §597	$12,669,000 for each of FY2018-FY2022
Peer Support TA Center	PHSA §547A	$1,000,000 for each of FY2019-FY2023
Treatment, Recovery, & Workforce Support	SUPPORT Act §7183	$5,000,000 for each of FY2019-FY2023
Emergency Department Alternatives to Opioids	SUPPORT Act §7091	$10,000,000 for each of FY2019-FY2021

Source: Public Health Service Act and SAMHSA, FY2021 Justification of Estimates for Appropriations Committees.

Notes: The FY2020 budget adds a new PRNS called "Grants to Develop Curricular for DATA Act Waivers" added by the SUPPORT for Patients and Communities Act of 2018 (P.L. 115-271).

[a] Previously listed under CSAP in FY2018.

Example: Building Communities of Recovery

In 2016, the Comprehensive Addiction and Recovery Act (CARA; P.L. 114-198) authorized funding for recovery community organizations through a new Section 547 of the PHSA(within the authorizations for the Substance Abuse Treatment PRNS). This Building Communities of Recovery (BCOR) program provides funding for the development, enhancement, expansion, and delivery of peer recovery support services for substance abuse disorders. Grant support also enables links between recovery networks and other community organizations such as health care providers, the criminal justice system, and housing and employment services. The BCOR program supplanted previous SAMHSA peer professional workforce development programs.

Substance Abuse Prevention PRNS

The substance abuse prevention PRNS support states and communities in carrying out activities related to the prevention of substance use. PHSA Section 516 authorizes the substance abuse prevention PRNS generally. Subsequent

PHSA sections authorize specific substance abuse prevention PRNS programs. PHSASection 516(f) authorizes to be appropriated $211 million (rounded) annually for each of FY2018–FY2022 to carry out substance abuse prevention PRNS.

Table 2 lists FY2020 grants and activities categorized as substance abuse prevention PRNS; additional details (e.g., program descriptions and funding levels) are available in SAMHSA's FY2021 budget request.[120]

Table 2. FY2020 substance abuse prevention PRNS

Program or Activity	Authorizing Law	Authorization of Appropriations
Substance Abuse Prevention PRNS General Authority	PHSA §516	$211,148,000 for each of FY2018-FY2022
Substance Abuse Prevention PRNS Capacity		
Strategic Prevention Framework	—	—
Federal Drug-Free Workplace	—	—
Minority AIDS	—	—
Sober Truth on Preventing Underage Drinking Act (STOP Act)	PHSA §519Ba	$1,000,000 for each of FY2018-FY2022; $5,000,000 for each of FY2018-FY2022; $5,000,000 for each of FY2008-FY2010; $3,000,000 for each of FY2018-FY2022
Tribal Behavioral Health Grants	—	—
Substance Abuse Prevention PRNS Science and Service		
Center for the Application of Prevention Technologies	—	—
Minority Fellowship Program	PHSA §597	$12,669,000 for each of FY2018-FY2022
Science and Service Program Coordination	—	—

Source: Public Health Service Act and SAMHSA, FY2021 Justification of Estimates for Appropriations Committees.

[a] PHSA §519B includes four authorizations of appropriations for various activities authorized in the provision. The authorization for appropriations for these are listed in the third column.

Example: Drug-Free Workplace and National Laboratory Certification

SAMHSA provides oversight of the Federal Drug-Free Workplace Program and the related National Laboratory Certification Program. The Federal Drug-Free Workplace Program aims to eliminate illegal drug use (and prescription

[120] Ibid.

drug misuse) in executive branch agencies and federally regulated industries by ensuring that employees are tested.[121] The National Laboratory Certification Program inspects and certifies the laboratories that conduct drug tests for executive branch agencies and federally regulated industries. Federally regulated industries include organizations receiving federal grants and organizations with federal contracts of $100,000 or more.[122] SAMHSA's Drug Testing Advisory Board (DTAB) advises the agency on its drug testing activities.[123]

Mental Health PRNS

The substance abuse treatment PRNS support states and communities in carrying out activities related to mental health prevention and treatment services. PHSASection 520A authorizes the mental health PRNS. PHSA Section 520A(f) authorizes to be appropriated $395 million (rounded) annually for each of FY2018–FY2022 to carry out mental health PRNS. *Table 3* lists FY2020 grants and activities categorized as mental health PRNS; additional details (e.g., program descriptions and funding) are available in SAMHSA's FY2021 budget request.[124]

Table 3. FY2020 mental health PRNS

Program or Activity	Authorizing Law	Authorization of Appropriations
Mental Health PRNS General Authority	PHSA §520A	$394,550,000 for each of FY2018-FY2022
Mental Health PRNS Capacity		
Seclusion and Restraint	—	—
Youth Violence Prevention	PHSA §581	$100,000,000 for each of FY2002-FY2003
Project AWARE	—	—
Mental Health First Aid[a]	PHSA §520J	$14,693,000 for FY2018-FY2022
Healthy Transitions	—	—
Infant and Early Childhood Mental Health	PHSA §399Z-2	$20,000,000 for FY2018-FY2022

[121] SAMHSA, Programs; Drug-free Workplace; Drug Testing, https://www.samhsa.gov/workplace/drug-testing, updated July 19, 2019.

[122] Drug-Free Workplace Act of 1988 (P.L. 100-690, Title V, Subtitle D, as amended) (41 U.S.C. §§701 et seq.).

[123] SAMHSA, *About Us; Advisory Councils; Drug Testing Advisory Board (DTAB)*, https://www.samhsa.gov/about-us/advisory-councils/drug-testing-advisory-board-dtab, Updated March 27, 2019.

[124] SAMHSA, FY2020 Justification of Estimates for Appropriations Committees.

Table 3. (Continued)

Program or Activity	Authorizing Law	Authorization of Appropriations
National Child Traumatic Stress Network	PHSA §582	$63,887,000 for each of FY2019-FY2023
Children and Family Programs	—	—
Consumer and Family Network Grants	—	—
Project LAUNCH	—	—
Mental Health System Transformation and Health Reform	—	—
Primary and Behavioral Health Care Integration	PHSA §520K	$51,878,000 for each of FY2018-FY2022
National Strategy for Suicide Prevention	PHSA §520L	$30,000,000 for FY2018-FY2022
Suicide Lifeline	PHSA §520E-3	$7,198,000 for each of FY2018-FY2022
GLS—Youth Suicide Prevention—States	PHSA §520E	$30,000,000 for each of FY2018-FY2022
GLS—Youth Suicide Prevention—Campus	PHSA §520E-2	$7,000,000 for each of FY2018-FY2022
GLS—Suicide Prevention Resource Center	PHSA §520C	$5,988,000 for each of FY2018-FY2022
AI/AN Suicide Prevention Initiative	—	—
Tribal Behavioral Health Grants	—	—
Homelessness Prevention Programs	—	—
Minority AIDS	—	—
Criminal and Juvenile Justice Programs	PHSA §520G	$4,269,000 for each of FY2018-FY2022
Assisted Outpatient Treatment for Individuals with SMI	P.L. 113-93 §224	$19,000,000 for each of FY2019-FY2020; $18,000,000 for each of FY2021-FY2022
Comprehensive Opioid Recovery Centers	PHSA §552	$10,000,000 for each of FY2019-FY2023
Assertive Community Treatment for Individuals with SMI	PHSA §520M	$5,000,000 for FY2018-FY2022
Strengthening Community Crisis Response Systems	PHSA §520F	$12,500,000 for FY2018-FY2022
Mental Health PRNS Science and Service		
Practice Improvement and Training	—	—
Consumer and Consumer Supporter TA Centers	—	—

Program or Activity	Authorizing Law	Authorization of Appropriations
Primary and Behavioral Health Care Integration Training and TA	PHSA §520K	$51,878,000 for each of FY2018-FY2022
Disaster Response	—	—
Homelessness	—	—
Minority Fellowship Programb	PHSA §597	$12,669,000 for each of FY2018-FY2022

Source: Public Health Service Act and SAMHSA, FY2021 Justification of Estimates for Appropriations Committees.

Notes:

[a] Originally part of Project AWARE, Mental Health First Aid provides mental health awareness training to grantees. "Mental health awareness training" was codified in its own section (Sec 520J) by Cures. Mental health awareness training activities—including the Mental Health First Aid program—are treated as distinct from Project AWARE in the SAMHSA FY2020 Justification of Estimates for Appropriations Committees.

[b] Minority Fellowship Program is included as a PRNS in three SAMHSA Centers: CMHS, CSAT, CSAP.

Example: Project LAUNCH

SAMHSA's Project Linking Actions for Unmet Needs in Children's Health (LAUNCH) is a national initiative aimed at promoting the wellness of children from birth to eight years old.

Project LAUNCH works "to ensure that the systems that serve them (including early childcare and education, home visiting, and primary care) are equipped to promote and monitor healthy social and emotional development" of young children.[125] It does this through behavioral health screenings for children, home visiting programs for families, and trainings for community providers. A multi-site evaluation completed in 2018 showed improved social and academic functioning among children, decreases in child problem behaviors, and enhanced community child and family-serving systems for participants in this program. Project LAUNCH operates under SAMHSA's general PRNS authorities—it does not have an explicit authorization in statute.

Other SAMHSA Grant Programs

In addition to the block grant programs and Programs of Regional and National Significance, SAMHSA also carries out several other statutorily required grant programs. These function similarly to statutorily required PRNS in that they target specific populations or substances of abuse. They are

[125] SAMHSA, FY2020 Justification of Estimates for Appropriations Committees, p. 47.

authorized in separate provisions from the PRNS in Title V of the PHSA, though SAMHSA will sometimes organize these programs with the PRNS when communicating about non-block-grant programs.

Children's Mental Health Services

The Children's Mental Health Services program supports services for children with serious emotional disturbance. The program also supports efforts to identify and serve children at risk. In recent years, SAMHSA has awarded competitive grants to help states, local governments, tribes, and territories develop and implement systems of care; cooperative agreements to sustain and expand systems of care; and contracts to provide technical assistance and conduct evaluations. The systems of care approach focuses on delivering evidence-based interventions in the least restrictive setting.

PHSA Title V, Part E (Sections 561–565) authorizes the Children's Mental Health Services program.[126] PHSATitle V, Part E, requires the HHS Secretary to award grants to support "comprehensive community mental health services for children with a serious emotional disturbance." It specifies reporting requirements, technical assistance requirements, and the ages of children to be served, among other factors. PHSASection 565 explicitly authorizes to be appropriated $119 million annually for each of FY2018-FY2022 to carry out the program.[127]

Projects for Assistance in Transition from Homelessness (PATH)

The Projects for Assistance in Transition from Homelessness (PATH) program supports services for people with serious mental illness (including those with co-occurring substance use disorders) who are homeless or at imminent risk of becoming homeless. The PATH program distributes funds to states (including the District of Columbia and specified territories) according to a formula. The states, in turn, make grants to local governments and private nonprofit organizations to support mental health and substance abuse treatment, case management, and other services. Up to 20% of the federal payments may be used for housing-related assistance. All services provided using PATH funding must be consistent with (and included in) the state's

---

[126] PHSA Title V, Part E (42 U.S.C. §§290ff-290ff-4).
[127] PHSA §565(f)(1) (42 U.S.C. §290ff-4(f)(1)).

comprehensive mental health services plan (as required for participation in the mental health block grant).[128]

Each state's allotment is based on its population living in urbanized areas (as a percentage of the total U.S. population living in urbanized areas). A minimum allotment for each state is prescribed in statute (with exceptions for specified territories). States must provide matching funds of at least $1 for every $3 of federal funds. The 21st Century Cures Act required the Assistant Secretary to conduct a study of the PATH grant allotment formula and to submit a corresponding report to Congress by January 2018.[129]

PHSA Title V, Part C (Sections 521-535) authorizes the Projects for Assistance in Transition from Homelessness program.[130] PHSASection 535 explicitly authorizes to be appropriated $65 million (rounded) annually for each of FY2018-FY2022.[131]

Public Health Emergencies and Disaster Response

SAMHSA plays a role in helping to ensure "the nation is prepared to address the behavioral health needs that follow" natural and human-caused disasters and emergent events, including public health emergencies.[132]

SAMHSA operates a Disaster Technical Assistance Center (DTAC) as the foundation of its disaster response initiatives.[133] SAMHSA DTAC assists states, territories, tribes, and local entities with all-hazards disaster behavioral health response planning. The intent of this program is to improve both preparedness and response to disasters and emergent events. SAMHSA partners with the Federal Emergency Management Agency (FEMA) to jointly fund DTAC. SAMHSA DTAC uses appropriated funds for programs that support survivors of disasters as well as organizations and providers administering aid. For example, through an interagency agreement with FEMA, SAMHSA operates the Crisis Counseling Assistance and Training Program (CCP), which provides community- based behavioral health

[128] The SAMHSA Charitable Choice provisions described on page 23 apply to the programs under PATH that provide substance abuse services. For more information, see HHS, "Charitable Choice Regulations Applicable to States," 68 *Federal Register* 56429-56449, September 30, 2003 and textbox footnotes on page 23.

[129] §9004(g)

[130] PHSA §§521-535 (42 U.S.C. §§290cc-21-290cc-35).

[131] PHSA §535 (42 U.S.C. §290cc-35).

[132] SAMHSA FY2020 Justification of Estimates for Appropriations Committees, p. 84.

[133] SAMHSA, Practitioner Training; Disaster Technical Assistance Center (DTAC), https://www.samhsa.gov/dtac.

outreach and psycho-educational services.[134] In addition to oversight of the CCP, SAMHSA offers technical assistance and program guidance. Other SAMHSA DTAC initiatives include immedia te crisis counseling via the Disaster Distress Helpline[135] and resource publication through the Disaster Behavioral Health Information Series (DBHIS) resource collections.[136]

For some public health emergencies—such as the opioid epidemic—SAMHSA plays a significant role in distributing grant funds for behavioral health prevention and treatment services; providing technical assistance to grantees and providers; and, in some cases, issuing rules and regulations. Provisions in the PHSA provide SAMHSA greater autonomy over grant management during public health emergencies. For example, PHSA Section 1957 allows states greater flexibility in meeting deadlines or other requirements for the MHBG, the SABG, PATH grant, or Protection and Advocacy for Individuals with Mental Illness grant in the case of a public health emergency. Funds made available for emergency response grants under PHSA Section 501 also remain available through the end of the fiscal year following the fiscal year for which the amounts are appropriated.

Treatment Systems for Homeless

The Treatment Systems for Homeless awards grants, contracts, and cooperative agreements to states, local governments, and communities to provide mental health and substance abuse services to individuals experiencing homelessness. Grants support activities such as the development and expansion of local systems that provide permanent housing or supportive services for adults, youth, families, and veterans. Some of the Treatment Systems for Homeless are joint initiatives managed by CMHS and CSAT.

PHSA Section 506 authorizes the Treatment Systems for the Homeless.[137] PHSASection 506 explicitly authorizes to be appropriated $41 million (rounded) annually for each of FY2018- FY2022.[138]

---

[134] SAMHSA, Practitioner Training; Disaster Technical Assistance Center (DTAC); Crisis Counseling Assistance Program (CCP), https://www.samhsa.gov/dtac/ccp.

[135] SAMHSA, Find Treatment; Disaster Distress Helpline, https://www.samhsa.gov/find-help/disaster-distress- helpline.

[136] SAMHSA, Practitioner Training; Disaster Technical Assistance Center (DTAC); DBHIS Collections, https://www.samhsa.gov/dtac/dbhis-collections.

[137] PHSA §506 (42 U.S.C. §§290aa-5).

[138] 42 U.S.C. §§290aa-5(e).

Protection and Advocacy for Individuals with Mental Illness (PAIMI)

The Protection and Advocacy for Individuals with Mental Illness (PAIMI) program supports state-designated protection and advocacy (P&A) systems mandated to protect individuals with mental illness residing in care or treatment facilities from abuse, neglect, and violations of their civil rights. The PAIMI program distributes funds to P&Asystems in the states (including the District of Columbia and specified territories) and the American Indian Consortium according to a formula.[139]

Unlike many of SAMHSA's other formula grants, for which formulas are prescribed in statute, PAIMI's formula is prescribed by the HHS Secretary, subject to statutory requirements.

Specifically, it must be based equally on (1) each state's population and (2) each state's population weighted by per capita income relative to the United States. A minimum allotment for each state is prescribed in statute. Exceptions to components of the formula and minimum allotment calculation are made for specified territories and the American Indian Consortium.[140]

State P&A systems were established under the Developmental Disabilities Assistance Act of 1975 (P.L. 94-103, as amended).[141] The PAIMI Act of 1986 (P.L. 99-319, as amended) authorized the formula grant to support P&Asystems in serving the mentally ill.[142] Section 10827 of the PAIMI Act explicitly authorized appropriations for the PAIMI program through FY2003. Since that time, the program has continued to operate under its general authorities and has continued to receive funding through the annual appropriations process. The Cures Act required GAO to submit a report on programs funded by PAIMI grants to specified congressional committees by July 2018.[143]

---

[139] For purposes of the PAIMI program, "State" is defined in statute as each of the 50 states, the District of Columbia, American Samoa, Guam, the Northern Mariana Islands, Puerto Rico, the U.S. Virgin Islands, and the "Trust Territory of the Pacific Islands" (42 U.S.C. §10802(7)). In some sections of the PAIMI Act, "Trust Territory of the Pacific Islands" has been replaced by "Marshall Islands, the Federated States of Micronesia, the Republic of Palau" (42 U.S.C. §10822(a)(1)(B), for example). The HHSSecretary is required to make an allotment to the American Indian Consortium (which represents the Navajo and Hopi Tribes in the Four Corners region of the Southwest) if the total amount appropriated for a fiscal year is at least $25 million (42 U.S.C. §10822(a)(2)(D)).

[140] 42 U.S.C. §10822.

[141] For example, see P.L. 106-402.

[142] P.L. 99-319 (42 U.S.C. §§10801-10827).

[143] §6023.

Minority Fellowship Program

The SAMHSA-administered Minority Fellowship Program provides grants to professional associations (e.g., the American Psychiatric Association and the American Nurses Association) to offer stipends to minority doctoral students who are studying for degrees in a mental or behavioral health profession.[144] PHSASection 597 requires the HHS Secretary to maintain a "Minority Fellowship Program" to award fellowships, which may include stipends, for post-baccalaureate training for mental health professionals in the fields of psychiatry, nursing, social work, marriage and family therapy, mental health counseling, and substance use disorder and addiction counseling. It authorizes to be appropriated $13 million (rounded) annually for each of FY2018-FY2022.[145]

Additional Opioid Grant Programs

State Targeted Response (STR) for the Opioid Crisis Grants

The State Targeted Response to the Opioid Crisis (Opioid STR) grant program provided nearly $1 billion to the states and territories over FY2017 and FY2018 to support activities related to the opioid epidemic. While the funds were appropriated to HHS generally, the responsibility for administering these grants was delegated to SAMHSA.[146] SAMHSA awarded grants to all 50 states, the District of Columbia, Puerto Rico, the Virgin Islands, the Northern Mariana Islands, Micronesia, Palau, and American Samoa.[147] The funds provided to each grantee were allocated based on a formula that considered two factors: (1) unmet need for opioid use disorder treatment and (2) drug poisoning deaths.

Section 7181 of the SUPPORT for Patients and Communities Act (SUPPORT Act; P.L. 115-271) reauthorized the Opioid STR grant for $500

---

[144] Of note, the Health Resources and Services Administration (HRSA) within HHS also provides workforce development programming for behavioral health providers. See, for instance, *HRSA; Grants; Behavioral Health* at https://bhw.hrsa.gov/grants/behavioral-health.

[145] 42 U.S.C. §290ll(c).

[146] U.S. Congress, House Committee of the Whole House on the State of the Union, *Departments of Labor, Health and Human Services, and Education, and Related Agencies Appropriations Bill, 2017*, To accompany H.R. 5926, 114th Cong., 2nd sess., July 22, 2016, 114-699, p. 4, available at https://www.gpo.gov/fdsys/pkg/CRPT-114hrpt699/pdf/CRPT-114hrpt699.pdf.

[147] HHS, SAMHSA, *FY2018 Justification of Estimates for Appropriations Committees*, p. 207 and HHS, SAMHSA, *FY2019 Justification of Estimates for Appropriations Committees*, p. 218.

million for each of FY2019 through FY2021. The SUPPORT Act was signed into law in October 2018 after the FY2019 Labor-HHS-Education appropriations bill (P.L. 115-245) was enacted, leaving the authorization for the STR grant expired when funding for FY2019 was appropriated. The grant program was not funded for FY2020.

State Opioid Response (SOR) Grants

Similar to the Opioid STR grants, the State Opioid Response (SOR) grants provided $1 billion in funding for states to address the opioid epidemic in FY2018.[148] The SOR grants sought to increase access to medication-assisted treatment and enhance state prevention, treatment, and recovery systems. The SOR grants followed similar distribution methods as the Opioid STR grants. The funds provided to each grantee were allocated based on a formula determined by the Secretary. The program included a 15% set-aside for the 10 states with the highest drug overdose mortality rates. The program also included a $50 million set-aside for tribes. For FY2019, the amount for the SOR grant program increased by $500 million—the same amount the Opioid STR grants were reduced. The grant program received level funding—$1.5 billion—for FY2020.

Data Collection and Related Activities

In addition to the activities described above, SAMHSA collects data and conducts related activities. Many of these activities are conducted—or coordinated—by the CBHSQ. Examples include the following:

- *Surveillance and data collection:* for example, the National Survey of Drug Use and Health (NSDUH), an annual household survey of drug use and other health information among the U.S. population age 12 or older.[149] Other examples include the National Survey of Substance Abuse Treatment Services (N-SSATS), an annual survey of all known substance abuse treatment facilities in the United States,[150] and the

---

[148] H.R. 1625.

[149] For more information about the NSDUH, see CRS Report R43047, Prevalence of Mental Illness in the United States: Data Sources and Estimates.

[150] SAMHSA, *National Survey of Substance Abuse Treatment Services (N-SSATS)*, https://www.samhsa.gov/data/data-we-collect/nssats-national-survey-substance-abuse-treatment-services.

Drug Abuse Warning Network (DAWN), a nationally representative public health surveillance system that monitors drug-related visits to hospital emergency departments.[151]

- *Statistical and analytic support:* for example, the Substance Abuse and Mental Health Data Archive (SAMHDA), a repository for public access data files that provides public access and analysis.[152]
- *Performance and quality information systems activities:* for example, the Evidence-Based Practices Resource Center (EBP Resource Center), a searchable online database of mental health and substance abuse information supported by scientific research.[153]153 The EBP Resource Center aims to "provide communities, clinicians, policy-makers, and others" with "the information and tools they need to incorporate evidence-based practices into their communities or clinical settings."[154] Launched in April 2018, the EBP Resource Center replaced the National Registry of Evidence-based Programs and Practices—in existence since 1997—after the Cures Act codified and amended the responsibilities of SAMHSA to publicly provide information on evidence-based program and practices.[155]
- *Agency-wide initiatives:* for example, SAMHSA's collaboration with the Health Resources and Services Administration (HRSA) to develop consistent methods of identifying and tracking behavioral health workforce needs.

PHSA Section 505 requires the HHS Secretary, acting through the SAMHSAAdministrator, to collect data on various topics. Specific requirements include conducting annual surveys and making summaries and

---

151 SAMHSA, *Substance Abuse & Mental Health Data Archive; Drug Abuse Warning Network*, https://www.datafiles.samhsa.gov/study-series/drug-abuse-warning-network-dawn-nid13516.

152 SAMHSA, Substance Abuse & Mental Health Data Archive, https://www.datafiles.samhsa.gov/.

153 SAMHSA, Programs; Evidence-Based Practices Resource Center, https://www.samhsa.gov/ebp-resource-center.

154 SAMHSA, *Programs; EBP Resource Center; About the Evidence-Based Practices Resource Center;* https://www.samhsa.gov/ebp-resource-center/about.

155 PHSA §543A (42 U.S.C. 290dd-2a). See also: SAMHSA, " Statement of Elinore F. Mccance-Katz, MD, PhD, Assistant Secretary for Mental Health and Substance Use Regarding the National Registry of Evidence-Based programs and Practices and SAMHSA's New Approach to Implementation of Evidence-Based Practices (EBPs)," press release, January 11, 2018, https://www.samhsa.gov/newsroom/press-announce ments/201801110330.

analyses available to the public.[156] PHSA Title V includes numerous other references to collecting and disseminating data, embedded within larger programs. Under PHSA Title XIX, both block grant programs also require some data collection and evaluation activities.

National Mental Health Policy Laboratory

Through its National Mental Health Policy Laboratory, SAMHSA evaluates and disseminates information on best practices in the field. Title VII (Section 7001) of the Cures Act established within SAMHSA a National Mental Health Policy Laboratory.[157] The statute requires the laboratory to facilitate the implementation of policy changes likely to improve the prevention and treatment of mental illness and substance use disorders, disseminate information on evidence-based practices, and periodically review SAMHSA programs to reduce duplication and make recommendations to improve effectiveness, among other responsibilities. The statute also allows the Assistant Secretary to award grants for (1) evaluating promising service delivery models and (2) expanding the use of evidence-based programs. In January 2018, SAMHSA announced the launch of the Policy Laboratory by naming its first director and officially establishing it as one of SAMHSA's Offices and Centers.[158]

Publications

SAMHSA publishes guidance, clinical best practices, and other resources on treatment, prevention, and recovery for mental and substance use disorders. Through the SAMHSA online store, clinicians, patients, and policymakers can access downloadable materials on a variety of topics.[159] SAMHSA offers series of treatment-related resources such as Treatment Improvement Protocols, SAMHSAAdvisories, and Evidence-Based Practice Kits, among others. The SAMHSA Store, where many of these materials can be obtained, is managed through the Public Engagement Platform contract through the Office of Communications.[160]

---

[156] PHSA §505 (42 U.S.C. §290aa-4).

[157] PHSA §501A (42 U.S.C. 290aa-0).

[158] SAMHSA, "Leadership Announcement," press release, January 9, 2018, https://blog.samhsa.gov/2018/01/09/ leadership-announcement and SAMHSA, *About Us; Who We Are; Offices and Centers: NMHSUPL,* https://www.samhsa.gov/about-us/who-we-are/offices-centers/nmhsupl.

[159] SAMHSA, *Publications and Digital* Products, https://store.samhsa.gov/.

[160] SAMHSA, *FY2020 Justification of Estimates for Appropriations Committees*, p. 287-289.

Technical Assistance

SAMHSA provides technical assistance to help states, territories, tribes, and other behavioral health providers develop and strengthen behavioral health care services. Technical assistance typically includes instruction on the grant application process, consultation on grant management, and workforce development programs. SAMHSAmay provide this technical assistance directly, through contract, or through a grant. SAMHSAoperates several National Technical Assistance and Resource Centers to enhance grantee performance and improve quality of service delivery.[161] The agency also organizes and disseminates training and learning resources to facilitate the identification of evidence-based programs. Some of these activities are explicitly authorized in statute.

Appendix

Table A-1. Abbreviations used in this report

Abbreviation	Definition
ADAMHA	Alcohol, Drug Abuse and Mental Health Administration
ADMS	Alcohol, Drug, and Mental Health Services
AHRQ	Association for Health Care Research and Quality
Assistant Secretary	Assistant Secretary of Mental Health and Substance Use
BCOR	Building Communities of Recovery
BHSIS	Behavioral Health Services Information System
CARA	Comprehensive Addiction and Recovery Act
CBHSQ	Center for Behavioral Health Statistics and Quality
CMHS	Center for Mental Health Services
CSAP	Center for Substance Abuse Prevention
CSAT	Center for Substance Abuse Treatment
Cures	21st Century Cures Act
DAWN	Drug Abuse Warning Network
DTAB	Drug Testing Advisory Board
DTAC	Disaster Technical Assistance Center
EBP	Evidence-Based Practices
ED	Department of Education
GAO	Government Accountability Office

[161] SAMHSA, *SAMHSA's National Technical Assistance & Resource Centers*, Rockville, MD, https://www.samhsa.gov/sites/default/files/ta-center-brochure.pdf.

Abbreviation	Definition
HHS	Department of Health and Human Services
HRSA	Health Resources and Services Administration
IHA	Institute for Health and Aging
ISMICC	Interdepartmental Serious Mental Illness Coordinating Committee
LAUNCH	Linking Actions for Unmet Needs in Children's Health
MHBG	Community Mental Health Services Block Grant
NASEM	National Academies of Science, Engineering, and Medicine
NIAAA	National Institute on Alcohol Abuse and Alcoholism
NIDA	National Institute on Drug Abuse
NIH	National Institutes of Health
NIMH	National Institutes of Mental Health
N-MHSS	National Mental Health Services Survey
NSDUH	National Survey on Drug Use and Health
N-SSATS	National Survey of Substance Abuse Treatment Services
OBRA	Omnibus Budget Reconciliation Act
OCMO	Office of the Chief Medical Officer
Opioid STR	State Targeted Response to the Opioid Crisis
P&A	protection and advocacy
PAIMI	Protection and Advocacy for Individuals with Mental Illness
PATH	Projects for Assistance in Transition from Homelessness
PHS	Public Health Service
PHSA	Public Health Service Act
PPHF	Prevention and Public Health Fund
PRNS	Programs of Regional and National Significance
SABG	Substance Abuse Prevention and Treatment Block Grant
SAMHDA	Substance Abuse and Mental Health Data Archive
SAMHSA	Substance Abuse and Mental Health Services Administration
SED	serious emotional disturbance
SMI	serious mental illness
SOR	State Opioid Response Grants
SUPPORT	Substance Use-Disorder Prevention that Promotes Opioid Recovery and Treatment Act
TEDS	Treatment Episode Data Set

Source: Table prepared by the Congressional Research Service.

Index

E

F

G

H

I

J

L

M

N

O

P

Q

R

Y